MATERNAL HEALTH AND CHILD MORTALITY

About the Editors

Dr. Nitish Mondal (b. 1984) received his M.Sc. (First Class First) (2007) and the Ph.D. degree in Anthropology (2014) from the University of North Bengal, West Bengal. Currently, Dr. Mondal is working as Associate Professor & Head in the Department of Anthropology, Sikkim University, Gangtok, Sikkim India. He is the recipient of UGC-NET Junior (2008) and Senior Research Fellowship (2010) for the Doctoral Research and Gold Medal (in Anthropology, 2007) from the University of North Bengal. He has published number of research papers in different peer-reviewed international and national journals of repute and two edited books and also engages as reviewer for several international and national journals. His research interest lies in Biological Anthropology, Anthropometry and Public Health, Human Growth, Nutrition and Body Composition Assessment and Bio-statistics.

Prof. Kh. Narendra Singh (b. 1966) is currently the Professor and Head of the Department of Anthropology, Assam University: Silchar (Diphu Campus), Assam. He did his Master's and Doctoral degrees in Anthropology from the Sabitribai Phule Pune University (formerly University of Pune), Pune. Besides anthropological field studies, Prof. Singh has vast experience of conducting various large-scale national level health survey including, DLHS-RCH, NFHS and GATS India. He is also the reviewer and joint editors of several international journals. Professor Singh has authored several edited volumes and published numerous articles/research papers in international journals of repute. He has guided dozens of research scholars for Ph.D. degree. His special areas of interest are Anthropology of Health, Tribal Studies and Nutrition and Health Communication.

MATERNAL HEALTH AND CHILD MORTALITY

Condition, Vision and Challenges

Editors

Nitish Mondal

Kh. Narendra Singh

CONCEPT PUBLISHING COMPANY PVT. LTD.

NEW DELHI-110 059

ISBN : 978-93-5594-530-3

First Published 2022

Published and Printed by

Concept
Since 1974

Concept Publishing Company Pvt. Ltd.
A/15-16, Commercial Block, Mohan Garden,
New Delhi-110059 (INDIA)
T: +91 11 41101460
E: publishing@conceptpub.com, *W*: www.conceptpub.com

Cataloging in Publication Data—Courtesy: D.K. Agencies (P) Ltd. <docinfo@dkagencies.com>

Maternal health and child mortality : condition, vision and challenges/editors, Nitish Mondal, Kh. Narendra Singh.
pages cm
Contributed articles.
Includes bibliographical references and index.
ISBN 9789355945303

1. Mothers—Health and hygiene—India. 2. Children—Health and hygiene—India. 3. Tribes—Health and hygiene—India. 4. Mothers—Nutrition—India. 5. Children—Nutrition—India. 6. Children—Mortality—India. 7. Maternal health services—India. I. Mondal, Nitish, 1984- editor. II. Singh, Narendra (Associate professor), editor.

LCC RG530.3.I4M38 2022 | DDC 362.198200954 23

FOREWORD

It gives me great pleasure to write a Foreword for the book *Maternal Health and Child Mortality: Condition, Vision and Challenges*, a volume edited by two young anthropologists of Diphu Campus of Assam University.

Freedom from hunger is basic human right. Nutrition is a state of health conditioned by the ecology of food, and of all factors influencing the health status of the individual members of the society, nutrition exerts the greatest influence. In a country like ours, malnutrition with a high incidence of infection is a major health problem. India shows the highest occurrence of childhood undernutrition in the world and it has been estimated that nearly half of the Indian children are undernourished. Malnutrition is the significant underlying factor for high incidence of infant and child mortality, growth retardation and reduced mental efficiency. The worst victims of malnutrition are not only the economically vulnerable segments of the society but more particularly, the biologically vulnerable groups like infants, pre-school children, expectant mothers and lactating mothers. The Census of India (2011) has recorded that 41.3 per cent of the girls in India get married before attaining 19 years of age. In rural India, 47.3 per cent of girls get married before attaining the age of 19 year, while in urban areas, the corresponding figure was found to be 29.2 per cent. Marriage at adolescent age has an adverse effect on the health status of the girl. All these proximate causes are ultimately linked to a host of underlying factors, specifically poverty and ignorance being the most significant determinants. Culture plays a great role on the mother-child health in India.

India is now committed to achieving universal health coverage, and that the Government of India launched the Ayushman Bharat Yojana on September 23, 2018, which rest on the twin pillars of health and wellness centres, and the National Health Protection Mission (AB-NHPM) has a target for 100 million families covering 500 million individuals. It is not impossible to achieve the target within a reasonable period of time with concerted efforts, but the problem we are facing is shortage of medical practitioners particularly in the villages, that puts a strain on the public health facilities, and coupled with it is the poor infrastructure development programmes at the village/block level. There also lies lack of desired specific training programmes for health care workers at the village level. Hope in near future the prevailing situations will change greatly towards providing a much better all-round health care facilities to the rural people of the villages in India.

In rural areas of India, the greatest need is of the primary health care facilities and the supporting infrastructure facilities in the region for running the primary health centres. Health centres must be supported with regular communication and transport facilities will all weather roads connectivity with villages and remote rural areas. Communication and road connectivity is in a very poor shape in rural areas that I have seen and experienced while conducting fieldworks in interior villages among the tribals of Ranchi and Hazaribagh districts when Jharkhand was not yet formed. However, health care facilities and connectivity have improved to some extent in rural areas only after the formation of the state of Jharkhand.

Apart from nutrition and health studies of the tribes and castes in India, the anthropologists in India are now more inclined in working on medical anthropology and medical economics, and other related parameters in rural and urban areas to understand the health and nutritional status and related aspects of the people in a holistic way.

In the present volume, Dr. Nitish Mondal and Prof. Kh. Narendra Singh have presented a collection of articles with special focus on maternal and child health conditions in India, with a subtitle on 'risk and challenges'. The volume contains twenty-five articles mainly focusing on maternal and child health status in north-east India, specifically among some of the tribes and caste population groups of Assam, Meghalaya and Arunachal Pradesh. Socio-economic conditions, health care practices, birth spacing, and lifestyle determinants on maternal and child health and nutritional status have also been presented by researches on communities sampled from West Bengal, Odisha, Uttar Pradesh, Punjab, Kerala and Tamil Nadu. Thus, communities from different socio-cultural regions of India have been covered.

A few articles, however, I feel do not fit well with the thrust area of the volume 'maternal and child health', like 'Ovarion endometriosis with or without—allied adenomyosis exert differential pain responses'; and the other one, 'Maternal inheritance—the burden of deficiency of Glucose-6-Phosphate Dehydrogenase enzyme in human'. These two articles discuss specific cases in specialized field of study and may not fit in a general way with the health status of mother and child directly, but the topics have their own importance in the study of human health.

Improvement in the maternal and child health cares, reducing the burden of maternal and child mortality, and working towards universal access to health care are the utmost priorities of the governments and several civil society organizations. We cannot emphatically say that maternity care and child birth in hospitals of rural areas have become safer in India over the last 20 years despite many initiatives taken for safe maternal and child care programmes at the national level. The situation has improved to some extent but yet not so assuring and smooth as it should be. Keeping all these aspects in mind, Dr. Nitish Mondal and Prof. Narendra Singh present in this volume a collection of articles based on empirical studies on mother and child health status and health care practices in some rural and urban areas of India.

This edited volume containing articles on mother and child gives a fragment of a total vision on the prevailing situation of the health status of mother and child in India. I feel the issues raised in this volume by authors will lead to a greater understanding of the challenges faced on mother and child health care particularly in rural areas. I congratulate the editors for their hard and dedicated works for the publication of this volume.

P. Dash Sharma
Retired Professor of Anthropology,
University of Ranchi, Jharkhand

PREFACE

During the past few decades there has been a growing recognition that addressing of the appropriate maternal and child health issues requires organising services in a continuum of health care that encompasses these health problems. Most of the health problems encountered in mothers and children of the developing countries could be prevented either by immunization or health education. Maternal health is one of the most crucial elements, has long been ignored in public health care and the maternal mortality rate (MMR) remains quite high in our country and contributes almost a quarter of the global estimates of maternal morbidity and mortality, however, a slight declining trend over two decades has been observed.

The World Health Organization (WHO) estimates that of 5,36,000 maternal deaths occurring globally each year, out of which 1,36,000 deaths take place in India. India's MMR has been reduced from 212 deaths per 1,00,000 live births in 2007 to 167 deaths per 1,00,000 live births in 2013. Improvement in the maternal and child health care, reducing the burden of maternal and child mortality, and working towards universal access to health care are the utmost priorities of the governments and several civil society organizations. The adolescent and illiterate mothers and those living in hard to reach areas still have a much greater chance of dying during childbirth. Adolescent girls living in rural areas of the country are vulnerable to teenage marriage and pregnancies. India has the highest number of child marriages in the world.

The National Census (2011) estimated that 41.3 per cent of the girls in India are married before 19 years of age. In rural India, 47.3 per cent of 19-year-old girls got married and in the urban areas, the corresponding figure was 29.2 per cent. Available data suggested that for every 1,000 girls aged 15 to 19 years, there were 76 adolescent births in India in 2010 compared to 49 worldwide and 53 in less developed regions. There is little evidence that maternity has become safer in India over the last 20 years despite the safe motherhood policies and programmatic initiatives at the national level. The status of women is being low in India, except in the southern and eastern states. The female literacy rate is observed to be unsatisfactory and women lack the empowerment to decide, including the decision to use reproductive health services and childcare.

Malnutrition among children is a major public health problem in India and it has been estimated that more than half of the Indian children are undernourished. Maternal and child mortality are being recognised as a human rights issue due to its vulnerability and preventability. Integration of a human rights perspective in maternal and child health programmes could contribute to eliminating avertable maternal and child deaths. The maternal and child health issues are much higher in the rural areas and attributed to lack of adequate health care facilities, lack of knowledge about health, hygiene and lack of awareness about health care services, institutional delivery and acute shortage of doctors and medical staff in the hospitals. The health system's conscious effort to improve maternal and child health, normative elements of human rights approach to maternal health (i.e. availability, accessibility, acceptability, and quality of maternal health services) were not upheld. The Government of India has made significant advancements to improve the maternal and health and show an increase in institutional delivery and immunization coverage but the desired target is yet to be achieved. Given the multiple efforts of the Government to improve maternal health why have the maternal health indicators not improved in the past decade? Due to lack of the managerial capacity, clear overall programme objectives, and evidence-based strategies, the schemes were implemented as an unconnected patchwork of efforts and, hence, did not lead to the desired improvement in the performance and achievement of objectives of the health system.

The edited volume highlights and discusses the major issues related to the maternal and child health in India with the following broad sub-themes:

1. Socio-Economic, Demographic and Double Burden of Maternal and Child Health.
2. Maternal Health Status, Child Mortality and Human Right Issues.

3. Reproductive Health, Indigenous Healthcare Practices and Health Services in India.
4. Changing Perspectives of Maternal and Child Health and Nutrition Status in India.
5. Recent Trends and Developments in Maternal and Child Healthcare.

In order to control the maternal and child deaths in India, concentrated efforts need to be put to identify the major determinants of the population, better health education, women's empowerment, and strengthening health care system to provide timely and quality services, including emergency and obstetric care. The present volume brings together scholars and academicians from various disciplines and health professionals, policy makers and social scientists under the same umbrella for discussion and critical evaluation of current health situation and efficacy and role of healthcare programme related to maternal and child health in India. The present volume focuses to identify the major socio-economic, demographic and cultural factors affecting the maternal and child health issues especially among the vulnerable segments living in rural India.

We hope this edited volume may be helpful for effective planning and operationalizing maternal and child health services in the country.

Nitish Mondal
Kh. Narendra Singh,

ACKNOWLEDGEMENTS

We are grateful to many individuals for their encouragement and valuable suggestions to publish this volume. First of all, we are very much thankful to Prof. P. Dash Sharma, Retd. Professor, Department of Anthropology, Ranchi University, Ranchi, an eminent biological anthropologist and great scholar for accepting our request to write the foreword of this edited volume. The editors gratefully acknowledge all the authors for their valuable contributions without which the publication of the present volume would not have been possible. The present volume contains twenty five well postulated research manuscripts contributed by eminent anthropologists, sociologists, social scientists and health professionals to acquaint the book readers on health and nutrition with special focus on maternal and child health in India. The topics contributed by the authors in the book are incredibly diverse and in-depth content and the authors offered their sincere efforts to explore and address the specific public health issues. The volume features with abundance of materials and wide ranging analysis which is extremely stimulative, useful and certainly serves the interest on the maternal and child health and nutritional issues.

Last but not the least, we deeply express our thankfulness to the Concept Publishing Company Pvt. Limited, New Delhi, India for extending their cooperation and support to publish this edited volume with professional dedication. We hope the present volume may be helpful to anthropologists, social scientists and other teaching community, researchers and policy makers especially focusing health issues of the tribal population of India.

Nitish Mondal

Narendra Singh

CONTENTS

LIST OF THE CONTRIBUTORS

Ms. Adrija Tripathy, Department of Bio-Medical Laboratory Science and Management, Clinical Nutrition and Dietetics, Vidyasagar University, Midnapore, West Bengal-721102, India.

Dr. Ajit K. Tamuli, Associate Professor, Department of Life Science and Bioinformatics, Assam University: Diphu Campus, Karbi Anglong, Assam-782460, India.
E-mail: arlappan@yahoo.com.

Mr. Amlan K. Ray, Spectrum Clinic and Endoscopy Research Institute, 28B, Shakespeare Sarani, Kolkata-700017, India.
E-mail: humanedestiny@gmail.com.

Ms. Arti Muley, Symbiosis Institute of Health Sciences, Symbiosis International (Deemed University), Lavale, Pune-412115, India.

Mrs. Chhandika Roy, Department of Anthropology, Rajiv Gandhi University, Rono Hills, Doimukh, Arunachal Pradesh-791112, India.
E-mail: chhandikaroy@gmail.com.

Dr. Chitradip Bhattacherjee, Post Doctoral Fellow, Indian Council of Social Science Research, West Bengal State University, Barasat, Kolkata, West Bengal-700126, India.

Prof. Debidas Ghosh, Department of Bio-Medical Laboratory Science and Management, Clinical Nutrition and Dietetics, Vidyasagar University, Midnapore-721102, India.
E-mail: debidas_ghosh@yahoo.in.

Mr. Dibya Pal, Department of Bio-Medical Laboratory Science and Management, Clinical Nutrition and Dietetics, Vidyasagar University, Midnapore-721102, India.

Ms. Farhin Ara, Department of Bio-Medical Laboratory Science and Management, Clinical Nutrition and Dietetics, Vidyasagar University, Midnapore-721102, India.

Dr. G. Sarika, Scientist-B (Medical), UNICEF Project, Public Health Nutrition, ICMR—National Institute of Nutrition, Hyderabad-500007, Telangana, India.

Mrs. Himangi Kalita, Research Scholar, Department of Anthropology, Assam University (Diphu Campus), Karbi Anglong-782462, Assam, India.
E-mail: himangikalita1@gmail.com.

Mr. Hriday Ranjan Gogoi, Department of Life Science and Bioinformatics, Assam University: Diphu Campus, Karbi Anglong-782460, Assam, India.

Dr. Huidrom Suraj Singh, Department of Anthropology, Manipur University, Canchipur, Imphal-795003, India.
E-mail: huidromsurajsingh@gmail.com.

Prof. Jaydip Sen, Department of Anthropology, University of North Bengal, Raja Rammohunpur, Darjeeling, West Bengal-734013, India.
E-mail: jaydipsen@gmail.com.

Dr. Junali Kropi, Department of Anthropology, Dibrugarh University, Dibrugarh-786004, India.
E-mail: junali09@hotmail.com.

Dr. Juri Borah, Assistant Professor, Department of Anthropology, Gurucharan College, Silchar-788004, Assam, India.
E-mail: juriborah571@gmail.com.

Dr. Jyoti Ratan Ghosh, Department of Anthropology, Visva-Bharati, Santiniketan-731235, West Bengal, India.
E-mail: jrghosh@rediffmail.com.

Dr. Kasturi Chatterjee, Cancer Biology and Inflammatory Disorder Division, CSIR-Indian Institute of Chemical Biology, Kolkata-700032, India.

Prof. Kaushik Bose, Professor, Department of Anthropology, Vidyasagar University, Midnapore-721102, West Bengal, India.
E-mail: kaushikbose@cantab.net.

Dr. Kavitha Menon, Professor, Symbiosis Institute of Health Sciences, Symbiosis International (Deemed University), Lavale, Pune-412115, India.
E-mail: kavitha.menon3@gmail.com.

Prof. Kh. Narendra Singh, Professor, Department of Anthropology, Assam University (Diphu Campus), Karbi Anglong-782462, Assam, India.
E-mail: kh.singh@gmail.com.

Dr. Mitravinda Aneesh, Assistant Professor, Department of Nutrition and Dietetics, Mount Carmel College, Bangalore-560052, India.
E-mail: mitrasav@gmail.com.

Ms. Madhushree Dey, Research Scholar, Department of Anthropology, Dr Harisingh Gour University, Sagar-470003, India.
E-mail: madhushreedey94@gmail.com.

Dr. Manoranjan Pal, Professor (Retd.), Indian Statistical Institute, 203 B.T. Road, Kolkata-700108, India.
E-mail: manoranjan.pal@gmail.com.

Dr. Nimmathota Arlappa, Scientist-F, Division of Public Health Nutrition, ICMR-National Institute of Nutrition, Hyderabad-500007, Telangana, India.
E-mail: arlappan@yahoo.com.

Dr. Nitamoni Bharali, Research Scholar, Department of Anthropology, Assam University (Diphu Campus), Karbi Anglong, Assam-782462, India.
E-mail: nbharali@gmail.com.

Dr. Nitish Mondal, Associate Professor, Department of Anthropology, Sikkim University, Gangtok-737102, Sikkim, India.
E-mail: nitishanth@gmail.com.

Ms. Pikli Khanra, Department of Anthropology, Vidyasagar University, Midnapore-721102, West Bengal, India.

Ms. Pooja Panchal, Symbiosis Institute of Health Sciences, Symbiosis International (Deemed University), Lavale, Pune-412115, India.

Dr. Pramathes Das Mahapatra, Spectrum Clinic and Endoscopy Research Institute, 28B, Shakespeare Sarani, Kolkata-700017, India.

Prof. Premananda Bharati, Professor (Retd.), Indian Statistical Institute, 203, B.T. Road, Kolkata-700108, India.
E-mail: pbharati@gmail.com.

Dr. Rajeshwari Sinha, Independent Researcher, New Delhi, India.
E-mail: rajeshwari.sinha@yahoo.com.

Dr. Ramanpreet Randhawa, Department of Human Genetics, Guru Nanak Dev University, Amritsar-143005, Punjab, India.
E-mail: raman.randhawa19@gmail.com.

Dr. Ramie H. Begum, Assistant Professor Department of Life Sciences and Bioinformatics, Assam University: Diphu Campus, Karbi Anglong-782460, Assam, India.
E-mail: ani.ara73@gmail.com.

Dr. Rita Patil, Associate Professor, Department of Food and Nutrition, Maniben Nanavati Women's College, Mumbai-400056, Maharashtra, India.
E-mail: rita.spatil@gmail.com.

Prof. Rajesh K. Gautam, Professor, Department of Anthropology, Dr Harisingh Gour University, Sagar-470003, India.
E-mail: goutamraj2006@gmail.com.

Dr. Sanghamitra Pati, Indian Council of Medical Research-Regional Medical Research Centre, Department of Health Research, Bhubaneswar-751023, Odisha, India.
E-mail: drsanghamitra12@gmail.com.

Prof. Sarthak Sengupta, Professor (Retd.), Department of Anthropology, Dibrugarh University, Dibrugarh-786004, Assam, India.
E-mail: rita.spatil@gmail.com.

Mr. Sarvendra Yadav, Research Scholar, Department of Anthropology, Dr. Harisingh Gour University, Sagar-470003, India.
E-mail: sarvendra2u@gmail.com.

Dr. Sayantan Jana, Cancer Biology and Inflammatory Disorder Division, CSIR-Indian Institute of Chemical Biology, Kolkata-700032, India.

Prof. Sharda Sidhu, Professor (Retd), Department of Human Genetics, Guru Nanak Dev University, Amritsar-143005, Punjab, India.
E-mail: shardasidhu@hotmail.com.

Ms. Shreyasi Roy, Research Fellow, Department of Anthropology, University of North Bengal, Raja Rammohunpur, Darjeeling-734013, West Bengal, India.
E-mail: shreyasiroy93@rediffmail.com.

Ms. Snehasikta Swarnakar, Cancer Biology and Inflammatory Disorder Division, CSIR-Indian Institute of Chemical Biology, Kolkata-700032, India.

Ms. Soma Pal, Department of Anthropology, Vidyasagar University, Midnapore-721102, West Bengal, India.

Dr. Subal Das, Department of Anthropology & Tribal Development, Guru Ghasidas Vishwavidyalaya, Bilaspur-495009, Chhattisgarh, India.
E-mail: dsubalvu@gmail.com.

Prof. Subir Biswas, Professor, Department of Anthropology, West Bengal State University, Barasat, Kolkata-700126, West Bengal, India.
E-mail: gargisubir@gmail.com.

Dr. Sudipta Ghosh, Assistant Professor, Department of Anthropology, North-Eastern Hill University, Shillong-793022, India.
E-mail: ghosh.sudipta@gmail.com.

Ms. Sujata Bhowmick (Ganguly), Department of Bio-Medical Laboratory Science and Management, Clinical Nutrition and Dietetics, Vidyasagar University, Midnapore-721102, West Bengal, India.

Mr. Surabhi Singh Yadav, Symbiosis Institute of Health Sciences, Symbiosis International (Deemed University), Lavale, Pune-412115, India.

Dr. Susmita Bharati, Professor, Indian Statistical Institute, 203, B.T. Road, Kolkata-700108, India.
E-mail: susmitabharati60@gmail.com.

Ms. Swastika Roy, Department of Anthropology, Visva-Bharati, Santiniketan-731235, West Bengal, India.

Dr. Thangjam Chitralekha Devi, Department of Anthropology, Manipur University, Canchipur, Imphal–795003, India.

Dr. Tiluttoma Baruah, Associate Professor, Cotton University, Guwahati-781001, Assam, India.
E-mail: tiluttomabaruah2019@gmail.com.

Dr. Viserano Peseyie, Research Scholar, Department of Anthropology, North-Eastern Hill University, Shillong-793022, India.
E-mail: avise_peseyie@yahoo.com.

SECTION-I

Socio-Economic, Demographic and Double Burden of Maternal and Child Health

1

Double Burden of Maternal and Child Malnutrition

An Indian Perspective

Nimmathota Arlappa and G. Sarika

Introduction

The world has transitioned from an era when underweight prevalence was more than double that of obesity, to one in which more people are obese than underweight (Lancet- NCD Risk Factor Collaboration, 2016). With the recent adoption of UN resolution of Decade of Action on Malnutrition (2016 to 2025) and the Sustainable Development Goals shifting focus from predominantly undernutrition (single sides of malnutrition) to end hunger and eradicate all forms of malnutrition, came to the forefront, the new nutrition reality, i.e. there are multiple forms of malnutrition that overlap in different ways and in different places (Global Nutrition Report, 2018). This coexistence of undernutrition along with overweight, obesity or diet-related non-communicable diseases (DR-NCDs) is referred as Double Burden of Malnutrition (DBM) (United Nations Decade of Action on Nutrition, 2015), which manifests at different levels i.e., of individuals (a child being stunted and overweight simultaneously or temporally separated), households (obese mother with a wasted child) and populations, and across the life-course (Food and Nutrition Paper 84. Rome; UN, 2006). The causes leading DBM relate to a sequence of epidemiological changes known as the nutrition transition (describes shift in dietary patterns, consumption and energy expenditure associated with economic development over time), epidemiological transition (describes the changes in overall population disease burden) and the demographic transition which describes the shift in population structure and lengthening life spans (Shrimpton and Rokx, 2012).

DBM and Its Prevalence

Today, globally one in every three persons suffers from at least one form of malnutrition: wasting, stunting, vitamin and mineral deficiency, overweight or obesity and diet-related NCDs. This simultaneous manifestation of both undernutrition and overweight and obesity predominantly affects most low-income and middle-income countries (LMICs) especially prevalent in sub-Saharan Africa, South Asia, and East Asia and the Pacific (Popkin *et al.*, 2019).

Life Course Manifestations of DBM

Malnutrition has adverse effects on health throughout life, but its early emergence has particularly harmful consequences, because early childhood development is characterized by critical sensitive periods which are responsive to nutritional influences (both inadequate and excesses of nutritional supply) in early life and contribute to intergenerational effects in both contexts. Such physiological sensitivity explains why early nutrition and growth have major implications for immediate survival, long-term health, and human capital (Victora *et al.*, 2008; Adair *et al.*, 2013).

Malnutrition often increases disease susceptibility, while ill health exacerbates poor nutrition. Inadequate or poor nutrition during fetal development or in early childhood causes malnutrition in the form of multiple micronutrient deficiencies, severe and irreversible cognitive and physical damage, e.g.: It is observed that early childhood stunting is closely associated with poor cognitive and educational performance in children (Ernesto Pollitt *et al.*, 2004). Iron deficiency affects pregnancy, impairs cognitive development, and reduces work productivity. Severe iron-deficiency anaemia may even result in death among women of childbearing age (World Bank, Repositioning Nutrition as Central to Development, 2005). Although stunting has been decreasing for the past four decades, the other end of the spectrum of DBM, i.e. obesity has seen an exponential increase. A study on Global

Ageing population by WHO observed that with about 1.9 billion adults overweight and 600 million adults obese global prevalence of overweight and obesity has more than doubled in 2014 from that of 1980. An estimate by the same organization said that around two-thirds of global burden of disease will be accredited to chronic NCDs, most of them strongly associated with diet (WHO, 2008).

Rapid urbanization and globalization of unhealthy lifestyles have resulted in changed social, economic, and structural factors which have fuelled a global crisis of obesity and NCDs (Popkin *et al.*, 2004). Women are more vulnerable to this double burden of "dysnutrition", because of their high nutritional requirements for pregnancy and lactation and also because of gender inequalities in poverty. Studies from LMICs indicate that high consumption of processed foods is associated with lower micronutrient intake, micronutrient deficiencies in children and the coexistence of child stunting and maternal overweight (Aitsi-Selmi *et al.*, 2015). This combination of overweighed mother and undernourished/stunted children is the most prevalent form of household level DBM and is called maternal and child double burden of malnutrition. It is of serious concern as maternal obesity is often associated with elevated fetal adiposity, especially when compounded by gestational diabetes.

Women who are overweight are more likely to develop gestational diabetes which often results in greater gestational weight gain, higher birth weight, faster post-natal weight gain and studies suggest that this high amount of nutrition in early life is associated with greater risk of obesity, abdominal adiposity, and insulin resistance in adulthood (Barquera *et al.*, 2007). When an overweighed mother is also previously stunted, the combined effect is predicted to increase the risk of gestational diabetes and of obstructed labour. The consequences of maternal obesity for the next generation, therefore, depend on the mother's own developmental experience. In a Swedish study, the intergenerational transmission of obesity was three times greater among mothers who were obese and born small for gestational age than in mothers of normal birth weight (Wells, 2017). Therefore, DBM might affect health outcomes of mothers and offspring related to childbirth (Taylor *et al.*, 2014).

A 2008 Lancet study has acknowledged that early exposure to undernutrition in childhood followed by later overweight during the course of life increases the risk of NCDs, by involving imbalance of the gut microbiome, inflammation, imposing a high metabolic load on a depleted capacity for homoeostasis, impaired insulin signalling and in women increases the risk of childbirth complications (WHO Expert Consultation, 2004). Children born with low birth weight due to intrauterine growth retardation or stunted in the first two years of life face a greater risk of obesity and/or NCDs like diabetes, hypertension, stroke, cardiovascular disease, and some forms of cancer in adulthood (World Bank, 2005). A 2006 report by World Health Organization emphasized that there was higher risk of high blood pressure, heart disease, and type-2 diabetes at an earlier age among people who were undernourished in younger age and obese in adulthood.

Economic Implications

Malnutrition not only requires for high budget outlays for health services but also results in loss in gross domestic product (GDP) due to diminished productive potential. It is estimated that an average of 0.6 per cent of GDP is lost to iron deficiency in adults in LMICs. When the damage to children's cognitive and motor development due to Iron deficiency anaemia is also counted, the economic loss increases to 4 per cent of GDP (Horton and Ross, 2003). It is estimated that the economic cost of obesity to LMICs is 2 per cent to 5 per cent of GDP (Barry *et al.*, 2004). NCDs lead to high healthcare costs, productivity losses, the need for long-term care, out of pocket expenditure and strained economies. A study released by World Economic Forum at the UN summit on NCDs in New York warns that five common chronic diseases—heart disease, chronic respiratory disease, cancer, diabetes and mental health woes will cost the world $47 trillion by 2030. In addition, addressing maternal mortality, infant mortality and morbidity, NCDs and mental health conditions require an ever-growing share of resources, increasing demand on the health system and thus reducing government's ability to invest on other development goals (Bloom *et al.*, 2014).

Indian Scenario

In spite of implementation of several national nutrition intervention programmes for more than four decades, the prevalence of undernutrition continues to be a major public health problem in India wherein it is home to about 50 per cent of world's undernourished children. Unfortunately, undernutrition still remains a leading cause of childhood morbidity and mortality in India and in many parts of the world. The Global Nutrition Report (2019) found that India has the world's largest number of stunted (46.6 million) and wasted children (25.5 million). Barring Puducherry, Delhi, Kerala and Lakshadweep, all other states have a higher proportion of stunted children in rural areas than the urban (NFHS-4) (Kurian *et al.*, 2019). As reported by the NNMB (2011-12), the prevalence of underweight, stunting and wasting among under 5 year rural children in 10 major states of India was 45 per cent, 48 per cent and 21 per cent, respectively. Similarly, the latest round of NFHS-4 (2014-15) reported the prevalence of underweight and stunting as 36 per cent and 38 per cent respectively, with wide variation between the states and regions.

Though the proportion of children who are stunted and underweight has been decreasing over a period of time, the prevalence of same is still very high in India at 39 per cent and 33 per cent respectively in 2017. However, the prevalence of child overweight has increased considerably in India in the past decade to 12 per cent in 2017. If these trends continue, achieving the UN Sustainable Development Goals (SDGs) of elimination of all forms of malnutrition by 2030 is highly impossible in India.

It is well established that malnourished children, particularly those with severe acute malnutrition, have a greater risk of death from common childhood illness such as diarrhoea, pneumonia, and malaria. Undernutrition contributes to about 45 per cent of deaths in children under 5 years of age (WHO, 2013). However, the latest Lancet publication attributes 68.2 per cent of under 5 deaths in India in 2017 due to undernutrition (United Nations Department of Economic and Social Affairs, 2019). Eliminating malnutrition would remove one-third of the global burden of disease and increase child survival (Mason *et al.*, 2003).

As reported by the NNMB periodic nutrition survey and NFHS surveys, the magnitude of dual nutrition burden has increased in India. Over the period of time, the prevalence of undernutrition decreased marginally, whereas that of overweight/obesity increased at alarming rates which could be attributed to rapid nutrition, demographic, and epidemiological transition in

India. As per NFHS-4, the prevalence of overweight/obesity among men and women has doubled in the last two decades from 1998-99 to 2015-16 in India. A swift increase in the overweight/ obesity has been observed in all the states of India in both rural and urban areas, where it has escalated to epidemic proportions. Among urban women, the prevalence of overweight/obesity has reached an alarming level. In 1998-99, 13 states had more than 20 per cent overweight/obesity prevalence which increased to 14 states in 2005-06 (with 10 states had more than 25% prevalence) and there were 28 states in India in 2015-16, where prevalence was more than 20 per cent.

In rural areas also, the prevalence of overweight/obesity among women increased substantially. In 1998-99, only four states had more than 15 per cent overweight/obesity prevalence which increased to more than 20 per cent in 2005-06 and there were 14 states with more than 15 per cent prevalence of overweight/obesity among rural women in 2015-16 (Shannawaz and Arokiasamy, 2018). It was found that overweight and obesity have become substantial problems among different socio-economic spectrum of women and men in India, particularly in older ages, not just in people living in urban areas, well-educated and households of highest wealth quintile but also among people living in poorer wealth quintile, uneducated and people belonging to socio-economically less developed states.

NCDs have become a major public health problem in India accounting for 62 per cent of the total burden of foregone DALYs and 53 per cent of total deaths. Out of pocket expenditure associated with the acute and long term effects of NCDs is high resulting in very high health expenditure for the households. A study in India showed that about 25 per cent of families with a member with CVD and 50 per cent of families with cancer experience catastrophic expenditure and 10 per cent and 25 per cent, respectively, are driven to poverty (Kundu *et al.*, 2018). In 2010, NCDs accounted for more disability-adjusted life years (DALYs) in India than communicable diseases – approximately 235 million *versus* 222 million DALYs, respectively (Institute for Health Metrics and Evaiuation, 2013). India is indeed undergoing simultaneous transitions. Research has shown that the multiple burdens of persistent undernutrition, micronutrient deficiencies, and rising overnutrition contributing to disease load predominantly DR-NCDs.

Table 1.1: Prevalence of Undernutrition among Rural under5 children according to SD (standard deviation) Classification (WHO Growth Standards) NFHS-4

S.No.	*State*	*Underweight*	*Stunting*	*Wasting*
1.	Andaman and Nicobar Islands	21.6	23.3	18.9
2.	Andhra Pradesh	31.9	31.4	17.2
3.	Arunachal Pradesh	19.5	29.4	17.3
4.	Assam	29.8	36.4	17
5.	Bihar	43.9	48.3	20.8
6.	Chandigarh	24.5	28.7	10.9
7.	Chhatisgarh	37.7	37.6	23.1
8.	Dadra and Nagar Haveli	38.9	41.7	27.6
9.	Daman and Diu	26.7	23.4	24.1
10.	Goa	23.8	20.1	21.9
11.	Gujarat	39.3	38.5	26.4
12.	Haryana	29.4	34	21.2
13.	Himachal Pradesh	21.2	26.3	13.7
14.	Jammu & Kashmir	16.6	27.4	12.1
15.	Jharkhand	47.8	45.3	29
16.	Karnataka	35.2	36.2	26.1
17.	Kerala	16.1	19.7	15.7
18.	Lakshadweep	23.4	27	13.8
19.	Madhya Pradesh	42.8	42	25.8
20.	Maharashtra	36	34.4	25.6
21.	Manipur	13.8	28.9	6.8
22.	Meghalaya	29	43.8	15.3
23.	Mizoram	11.9	28	6.1
24.	Nagaland	16.8	28.6	11.2
25.	Delhi	27	32.3	17.1
26.	Puducherry	22	23.7	23.6
27.	Punjab	21.6	25.7	15.6
28.	Rajasthan	36.7	39.1	23
29.	Sikkim	14.2	29.6	14.2
30.	Tamil Nadu	23.8	27.1	19.7
31.	Telangana	28.5	28.1	18
32.	Tripura	24.1	24.3	16.8
33.	Uttar Pradesh	39.5	46.3	17.9
34.	Uttrakhand	26.6	33.5	19.5
35.	West Bengal	31.5	32.5	20.3
36.	Odisha	34.4	34.1	20.4
	India	**38.3**	**41.2**	**21.5**

India is in "severe public health concern" category with a high prevalence of more than forty per cent of rural under5 stunting and prevalence of wasting being more than 15 per cent. Bihar is reportedly having the highest (48.3%) proportion of stunted under 5 children and lowest (19.7%) in Kerala. The percentage of underweight children ranging from 11.9 per cent (least) in Mizoram to 47.8 per cent in Jharkhand and prevalence of wasting ranging from a low 6.1 per cent in the state of Mizoram to a high 27.6 per cent in the UT of Dadra and Nagar Haveli (NFHS 4) **(Table 1.1).**

Table 1.2: Time trends in prevalence (%) of undernutrition (<median-2 SD) among rural pre-school children (1-5 years) according to SD Classification (WHO Growth Standards)

States	*Period*	*N*	*(Undernutrition—Per cent)*		
			Underweight	*Stunting*	*Wasting*
Kerala	1975-79	418	71.6	78.5	33.0
	1996-97	886	21.5	27.5	12.3
	2011-12	523	23.5	27.3	12.0
Tamil Nadu	1975-79	744	71.2	81.7	24.7
	1996-97	819	36.0	44.7	16.4
	2011-12	600	31.5	24.6	20.9
Karnataka	1975-79	1784	76.0	80.4	27.2
	1996-97	1681	51.6	50.2	24.5
	2011-12	676	43.1	45.4	15.3
Andhra Pradesh	1975-79	650	75.8	82.2	31.3
	1996-97	1962	55.6	55.7	30.1
	2011-12	773	38.5	48.0	12.3
Maharashtra	1975-79	627	82.1	89.5	25.3
	1996-97	1010	54.1	67.9	17.0
	2011-12	702	37.5	48.1	09.6
Gujarat	1975-79	1011	77.1	83.3	29.1
	1996-97	639	59.0	64.8	33.3
	2011-12	808	57.4	57.2	23.3
Odisha	1975-79	451	70.0	78.0	25.3
	1996-97	1650	50.6	55.4	19.0
	2011-12	764	46.0	52.1	13.8
Pooled	**1975-79**	**5685**	**75.5**	**82.0**	**27.0**
(for 7 States)	**1996-97**	**8647**	**48.6**	**52.8**	**22.5**
	2011-12	**4846**	**41.1**	**44.3**	**15.5**

In the last three decades, overall decrease of about forty five per cent is reported in under 5 undernutrition in Rural India. More than sixty per cent decrease in the prevalence of undernutrition in rural pre-school children is seen in the state of Kerala and Gujarat with highest proportion of underweight, stunted and wasted rural school children has seen the least fall of about twenty per cent. Almost all the states have seen a consistent fall, except for Tamil Nadu which has seen an increase in under 5 wasting in the last decade **(Table 1.2).**

Unlike the consistent fall over the time, seen in rural under 5 undernutrition, a good number of states like West Bengal (35%), Odisha (25%) , Maharashtra (20%) and Karnataka have seen an alarming trend of increase in the prevalence of tribal under 5 wasting, with few other states showing very slight fall or no change. With more than half of tribal under 5 children being underweight and stunted and about one-fifth of them being wasted, it is evident that the prevalence of all forms of undernutrition is higher when compared to rural children. It reflects upon poor penetration of Governmental Nutrition Intervention programmes **(Table 1.3**).

Table 1.3: Time trends in prevalence (%) of undernutrition (<median-2 SD) among tribal pre-school children (1-5 years) according to SD Classification (WHO Growth Standards)

States	*Period*	*N*	*(Undernutrition-Per cent)*		
			Underweight	*Stunting*	*Wasting*
Kerala	1998-99	868	43.5	51.0	15.8
	2007-08	1127	43.6	53.7	15.4
Tamil Nadu	1998-99	1346	60.2	50.3	30.8
	2007-08	1356	47.2	46.1	19.0
Karnataka	1998-99	1059	47.3	46.4	18.8
	2007-08	889	42.6	39.4	21.7
Andhra Pradesh	1998-99	1312	51.5	48.8	26.4
	2007-08	1377	50.7	52.1	19.2
Maharashtra	1998-99	1458	68.0	68.8	24.6
	2007-08	1751	63.7	60.7	29.3
Gujarat	1998-99	1421	56.9	58.1	28.8
	2007-08	1488	46.9	53.8	23.8
Madhya Pradesh	1998-99	1514	61.6	66.7	23.7
	2007-08	1164	52.4	52.0	21.0
Odisha	1998-99	1946	60.7	68.5	15.8
	2007-08	1915	57.7	64.6	19.9
West Bengal	1998-99	888	49.4	49.7	20.1
	2007-08	891	52.3	45.9	27.2
Pooled	**1998-99**	**11830**	**56.9**	**58.1**	**22.9**
(for 9 States)	**2007-08**	**11958**	**51.9**	**54.7**	**21.9**

Urban India has fared slightly better with about twenty five per cent of under 5 children being underweight, one-third of the children stunted and about fifteen per cent wasted. In spite of these figures, India needs to increase the intensity with which interventions have to be targeted to reach global standards of nutritional status among under 5 children **(Table 1.4)**.

Table 1.4: Prevalence (%) of Undernutrition among Urban under 5 year children according to SD Classification (WHO Growth Standards) NFHS-4

Urban under 5 years	*N*	*Under Weight*	*Stunting*	*Wasting*	*Overweight and Obesity*
Boys	6279	25.3	29.8	15.9	4.2
Girls	5818	24.7	27.6	15.2	4.3
Pooled	**12097**	**25.1**	**28.7**	**15.6**	**4.3**

In the age group of 5-17 years, the highest prevalence of thinness is seen in adolescent age band of 10-13 years in both rural boys and girls (the period of second growth spurt, period of rapid growth with increased nutritional needs). Tamil Nadu, with half of 5-9 year old boys and about two thirds of 10-13 years of age being thin (WAZ<-2SD) and Karnataka with about one in three among 14-17 years being WAZ<-2SD, have the highest proportion of thinness (WAZ<-2SD) among rural boys for the respective age groups. The highest proportion of thinness among rural girls in age bands of 5-9 and 14-17 years is seen in the state of Kerala and for rural girls of age 10-13 years, Gujarat has the highest proportion (45%). Kerala has least proportion of school age boys (about 28%) and girls (about 20%) who are WAZ<-2SD **(Tables 1.5 and 1.6).**

On an average one in every 4 school/adolescent boys is thin (WAZ<-2SD) ranging from a low of 14 per cent in Assam to a high of about 36 per cent in Andhra Pradesh. Andhra Pradesh has the highest prevalence of thin boys in all age bands. Highest proportion of thinness is seen in the age band of 10-13 years, also with a pooled average of 12.5 per cent, it is the same age band that has more children who are overweight/obese, with a range of 4.3 per cent in the state of Uttar Pradesh to 20.4 per cent in Kerala (**Table 1.7**).

Table 1.5: Prevalence (%) of Undernutrition (Thinness) among rural boys of age 5-17 years by BMI-Z scores

State	*5-9 years*	*10-13 years*	*14-17 years*
Kerala	26.6	33.2	25.9
Tamil Nadu	51.1	62.3	45.4
Karnataka	43.8	56.0	59.8
Andhra Pradesh	38.7	52.3	43.7
Maharashtra	33.5	48.1	47.5
Gujarat	43.6	51.2	50.5
Madhya Pradesh	39.4	33.8	34.7
Odisha	36.4	49.7	34.1
West Bengal	30.0	42.5	24.8
Uttar Pradesh	27.5	42.9	36.1
Pooled	**36.5**	**46.9**	**41.1**

Table 1.6: Prevalence (%) of Undernutrition (Thinness) among rural girls of age 5-17 years by BMI-Z scores

State	*5-9 years*	*10-13 years*	*14-17 years*
Kerala	22.0	21.1	16.8
Tamil Nadu	36.4	43.3	30.1
Karnataka	36.8	44.4	32.7
Andhra Pradesh	27.4	33.9	26.4
Maharashtra	32.0	32.4	26.3
Gujarat	36.3	44.9	26.3
Madhya Pradesh	36.8	44.0	20.3
Odisha	29.1	35.2	13.3
West Bengal	28.6	27.9	13.6
Uttar Pradesh	24.2	34.0	20.1
Pooled	**30.9**	**36.1**	**22.7**

Table 1.7: Distribution (%) of Urban School Age Children and Adolescents Boys According to BMI-Z scores by SD Classification (with 95% C.I)

State	*Age Group*	*N*	*Thinness WAZ <-2SD*	*Overweight and Obesity WAZ >+1SD*
Kerala	5-9	340	23.5	11.2
	10-13	303	22.1	20.4
	14-17	293	21.5	17.4
Tamil Nadu	5-9	504	24.6	9.4
	10-13	394	24.4	17
	14-17	376	28.7	9.3
Karnataka	5-9	491	26.7	6.3
	10-13	364	33.0	11
	14-17	337	26.4	6.6
Andhra Pradesh	5-9	467	36.2	6.4
	10-13	361	36.8	10.8
	14-17	362	36.7	6.4
Maharashtra	5-9	522	28.9	4.7
	10-13	453	33.6	10.4
	14-17	424	33.5	10.4
Gujarat	5-9	455	23.7	8.0
	10-13	386	21.8	18.1
	14-17	356	23.3	18.8
Madhya Pradesh	5-9	546	24.7	3.6
	10-13	454	35.2	5.3
	14-17	435	31.3	4.8
Odisha	5-9	488	20.5	12.7
	10-13	365	21.4	14.3
	14-17	276	19.9	10.5
West Bengal	5-9	515	22.3	10.3
	10-13	446	29.8	10.5
	14-17	377	30.0	6.9
Uttar Pradesh	5-9	686	27.3	2.8
	10-13	657	34.7	4.3
	14-17	549	28.8	4.0
Andaman & Nicobar	5-9	574	19.5	12.4
	10-13	456	20.4	18.8
	14-17	455	25.4	13.7
Assam	5-9	143	14.7	14
	10-13	107	18.7	18.7
	14-17	81	22.2	14.8
Bihar	5-9	496	15.3	5.8
	10-13	461	19.7	4.6
	14-17	508	13.2	4.7
Delhi	5-9	261	16.1	10.7
	10-13	209	16.7	15.7
	14-17	254	18.9	15.8
Puducherry	5-9	399	26.8	11.8
	10-13	381	22.8	20.2
	14-17	287	26.1	12.2
Rajasthan	5-9	209	19.1	7.1
	10-13	196	19.4	18.9
	14-17	235	23.0	16.2
Pooled	**5-9**	**7096**	**23.9**	**8.0**
	10-13	**5993**	**26.9**	**12.5**
	14-17	**5605**	**26.0**	**9.8**

Similar to the distribution among rural school age children, the prevalence of thinness is seen to be highest in 10-13 years of age in the urban school girl children with about one-fifth of them being thin (WAZ<-2SD), prevalence in states ranging from about 7 per cent to 25 per cent. Interestingly, it is the same age group of 10-13 years, where with pooled proportion of 10.8 per cent most of overweight and obesity among urban school/adolescents is seen **(Table 1.8)**.

Table 1.8: Distribution (%) of Urban School Age Girl Children and Adolescents according to BMI-Z Scores by SD Classification (with 95% C.I).

State	*Age group*	*N*	*Thinness WAZ <-2SD*	*Overweight/ Obesity WAZ >+1SD*
Kerala	5-9	327	18.0	11.1
	10-13	312	18.9	11.9
	14-17	297	14.8	12.1
Tamil Nadu	5-9	483	17.2	8.1
	10-13	387	20.7	14.2
	14-17	383	18.5	18.1
Karnataka	5-9	487	23.0	6.7
	10-13	381	20.5	7.1
	14-17	375	16.3	9.6
Andhra Pradesh	5-9	466	24.5	6.2
	10-13	329	23.1	11.8
	14-17	370	18.9	8.3
Maharashtra	5-9	436	23.2	3.0
	10-13	394	26.9	8.4
	14-17	415	14.0	11.8
Gujarat	5-9	385	17.4	7.1
	10-13	316	15.8	13
	14-17	341	17.6	12.9
Madhya Pradesh	5-9	484	24.4	4.3
	10-13	393	24.9	7.7
	14-17	442	14.7	7.1
Odisha	5-9	424	16.5	9.4
	10-13	369	13.6	11.7
	14-17	323	6.2	13
West Bengal	5-9	552	17.2	5.6
	10-13	438	19.6	8.9
	14-17	428	10.7	8.4

(Table 1.8 contd.)

(Table 1.8 contd.)

State	*Age Group*	*N*	*Thinness WAZ <-2SD*	*Overweight/ Obesity WAZ >+1SD*
Uttar Pradesh	5-9	670	25.4	3.3
	10-13	572	25.5	5.4
	14-17	690	14.5	5.2
Andaman & Nicobar	5-9	506	13.2	11.7
	10-13	453	12.6	15.9
	14-17	433	16.8	10.2
Assam	5-9	120	9.2	12.5
	10-13	91	18.7	17.7
	14-17	103	7.8	11.7
Bihar	5-9	395	17.7	3.8
	10-13	416	17.6	5.5
	14-17	467	10.9	4.9
Delhi	5-9	225	9.8	14.2
	10-13	215	12.1	12.1
	14-17	205	9.7	11.3
Puducherry	5-9	415	16.1	11.1
	10-13	309	16.5	20.4
	14-17	311	10.9	16.1
Rajasthan	5-9	196	14.8	8.2
	10-13	181	17.7	8.3
	14-17	252	15.5	11.1
Pooled	**5-9**	**6571**	**19.1**	**7.2**
	10-13	**5556**	**19.5**	**10.8**
	14-17	**5835**	**14.1**	**10.1**

Table 1.9: Various Studies Showing Prevalence (%) of Overweight and Obesity among Urban Children in India

Author	*Year*	*Age Group (Y)*	*N*	*Overweight and Obesity*
Laxmaiah *et al.*	2011	12-15	2,257	15.0
Laxmaiah *et al.*	2008	12-17	8,142	9.6
Mohan B. *et al.*	2004	11-17	2,467	14.2
Khadikar *et al.*	2004	10-15	1,228	25.6
Laxmaiah *et al.*	2003	12-17	1,208	14.9
Subramaniam *et al.*	2003	10-15	707	16.0
Kapil U. *et al.*	2002	10-16	870	32.1
Ramchandran A. *et al.*	2002	13-18	4,700	19.9

Chronic energy deficiency (CED) in rural Indian women is 26.7 per cent with Sikkim reportedly having lowest proportion of 6.4 per cent and Dadra and Nagar Haveli the highest proportion of 28.5 per cent. The percentage of rural women being obese/ overweight ranges from a low of 11.7 per cent in Bihar to 41.5 per cent in Chandigarh. From this data, it is pretty much evident that overweight and obesity are no longer a problem of urban nouveau riche/upper socio-economic echelons. With pooled average of about 15 per cent of rural men and women being obese/ overweight, it has become a substantial problem among different socio-economic spectrum of women and men in India **(Table 1.10).**

It has been observed that there is a consistent fall in the proportion of CED in rural adult women, with highest decrease of 63 per cent in Kerala to least of 7 per cent in Odisha. Overall every one in three rural adult women is chronic energy deficient, with a low proportion of 17.7 per cent in Kerala to high of 42.4 per cent in Odisha. Likewise, it is reported that there has been almost 400 per cent increase in prevalence of overweight/obesity in rural adult women across the states, with Andhra Pradesh reporting the prevalence to increase by 160 per cent in last three decades to an alarming 12 times rise in prevalence of overweight/obesity in the state of Kerala **(Table 1.11).** Like mentioned earlier, India is indeed undergoing simultaneous transitions with fall in prevalence of undernutrition and alarming rise in overweight/obesity. This could be attributed to rapid economic, social, lifestyle, demographic, nutrition as well as epidemiological transition in India.

Table 1.10: Prevalence (%) of Malnutrition [Chronic energy deficiency (CED) and Overweight] among Rural Adult Population According to SD Classification (WHO Growth Standards)

S.No.	State	CED		Overweight	
		Men	Women	Men	Women
1.	Andaman and Nicobar Islands	8.7	13.1	38.2	31.8
2.	Andhra Pradesh	14.8	17.6	33.5	33.2
3.	Arunachal Pradesh	8.3	8.5	20.6	18.8
4.	Assam	20.7	25.7	12.9	13.2
5.	Bihar	25.4	30.4	12.6	11.7
6.	Chandigarh	21.7	13.3	32	41.5
7.	Chhattisgarh	24.1	26.7	10.2	11.9
8.	Dadra and Nagar Haveli	19.7	28.5	22.9	19.2
9.	Daman and Diu	12	12.9	30.7	31.6
10.	Delhi	17.7	12.8	24.6	34.9
11.	Goa	10.8	14.7	32.6	33.5
12.	Gujarat	24.7	27.2	19.7	23.7
13.	Haryana	11.3	15.8	20	21
14.	Himachal Pradesh	18	16.2	22	28.6
15.	Jammu & Kashmir	11.5	12.1	20.5	29.1
16.	Jharkhand	23.8	31.5	11.1	10.3
17.	Karnataka	16.5	20.7	22.1	23.3
18.	Kerala	8.5	9.7	28.5	32.4
19.	Lakshadweep	7.4	12.5	24.6	41.4
20.	Madhya Pradesh	28.4	28.3	10.9	13.6
21.	Maharashtra	19.1	23.5	23.8	23.4
22.	Manipur	11.1	8.8	19.8	26
23.	Meghalaya	11.6	12.1	10.1	12.2
24.	Mizoram	7.2	8.3	21	21.1
25.	Nagaland	11.5	12.2	14	16.2
26.	Odisha	19.5	26.4	17.2	16.5
27.	Puducherry	10.2	11.3	37.1	36.7
28.	Punjab	10.9	11.7	27.8	31.3
29.	Rajasthan	22.7	27	13.2	14.1
30.	Sikkim	2.4	6.4	34.8	26.7
31.	Tamil Nadu	12.4	14.6	28.2	30.9
32.	Telangana	21.4	23.1	24.2	28.1
33.	Tripura	15.7	18.9	15.9	16
34.	Uttar Pradesh	25.9	25.3	12.5	16.5
35.	Uttarakhand	16.1	18.4	17.7	20.4
36.	West Bengal	19.9	21.3	14.2	19.9
	India	**23.0**	**26.7**	**14.3**	**15.0**

Table 1.11: Time-trends in Distribution (%) of Rural Adult Women by Chronic Energy Deficiency (CED) and Overweight and Obesity

State	*Period*	*N*	*CED*	*Overweight and Obesity*
Kerala	1975-79	2372	47.3	2.4
	1996-97	3480	24.6	15.8
	2011-12	3610	17.7	30.4
Tamil Nadu	1975-79	2197	50.9	4.6
	1996-97	1534	40.4	8.6
	2011-12	3173	25.7	23.2
Karnataka	1975-79	3560	57.4	2.4
	1996-97	3394	57.0	3.4
	2011-12	3375	36.6	11.8
Andhra Pradesh	1975-79	2478	52.7	4.8
	1996-97	2862	56.9	3.6
	2011-12	3218	32.8	12.7
Maharashtra	1975-79	2836	57.2	2.4
	1996-97	2022	50.2	3.2
	2011-12	3572	36.8	10.7
Gujarat	1975-79	2672	49.1	4.0
	1996-97	1691	55.9	4.0
	2011-12	3381	42.3	11.5
Odisha	1975-79	9650	45.7	2.4
	1996-97	3039	53.2	1.6
	2011-12	3160	42.4	7.2
Pooled (for 7 States)	**1975-79**	**17080**	**52.4**	**3.2**
	1996-97	**18022**	**47.8**	**6.0**
	2011-12	**23489**	**33.3**	**15.5**

Conclusion

Historically undernutrition and overweight have been considered separate challenges affecting distinct populations, and with contrasting risk factors. Undernutrition was said to be associated with poverty, food insecurity, and infection, while obesity was linked with affluence, dietary richness, and sedentary behaviour. But growing evidences have suggested that increasingly, the two forms of malnutrition co-occur within communities, families, and even individuals and those different forms of malnutrition share common drivers and are characterised by multiple physiological connections and interactions (Swinburn *et al.*, 2019). Unfortunately actions to address these different manifestations of malnutrition are still isolated from each other and implemented through different governance and funding mechanisms. The fact that this isolated approach to address one form of malnutrition has inadvertently harmed the other is furthered by major international institutions (UN) and donors revisiting their strategies to reconsider the scope of nutrition priorities, developing strategy documents, and formulating initiatives to focus on overweight and obesity as well as undernutrition (UN Children's Fund, 2019).

DBM needs interventions that simultaneously prevent or reduce the risk of both nutritional deficiencies leading to underweight, wasting, stunting and micronutrient deficiencies, and problems of obesity and diet related NCDs. "Double-duty actions" coined in the 2015 Global Nutrition Report are such strategies, programmes and policies which are designed to effectively address malnutrition in all its forms in a more holistic way (IFPRI—Global Nutrition Report 2015). They are a means of leveraging shared opportunity and reducing risks of established programmes and policies currently addressing undernutrition. Emphasis should be laid that all DBM strategies should incorporate malnutrition in all its forms and designed after a thorough risk benefit analysis and assessing the opportunities they provide to be qualified as double-duty actions. These actions must have inbuilt evaluations to ensure that their effects on outcomes can be assessed, including possible unintended consequences (WHO—Double-duty Actions for Nutrition: Policy Brief 2017). Funding should be modified in a way that these actions to deliver the strategy should be able to guide and justify the allocation of resources (Shekar *et al.*, 2017).

Double Duty Actions with Regard to Maternal and Child DBM

Nutrition in mothers during pregnancy and lactation in early life of infants and young children has profound implications for malnutrition in all its forms throughout the life course. Hence, programmes which consistently improve food environments by enhancing household access to nutritious foods, thereby leading to increased quality of mothers' and young children's diets are to be designed. For lactating mothers and their infants, one such intervention which is very widely adopted around the world is the protection, promotion, and support of optimal breastfeeding practices (World Health Organization, 2013).

Evidence shows that breastfeeding not only helps to prevent undernutrition, stimulates immunity and cognitive development, but also to reduce the risk of overweight in childhood, obesity and DR-NCDs in later life and, for the mother helps in spacing and reduces the risk of breast cancer (Horta *et al.*, 2015; Victora *et al.*, 2016; World Cancer Research Fund, 2017). Thus, interventions targeting mothers who are breastfeeding might simultaneously improve maternal health while also mitigating the DBM in the next generation.

Another such intervention could be timely introduction of sufficient diverse, nutritious and fresh foods as complementary foods, which helps in child's growth and cognitive development and also to prevent overweight/obesity during early childhood, and obesity and DR-NCDs at adulthood (WHO 2013; Global action plan for the prevention and control of NCDs 2013-2020). But for these interventions to be successful, major societal shifts are required regarding nutrition and public health. Capacity strengthening at individual as well as institutional level will be needed to change mindsets and enable action. Sense of ownership among the stakeholder community needs to be inculcated to adopt a new paradigm and mindset that favours an approach to design actions which simultaneously address the whole spectrum of problems related to malnutrition. It is only through this holistic approach to implement a comprehensive change that is sustained over decades, attaining the Sustainable Development Goal (SDG) of ending malnutrition in all its forms can be hoped for.

REFERENCES

Adair, L.S., Fall, C.H., Osmond, C., *et al.* 2013. "Associations of linear growth and relative weight gain during early life with adult health and human capital in countries of low and middle income: findings from five birth cohort studies." *Lancet* **382:** 525-34. doi: 10.1016/S0140-6736(13)60103-8.

Aitsi-Selmi, A. 2015. "Households with a stunted child and obese mother: trends and child feeding practices in a middle-income country, 1992–2008." *Matern Child Health* J. **19**(6):1284-91. doi: 10.1007/s10995-014-1634-5.

Barquera, S., Peterson K.E., Must, A. *et al.* 2007. "Coexistence of maternal central adiposity and child stunting in Mexico." *Int J Obes (Lond)* **31**(4):601-7. doi: 10.1038/sj.ijo.0803529.

Bloom, D.E., Cafiero-Fonseca, E.T., Candeias, V., Adashi, E., Bloom, L., Gurfein, L., Jané-Llopis, E., Lubet, A., Mitgang, E., Carroll, O'Brien J., Saxena, A. 2014. "Economics of Non-Communicable Diseases in India: The Costs and Returns on Investment of Interventions to Promote Healthy Living and Prevent, Treat, and Manage NCDs." World Economic Forum, Harvard School of Public Health.

Cnattingius, S., Villamor, E., Lagerros, Y.T., Wikström, A.K., Granath, F. 2012. "High birth weight and obesity—a vicious circle across generations." *Int J Obes (Lond).* **36**:1320-4. doi: 10.1038/ijo.2011.248.

Food and Agriculture Organization. 2006. The double burden of malnutrition. Case studies from six developing countries. *FAO Food and Nutrition Paper 84.* Rome: Food and Agriculture Organization of the United Nations, 2006.

Grantham-McGregor, S., Cheung, Y.B., Cueto, S., *et al.* 2007. "Developmental potential in the first 5 years for children in developing countries." *Lancet.* **369**:60—70. doi:10.1016/S0140-6736(07)60032-4.

Global Nutrition Report independent expert group 2018 global nutrition report: shining a light to spur action on nutrition.

Horta, B.L., Loret de Mola, C., Victora, C.G. 2015. "Long-term consequences of breastfeeding on cholesterol, obesity, systolic blood pressure and type 2 diabetes: a systematic review and meta-analysis." *Acta Paediatr.* **104**:30 37. doi:10.1111/apa.13133.

IFPRI-Global Nutrition Report 2015: Actions and accountability to advance nutrition and sustainable development. International Food Policy Research Institute.

Institute for Health Metrics and Evaluation [IHME], 2013.

John, B. Mason *et al.*, "At Least One-Third of Poor Countries ' Disease Burden Is Due to Malnutrition", Disease Control Priorities Project Working Paper 2003.

Kundu, M.K., Hazra, S., Pal, D., Bhattacharya, M. 2018. "A review on Non-communicable Diseases (NCDs) burden, its socio-economic impact and the strategies for prevention and control of NCDs in India." *Indian J Public Health.* **62**(4):302-304.

Kuper, H., Taylor, A., Krishna, K.V., *et al.* "Is vulnerability to cardiometabolic disease in Indians mediated by abdominal adiposity or higher body adiposity." *BMC Public Health.* 2014; **14**:1239. Published 2014 Dec 1. doi:10.1186/1471-2458-14-1239.

Mohd. Shahnawaz, P. 'Arokiasamy. 2018. *Overweight/Obesity: An Emerging Epidemic in India Journal of Clinical and Diagnostic Research,* **12**(11): LC01-LC05.

NCD Risk Factor Collaboration (NCD-RisC). Trends in adult body-mass index in 200 countries from 1975 to 2014: a pooled analysis of 1698 population-based measurement studies with 19·2 million participants [published correction appears in Lancet. 2016 May 14;387(10032):1998]. *Lancet.* 2016; **387**(10026):1377-1396. doi:10.1016/S0140-6736(16)30054-X.

Oommen, C. Kurian and Shoba Suri, "Weighed Down by the Gains: India's Twin Double Burdens of Malnutrition and Disease", Observer Research Foundation. *Occasional Paper No. 193,* May 2019.

Pollitt, E., Gorman, K.S., Engle, P.L., Rivera, J.A., Martorell, R. 1995. "Nutrition in early life and the fulfilment of intellectual potential." *J Nutr* **125**:1111S-1118S.

Popkin, B.M., Corvalan, C., Grummer-Strawn, L.M. "Dynamics of the double burden of malnutrition and the changing nutrition reality." *Lancet,* 2020; **395**(10217):65-74. doi:10.1016/S0140-6736(19)32497-3

Popkin, B.M., Gordon-Larsen, P. "The nutrition transition: worldwide obesity dynamics and their determinants." *Int J Obes Relat Metab Disord.* 2004; 28 Suppl **3**:S2 S9. doi:10.1038/sj.ijo.0802804.

Shekar, M., Kakietek, J., Dayton Eberwein, J., Walters, D.: *An investment framework for nutrition: reaching the global targets for stunting, anaemia, breastfeeding, and wasting.* The World Bank, 2017.

Shrimpton, R., Rokx, C. "The double burden of malnutrition: a review of global evidence." *Health, Nutrition and Population (HNP) discussion paper.* Washington DC: World Bank; 2012.

Sue, Horton and Jay Ross, "The Economics of Iron Deficiency", *Food Policy,* 28, no. 1, 2003.

Swinburn, B.A., Kraak, V.I., Allender S., *et al.* 2019. The Global Syndemic of Obesity, Undernutrition, and Climate Change: *The Lancet Commission report* [published correction appears in Lancet. **393**(10173):746]. *Lancet.* 2019; **393**(10173):791-846. doi:10.1016/S0140-6736(18)32822-8.

UN Children's Fund (Implementing taxes on sugar-sweetened beverages: an overview of current approaches and the potential benefits for children, 2019.

United Nations Decade of Action on Nutrition. In: Seventieth session of the United Nations General Assembly, New York, 15–28 September, 2015. Agenda item 15.

United Nations Department of Economic and Social Affairs. Sustainable development goal 2. United Nations, 2019.

Victora, C.G., Adair, L., Fall, C., *et al.* Maternal and child undernutrition: consequences for adult health and human capital [published correction appears in Lancet. **371**(9609):302]. *Lancet.* 2008; **371**(9609):340-357. doi:10.1016/S0140-6736(07)61692-4.

Victora, C.G., Bahl, R., Barros, A.J., *et al.* "Breastfeeding in the 21st century: epidemiology, mechanisms, and lifelong effect." *Lancet.* 2016; **387**(10017):475-490. doi:10.1016/S0140-6736(15)01024-7.

Wells, J.C. 2017 The New "Obstetrical Dilemma": Stunting, Obesity and the Risk of Obstructed Labour. *Anat Rec (Hoboken).* 2017; **300**(4):716-731. doi:10.1002/ar.23540.

WHO : Global action plan for the prevention and control of non-communicable diseases 2013-2020. World Health Organization (WHO), Geneva, Switzerland, 2013.

World Bank, Repositioning Nutrition as Central to Development: 49, 2005.

World Cancer Research Fund : American Institute for Cancer Research, Diet, nutrition, physical activity and breast cancer, 2017.

World Health Organization (Double-duty actions for nutrition: policy brief. 2017.

World Health Organization. *WHO Study on global Ageing and adult health* (SAGE). Geneva: WHO. 2008

World Health Organization: *Essential nutrition actions. Improving maternal, newborn, infant and young child health and nutrition.* Geneva. 2013.

2

Socio-Economic Determinants of Maternal Health

Rita Patil

Introduction

Maternal health is a broad term that usually considers health prior to, during and after pregnancy. It is important for ensuring good maternal health as they carry the health of the next generation with them. Girls and women who are healthy, have a good pregnancy and healthy offsprings and children. Eight Millennium Development Goals (MDGs) were framed in 2000 to improve health of human beings all over the world (UNDP). Goal 5 was to improve maternal health. Several health schemes and policies have been introduced and implemented in order to improve health status of people. Maternal deaths in developing and under-developed countries have been common occurrences. This is because of several programme interventions conducted all over the world. Maternal mortality in the world has dropped significantly. It reduced by 44 per cent over the last 25 years from 1990 to 2015. Most of these maternal deaths were reported from developing countries. Both the World Health Organisation and UNICEF have reported that in 2015, India alone contributed to 15 per cent of the global maternal deaths (Chauhan and Kumar, 2016). This is quite a high rate of maternal mortality considering the economic growth and development being seen in India. It was unfortunate that India's maternal mortality ratio was 7 times higher than Russia, six times higher than China and about 4 times higher than that of Brazil in 2015 (World Bank, 2015).

This chapter has tried to draw attention to factors related to maternal health services and the use of maternal health care services in different socio-economic groups. India though developing fast has the worst performance in the health sector compared to other countries in the South and East Asian region. The Indian health policies have been unable to markedly reduce maternal mortality rate. Also, the maternal mortality rate is highly varied in different states. It was as high as 237 in Assam and as low as 46 in Kerala in 2014-16. Joe *et al.* (2015) have reported that maternal deaths were associated with haemorrhage (38%) and infection (11%). They also stated that anaemia and hypertension were causes of maternal mortality in different states of India. The reasons mentioned are avoidable with awareness programmes and schemes. Several studies in India have studied the developments in maternal health care (Filippi *et al.*, 2006; Sunil *et al.*, 2006; Gage and Calixte, 2006; Ram and Singh, 2006; Pathak *et al.*, 2010). Education and SES have shown to be important determinants for maternal health care. Urban and rural differences also have been reported by different researchers (Verma *et al.*, 2001; Mistry *et al.*, 2009; Saikia and Singh, 2009).

Becker *et al.* (1993) reported that mother's education, was a significant factor for use of prenatal care among urban women. Education gives women a greater understanding of their well-being and so they utilize available health care facilities. Socio-economic status also determined the use of contraceptives, appropriate immunization in the urban areas but not in rural. Most of the states in India have been and are a patriarchal society. The inequalities due to this have caused women to be the underprivileged sex for many issues; particularly the health issues. Anaemia, undernutrition, micronutrient deficiencies are commonly seen among women due to the poor access to health care and lack of adequate food (Muzaffar, 2015). Women have also been marginalised in education, financial support and job opportunities.

There is a huge overlap between the factors affecting maternal health care. Figure 2.1 shows various social, economic, cultural and environmental factors related to each other. These factors affect the usage and availability of good food and health care. This chapter has discussed some noticeable factors herein.

- Delay in receiving adequate and appropriate care
- Delay in recognising need for maternal health services.
- Delay in reaching a medical facility that provides care

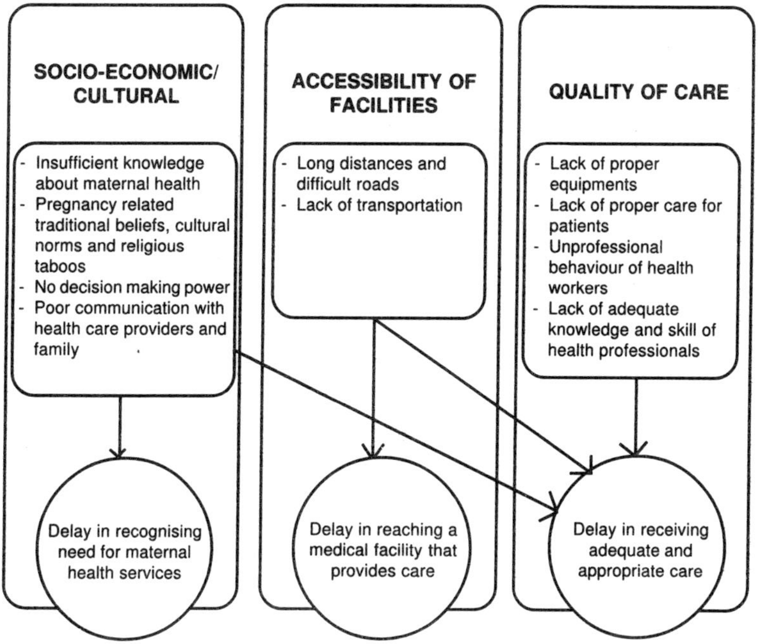

Fig. 2.1: Factors affecting Maternal Health care Services.

Education

A woman's education is an important factor related to prenatal care all over the world. Education empowers women and helps them understand the importance of health care and the usage of available facilities in prenatal and post-natal situations. Earlier studies have suggested the need to pay attention towards less educated women as they may miss significant health programmes (Caldwell, 1981). A study in Jammu & Kashmir reported women who were educated sought health care services compared to women who were lesser educated or illiterate (Muzzafar, 2015). Also, as education level was raised utilisation of government health care facilities reduced and private health care was preferred. Individual and husband's education has positive influence on the use of services in both urban and rural areas. Results have reported that education of women and even husband's, is an important factor for use of necessary health care services among both urban and rural women. A study in Nigeria reported that with education there was better awareness and utilization of health services. For rural women too, education was an important factor for responsiveness to health services (Agunwa *et al.*, 2017).

In urban areas, the odds ratios of availing full antenatal care among women with secondary education and above was higher. Similar result was obtained in rural areas. Husband's education was also found to influence the use of full antenatal care in the same way. Literacy was positively associated with haemoglobin levels in the study of Dutta and Sengupta (2017). Their results were consistent with reports from other studies too (Bisoi *et al.*, 2011; Chowdhury *et al.*, 2015; Balasubramanian *et al.*, 2016; Mangla and Singla, 2016).

Socio-economic Status

Education, food availability, accessibility to other facilities and possession of materialistic things, all depend on socio-economic status. Economic status of households, birth order of mother, interval between children and the area of residence also impact availability and use of health care services. Being able to obtain health information depends on access to televisions or radios which may make valuable information available to women (Acharya *et al.*, 2015). They reported that subjects were exposed to radio (60%) and television (43.1 %) once a week, respectively. Women with exposure to media made a greater use of full services (more antenatal visits, regular nutritional supplementation as per advice, tetanus immunization etc.) compared to women who were not exposed to any form of media. Socialising and freedom of movement (going to the market and visiting relatives and friends) was positively associated with the use of health care services (Chauhan and Kumar, 2016).

Urban and rural differences are prominent in various SES groups. A study reported that 38 per cent women in urban areas possessed a television and a lesser percentage (23) of rural women possessed a TV. They also observed a positive association between owning a TV and use of prenatal care, immunizations and contraception (Acharya *et al.*, 2015). Physical access to health care, travel time and mode of transport are dependent on affordability. Utilisation of the health care services increases with improving household economic status (Patel *et al.*, 2018). Wealth index and education were the most significant variables that affected the use of maternal health care services in the study of Kumar and Gupta (2015). They also reported that household economic status had a significant positive effect on the use of antenatal care among rural women. Women from the richer wealth quintile and richest wealth quintiles were significantly using full antenatal care compared with women from the poorest wealth quintile. Standard of living is affected by SES and it is an important determinant which creates variances in utilization of maternal health services.

India is a country of vast cultural and regional diversity along with socio-economic and religious differences. In India, caste is an important element of determining socio-economic status. The health of people is not only affected by available medical facilities but also due to their social and economic status. Lower caste persons, most of whom are poor, migrate to cities in search of work. They may also be disadvantaged from getting clean water, proper sanitation, food and good housing. Scheduled Caste women living in rural areas were likely to use poor maternal services (12.4% full antenatal care, 32% safe delivery and 30.4% postnatal care) compared to women living in urban areas of the same caste (32% full antenatal care, 75% safe delivery and 62.2% postnatal care). Thus, it indicates that an exposure to urban life, interaction with other communities etc. improves the utilization of maternal health care facilities (Kumar and Gupta, 2015).

Health Care Access and Services

The socio-economic inequalities in maternal health care service use are a worldwide fact. A study in Ghana reported wealth-related inequalities in at least four antenatal clinics. They have suggested that the inequalities were pro-rich. The women from financially better households had the advantage of using health care services compared to poorer women. There are differences in the use of antenatal care, medical assistance at delivery and post-natal care between urban and rural women (Novignon, 2019). It was reported that maternal health care services were used by more urban (27%) women than the rural women (11%). Seventy six per cent of urban women had proper medical assistance at delivery compared to only 40 per cent of rural women. Similarly, for post-natal care more urban women (69%) received the benefit compared to rural women (29%). It was also observed that younger women used the maternal health care services compared to women older in age (Chauhan and Kumar, 2016). Health services for pregnant women include antenatal services, institutional deliveries and post-natal services. Singh *et al.* (2019) reported that these services were poorly utilised in their study conducted in UP. They suggested that the role of health workers is very crucial for antenatal and post-natal care.

The Integrated Child Development Services (ICDS) scheme was launched by Government of India in 1975. After a brief discontinuation in 1978, it was started again in the 1980s and still continues. This scheme was more for children than for women. Amidst most the objectives for children, there was one for women-to enhance the capability of the mother to look after the normal health and nutritional needs of the child through proper nutrition and health education. A study in 2005 reported that the ICDS programme had not helped to reduce malnutrition, mainly due to problems in executing the scheme. They found that the poorest states had received least funding. They found limited evidence of reduced child malnutrition due to the scheme. They suggested that efforts have to be made to ensure that funds are fully utilized by all states and also ensure proper allocation of funds to the ICDS scheme (Lokshin *et al.*, 2005). Chakrabarti *et al.* (2019) have also studied the performance of the scheme. They have concluded that due to certain policies, the scheme reaches more number of people than before. Also, the ones who need the scheme are actually not getting it. They have suggested that implementation of scheme needs to be better and it should include more households from the lower SES and women with poor education.

Government of India later launched the National Rural Health Mission (NRHM) scheme in 2005 which focused on improving health system performance and health status of people in rural areas. The main objective of NRHM was to reduce maternal and child mortality by providing access to equitable, affordable, accountable and effective primary health care services to the rural population (Kumar, 2005). Another scheme, Janani Suraksha Yojana (JSY) was also launched to encourage safe deliveries among rural women. It was estimated that implementation of these schemes would promote proper institutional deliveries and reduce maternal mortality among pregnant women of rural areas (Lim *et al.*, 2010). Kerala and Tamil Nadu are the two states who have regularly reported low maternal mortality. The success of Kerala lies in the high level of awareness in the community due to good literacy rates. Also there is good infrastructure and roads leading to easy access to health services, particularly in the urban areas. In Tamil Nadu, the decline in maternal mortality has been because of the Government initiatives offered to women. Tamil Nadu offered a scheme similar to Janani SurakshaYojana in which investments were made for appointing nurses and offering cash incentives for institutional delivery. They also monitored maternal deaths, analyzed medical and social causes. Their schemes and actions were planned according to the observations recorded (Jain, 2016).

The State Government of Gujarat introduced the Chiranjeevi Scheme and they have reported the success of this scheme. The Government collaborated with obstetricians-gynaecologists in private practice for being available to women in the rural areas. They planned and executed the consultations and financial provisions and formed a public-private partnership. They also appointed committed qualified officials who managed the programme (Vora *et al.*, 2009). The Reproductive, Maternal, New-born, Child and Adolescent Health (RMNCH+A) framework was initiated by Government of India in 2013. It aimed to—(1) tackle the causes of mortality and morbidity among women and children, and (2) to understand the problems in accessing and utilizing health care services. This framework was a landmark move in the country's health planning. Innovative steps were planned and included selecting poor-performing districts, prioritising health care interventions, collaborating with development partners and creating an effective system of delivering health care with improved efficiency. One hundred and eighty four high priority districts were identified across the country. Several interventions were identified at district, state and national level which would provide technical support to the respective health departments. However, the impact has not been visibly recognised and only the gaps were identified in mechanisms. Additionally, the Government realised the importance of social factors in achieving improvement in health care systems. Thus, 'Transformation of Aspirational

Districts' initiative was introduced in 117 districts across the country in 2018. This initiative included health and nutrition, education, agriculture and water resources, financial inclusion, skill development, basic infrastructure and operational and implementation components. The RMNCH+A framework were consistent with the sustainable development goals of the United Nations. The objectives of the initiative were to improve India's ranking in Human Development Index, raise living standards and ensure inclusive growth of all sectors (Taneja *et al.*, 2019).

Food and Nutrition

In India, food insecurity is a major concern, particularly for women. It is influenced by SES, availability of food and even caste. Also, Indian society is of patriarchal families wherein husbands are the decision makers. Thus, how to use the money for food and what to buy is not in a woman's hand. Within a given budget women are concerned about meeting food needs of the family. Thus, they tend to buy cheap foods and even limit their own food consumption to spare food for children, husband and others (Mohapatra, 2012; Sabar, 2014; Gupta *et al.*, 2015). Food insecurity is furthermore caused because of environmental conditions and gender bias. Some other factors affecting food insecurity are improper coordination, lack of political will, poorly monitored nutritional programmes and faulty public (Upadhyay and Palanivel, 2011). Payne *et al.* (2016) have reported their study of food insecurity in Indian women. They found that increased poverty, several coping mechanisms, lower dietary diversity, husband making decisions about how the money earned by a woman should be used and unable to save money to use for food expenses; all had significant high odds ratio for food insecurity.

Women's food consumption is dependent on many aspects and it differs with the socio-economic status. A study reports that vegetarianism, religion, and caste were the strongest predictors of poor food consumption in women in lower SES group compared to the higher SES group (Fledderjohann *et al.*, 2016). Add to that the distributional inequalities of food in the family where women are disadvantaged for the quantity of food and the consumption of milk, fruits and vegetables in the lower classes. The issues of food consumption and nutrition are complex and are influenced by the following:

(a) Physiological-taste, hunger and appetite.
(b) Economic-family income, cost of food and its availability.
(c) Physical-cooking skills, time available for cooking, ease of access to food and education.
(d) Social-caste, culture, peers, religious taboos and superstitions related to food.
(e) Psychological-stress, mood etc.
(f) Knowledge, attitudes and practices about food.
(g) Stage of life.

Physiological needs are important as we need energy and macronutrients to live a healthy life. Hunger, satiety and palatability of food controls food intake. It is very well known that macronutrients, carbohydrates, proteins and fats are responsible for signals of satiety. The volume of food or portion size consumed also determines satiety irrespective of energy and nutrient content. Sensory characteristics of food (taste, smell, texture and appearance) define palatability. Sweet and high-fat foods are desirable as compared to roasted or boiled foods. Poorer women may not consume adequate diets. Expensive foods like fruits and vegetables are missing in their diets or are rarely consumed. Accessibility to food depends on geographical location and transport available. Better purchasing power cannot ensure balanced diets (Shetty, 2002; Rao *et al.*, 2010).

Education and awareness largely is responsible for selecting and consuming appropriate foods. Due to rising food costs, nutrition knowledge alone cannot ensure selection of nutritious food. But it will definitely help to choose healthy foods whenever afforded. Education will also help read and understand food labels and other sources available. Nutrition labels were not read and followed due to illiteracy in the low and middle income household study in Delhi (Pradhan *et al.*, 2013). Pradhan *et al.* (2013) reported that along with income, food prices, likes and dislikes of family and seasonal availability affected food expenditure and consumption patterns. The households in the study reported to eat 2 or 3 times a day which was because of the work pattern.

Traditional beliefs, cultural specifications for food also impacted food selection and consumption. The superstitions of food particularly hot and cold foods were reported for food habits. Due to rising food costs, families were buying cheaper ingredients or even eating lesser. Also, women were the decision makers regarding food purchase and cooking. Similar to rural households, seasonal availability was preferred, may be because costs are lesser for seasonal foods. Socio-economic determinants are important for all aspects of health not only for women but for all. Families who have their own land in accessible locations have reported comparatively better conditions for maternal health. Considering the varied determinants for maternal health following steps should be taken:

(1) Prevent malnutrition, particularly micronutrient deficiencies in women.
(2) Promote kitchen gardening and animal husbandry to maintain sufficient food for the family.
(3) Educate the women to incorporate nutrient rich regional foods and a local variation of diet.
(4) Prevalence of anaemia is high among backward classes, particularly tribal women. They should be given iron supplements to combat anaemia (Biswas and Baruah, 2014).
(5) Educate women about danger signs during pregnancy and also prepare them for childbirth.
(6) Importance of eating fruits, vegetables and protein foods need to be emphasized in public health campaigns.

Conclusion

Maternal Health issues are a plethora of controllable and uncontrollable factors. These factors cannot be addressed one at a time. They need to be considered all together. All the possible maternal health care services should have a wide-ranging approach. Health issues like anaemia, infectious diseases, adolescent health and nutrition, reproductive tract infections, contraception, safe abortion services all have to be prioritised and made available to all women. Community and socio-cultural factors are directed towards benefits for good maternal health and are equally important. Social inequities towards Scheduled Castes and Scheduled Tribes have to be eliminated with education. Health care services should be made available in villages and tribal areas. Government policies need to be well regulated without corruption. Other factors like good roads and transport, food security and nutrition, as well as prevention of violence against women have to be tackled too. It is a fact that there is a huge disparity in the accessibility of free maternal health services for women. In rural areas, women have to walk long distances to avail free health care facilities. Providing these free services as near as possible to clusters of households is needed to ensure maternal health care for all women. Empowerment of women has to be recognized as a necessary factor for improving their health and for better maternal health outcomes. They should be involved in all decision making agencies that make policies for women. Robust recommendations are necessary to improve maternal health care services for women of lower SES group. Education is a must to change and improve economic status and accessibility to health services. Removing maternal health inequality within the social classes also needs to be addressed. All policies regarding maternal health should be focused on women of lower castes, uneducated and rural regions.

REFERENCES

Acharya, D., Khanal, V., Singh, J.K., *et al.* 2015. Impact of mass media on the utilization of antenatal care services among women of rural community in Nepal. *BMC Res Notes.* **8**:345.

Agunwa, C., Obi, I., *et al.* 2017. Determinants of patterns of maternal and child health service utilization in a rural community in south eastern Nigeria. *BMC Health Services Research.* **17**:715.

Balasubramanian, T., Aravazhi, M., Sampath, S.D. 2016. "Awareness of Anaemia among Pregnant Women and Impact of Demographic Factors on their Hemoglobin Status." *International Journal of Scientific Study,* **3**(2): 303-305.

Becker, S., Peters, D.H., Gray, R.H., *et al.* 1993. "The determinants of use of maternal and child health services in Metro Cebu, the Philippines." *Health Transition Review,* **3**(1): 77-89,

Bisoi, S., Haldar, D., Majumdar, T. *et al.* 2011. "Correlates of Anaemia Among Pregnant Women in Rural Area of West Bengal." *The Journal of Family Welfare,* **57**(1):72-78.

Caldwell, J.C. 1981. "Maternal education as a factor in child mortality." *World Health Forum* **2**: 75-78.

Chakrabarti, S., Raghunathan, K., Alderman, H. *et al.* 2019. "India's Integrated Child Development Services Programme: Equity and Extent of Coverage in 2006 and 2016." *Bulletin of the World Health Organization,* **97**: 270-282.

Chandrasekhar, S., Aguayo, V.M., Krishna, V., Nair, R. 2017. "Household food insecurity and children's dietary diversity and nutrition in India: Evidence from the comprehensive nutrition survey in Maharashtra." *Matern Child Nutr,* **13**(S2): e12447.

Chauhan, B.G., Kumar, A. 2016. "Rural-urban Differential in Utilization of Maternal Healthcare Services in India: A Decomposition Analysis." *Social Science Spectrum.* **2**(1): 49-62.

Chowdhury, H.A., Ahmed, K.R., Jebunessa, F. *et al.* 2015. "Factors associated with maternal anaemia among pregnant women in Dhaka city." *BMC Women's Health,* **15**(77): 1-6.

Do, N., Giang, H.T.T., Phonvisay, A., Oh, J. 2018. "Trends of socio-economic inequality in using maternal health care services in Lao People's Democratic Republic from year 2000 to 2012." *BMC Public Health* **18**:875.

Dutta, P., Sengupta, B. 2017. Socio-economic Determinants of Maternal Anaemia: A Disaggregated Level Analysis from Assam, India. Proceedings of the 3rd International Conference on Public Health, **3**:71-87.

Filippi, V., Ronsmans, C., Campbell, O. *et al.* 2006. "Maternal health in poor countries: the broader context and a call for action." *Lancet,* **9546**: 1535-1541.

Fledderjohann, J., Vellakkal, S., Stuckler, D. 2016. "Breastfeeding, pregnant, and non-breastfeeding nor pregnant women's food consumption: A matched within-household analysis in India." *Sexual Reproductive Healthcare,* **7**: 70–77.

Gage, A.J., Guirlène Calixte, M. 2006. "Effects of the physical accessibility of maternal health services on their use in rural Haiti." *Population Studies,* **60**(3): 271-288.

Jain, R., Desai, S., Vanneman, R. 2016. Janani Suraksha Yojana and Declining Socio-economic Inequalities in Maternal Health Care in Rural India. India Human Development Survey.

Joe, W., Sharma, S., Sharma, J. *et al.* 2015. Maternal Mortality in India: A Review of Trends and Patterns. Institute of Economic Growth, working paper number 353.

Kumar, P., Gupta, A. 2015. "Determinants of Inter and Intra Caste Differences in Utilization of Maternal Health Care Services in India: Evidence from DLHS-3 Survey." *Int Res J Social Sci.* **4**(1): 27-36

Kumar, S. 2005. "Challenges of Maternal Mortality Reduction and Opportunities under National Rural Health Mission—A Critical Appraisal." *Indian Journal of Public Health,* Vol. XXXXIX, No.3.

Lim, S.S., Dandona, L., Hoisington, J.A., *et al.* 2010. "India's Janani Suraksha Yojana, a conditional cash transfer programme to increase births in health facilities: An impact evaluation." *The Lancet* **375**: 2009-2023.

Lokshin, M., Das Gupta, M., Gragnolati, M., Ivaschenko, O. 2015. "Improving Child Nutrition? The Integrated Child Development Services in India." *Development and Change,* **36**(4): 613-640.

Mangla, M., Singla, D. 2016. "Prevalence of anaemia among pregnant women in rural India: a longitudinal observational study." *International Journal of Reproduction, Contraception, Obstetrics and Gynaecology,* **5**(10): 3500-3505.

Mistry, R., Galal, O., Lu, M. 2009. "Women's autonomy and pregnancy care in rural India: A contextual analysis." *Social Science Medicine,* **69**(6): 926-933.

Mohapatra, G. 2012. "Hunger and Coping Strategies among Kondh Tribe in Kalahandi District, Odisha (Eastern India)." *Transcience: a journal of global studies,* **3**(2): 51-60.

Muzaffar, N. 2015. "Maternal Health and Social Determinants: A Study in Jammu and Kashmir." *Public Health Research,* **5**(5): 144-152.

Novignon, J., Ofori, B., Tabiri, K.G. *et al.* 2019. "Socio-economic inequalities in maternal health care utilization in Ghana." *International Journal for Equity in Health,* volume **18**: 141.

Patel, P., Das, M., Das, U. 2018. "The perceptions, health-seeking behaviours and access of Scheduled Caste women to maternal health services in Bihar, India." *Reproductive Health Matters,* **54**:114-125.

Pathak, P.K., Mohanty, S.K. 2010. "Does the safe-motherhood programme reach the poor in Uttar Pradesh, India?" *Asian Population Studies* **6**(2): 173-191.

Pathak, P.K., Singh, A., Subramanian, S.V. 2010. "Economic inequalities in maternal health care: Prenatal care and skilled birth attendance in India, 1992–2006." PloSone, **5**(10): e13593.

Payne, H.E., Gray, B., Davis, S.F. *et al.* 2016. "Factors associated with food insecurity among women and children in rural Rajasthan, India." *Journal of Gender, Agriculture and Food Security,* **1**(3): 23-39.

Pradhan, M.R., Taylor, F.C., Agrawal, S. *et al.* 2013. "Food Acquisition and Intra-household Consumption Patterns: a study of low and middle income urban households in Delhi, India." *Indian J Community Health.* **25**(4): 391–402.

Ram, F. and Singh, A. (2006). "Is antenatal care effective in improving maternal health in rural Uttar Pradesh? Evidence from a district level household survey." *Journal of Biosocial Science,* **38**(4): 433-448.

Rao, K.M., Balakrishna, N., Arlappa, N. *et al.* 2010. "Diet and Nutritional Status of Women in India." *J. Hum Ecol,* **29**(3): 165-170.

Sabar, B. 2014. "Food Insecurity and Coping Strategies: A Tale of Two Particularly Vulnerable Tribal Groups in Karnataka." *Journal of Asian and African Studies,* 0021909614558953.

Saikia, N., Singh, A. 2009. "Does type of household affect maternal health? Evidence from India." *Journal of Biosocial Science,* **41**(03): 329-353.

Shetty, P.S. (2002). "Nutrition transition in India." *Public Health Nutrition,* **5**(1A): 175-182.

Singh R., Neogi S.B., Hazra A. *et al.* 2019. "Utilization of maternal health services and its determinants: a cross-sectional study among women in rural Uttar Pradesh, India." *J Health PopulNutr.*, **38**(1):13.

Sunil T.S., Rajaram S., Zottarelli L.K. 2006. "Do individual and programme factors matter in the utilization of maternal care services in rural India? A theoretical approach." *Social Science Medicine,* **62**(8), 1943-1957.

Taneja G., Sridhar V.S., Mohanty S., *et al.* 2019. "India's RMNCH+A Strategy: Approach, Learnings and Limitations." *BMJ Glob Health.* 4:e001162.

Do N., Tran H.T.G., Phonvisay A., Oh J. 2018. "Trends of socioeconomic inequality in using maternal health care services in Lao People's Democratic Republic from year 2000 to 2012." *BMC Public Health (2018)* **18**:875. https://doi.org/10.1186/s12889-018-5811-0

Upadhyay R.P., Palanivel C. 2011. "Challenges in achieving food security in India." *Iranian Journal of Public Health,* **40**(4), 31.

Verma K., Thomas A., Sharma A., Dhar A., Bhambri V. 2001. "Maternal mortality in rural India: A hospital based 10 year retrospective analysis." *Journal of Obstetrics and Gynaecology Research,* **27**(4): 183-187.

Vora K.S., Mavalankar D.V., Ramani K.V. *et al.* 2009. "Maternal Education as a Factor in Child Mortality." *J Health PopulNutr,* **27**(2):184-201.

3

Socio-economic, Demographic and Lifestyle Determinants of Overnutrition in Indian Children

Arti Muley, Surabhi Singh Yadav, Pooja Panchal and *Kavitha Menon*

Introduction

India has the second-largest child population which accounts closely for one-third of the total Indian population. The health and well-being of the children determine the country's economic output and development in addition to the lower adult disease burden (Hoddinott, 2013). The global child health scenario indicates a great divide between developed nations and developing countries. While developed nations have a high prevalence of overnutrition, overweight, and obesity, in developing countries including triple burden of malnutrition—coexist (i.e. chronic undernutrition and micronutrient deficiencies together with overnutrition). The aforementioned nutritional challenges remains as an unfinished agenda for India. The rising prevalence of overnutrition rates further add to the complexity to the management of these nutritional challenges. Gómez *et al.*, 2013). Globally about 38 million children (5.6%) under five were overweight, which is an increase of 8 million since 2000, and almost half of these children lived in Asia and a quarter in Africa (UNICEF/WHO/World Bank, 2020). Indian children have an unacceptably high prevalence of malnutrition, which includes overweight and obesity. In 2017, the prevalence of childhood overweight in India among 2-4 years was 11·5 per cent (95% CI

8·5–14·9), and it is projected to 17·5 per cent in 2030 (India State-Level Disease Burden Initiative Malnutrition Collaborators, 2019). However, there exist regional disparities in the prevalence and incidence of childhood overweight and obesity in India. According to the comprehensive national nutritional survey, 2016-18, the prevalence of overweight among 1-4 years, 5-9 years and 10-19 years (overweight or obese) was 1.8 per cent, 3.7 per cent and 4.8 per cent, respectively. The above data from the first of its kind survey provided nationally representative figures of Indian childhood prevalence of overweight and obesity among different age groups (young children, older children, and adolescents) (MoHFW, 2019).

There are challenges in the appropriate representation and interpretation of the data on malnutrition in India. While the data on the prevalence of undernutrition is abundant, definable, and comparable across different Indian regions, the same could not be applied to the overnutrition scenario. There are variations in the interpretation of data across the literature that makes it difficult to consolidate the childhood overweight and obesity prevalence in India. Childhood overweight and obesity are defined differently based on the age group of the child. The two age groups considered are—birth to age 5 years and 5 to19 years. In the birth to five years age group, children are overweight and obese if their Body Mass Index (BMI) is >2 standard deviations and BMI >3 standard deviations above the WHO growth standard median, respectively. On the other hand, among 5 to 19 years, children are overweight when BMI >1 standard deviation and obese when BMI >2 standard deviation above the WHO growth standard median (Onis *et al.*, 2007). Further, the Indian Association of Paediatrics (IAP) recommends the use of the WHO growth charts for young children below the age of 5 years, and for 5-18 years old Indian children sex-specific IAP growth curves (Khadilkar *et al.*, 2015). Also, there are studies that have used other growth standards such as CDC growth charts and other indicators to classify overweight and obesity. Despite the aforementioned challenges, the projected surge in the prevalence of childhood overweight in the coming years underscores the need to understand the determinants of these major childhood public health issues. Such an effort would be imperative to plan interventions and policies to address childhood overweight and obesity in India. Therefore, the present chapter aims to explore and summarise the prevalence of childhood overweight and obesity in India and identify the potential determinants from the available literature in this area over the last decade.

National Prevalence of Childhood Overweight and Obesity

The present chapter collated information from Indian studies published in the last decade. The studies included a systematic review of pooled studies on childhood overweight and obesity and primary studies on different age groups under 18 years of age. Over the last three decades, several national health surveys were conducted in India including the National Health and Family Welfare (NFHS) surveys—1 (1992-93), 2 (1998-99), 3 (2005-06) and 4 (2013-14) (IIPS, 1995; IIPS, 2000; IIPS, 2007; IIPS, 2017). Additionally, the District-Level Household and Facility Survey (DLHS), and the Annual Health Survey (AHS) (IIPS, 2009; MoHFW, 2014; Meenakshi, 2016). These surveys primarily focused on the nutritional status of under-five children and adults and information on older children was unavailable. The two surveys that focused on the different childhood indicators of overnutrition and the nutritional challenges of children were the Rapid Survey on Children (RSOC) and Comprehensive National Nutritional Survey (CNNS), 2016-18; both supported by the UNICEF (MoWCD/UNICEF, 2014; MoHFW GoI/UNICEF/Population Council, 2019). Additionally, several smaller studies investigated the prevalence and correlate of childhood overweight and obesity. Information from these studies was harnessed and presented below to identify the determinants of childhood overweight and obesity.

Multiple Indian studies reported childhood obesity prevalence over the last decade. In the absence of nationally representative data, the first information was reported in a systematic review on the epidemiology of childhood overweight and obesity in India for the different age groups of children in 2016. The data from the systematic review reported increasing trends for combined overweight and obesity in children and adolescents over the last decade. The pooled data after 2010 estimated a combined prevalence of 19.3 per cent of childhood overweight and obesity which was significantly higher (two-sample z-test, $p<0.01$) than the earlier prevalence of 16 per cent reported in 2001 (Ranjani *et al.*, 2016) (Table 3.1). The RSOC survey

(2013-14) on 28,000 adolescent girls aged 10-18 years reported that 4.5 per cent of 15-18 years old girls had BMI >25 kg/m^2. Three Indian states, namely Andhra Pradesh, Tripura, and Tamil Nadu (8% each) showed a higher proportion of overweight or obesity in 10-18-year-old Indian adolescent girls. Subsequently, the most recent survey, CNSS (2016-18) was the first national survey that assessed overweight and obesity in Indian children of different age groups (Table 3.1). The survey results indicated lower combined prevalence of overweight and obesity in 5-9 years (5.3%) and 10-19 years (4.8%) aged Indian children compared to the pooled analysis of the studies from India. These data collectively indicate the variations in the reported prevalence of overweight and obesity across the surveys. This could be partly being explained due to the variations in the indicators used for the studies, residence of the children, rural-urban differences and wealth status.

Regional Variations in the Prevalence Rates for Childhood Over-nutrition

India is a diverse country with great regional variations. These variations were evident in the prevalence of over-nutrition prevalence. The data from smaller Indian studies conducted over the last decade was collated, aggregated on a regional basis and the results are presented (Table 3.1). Studies from the Northern India—Jammu and Shimla reported similar prevalence rates in two different age groups of children. In the study from Jammu among 203 children (6-14 years) reported a combined prevalence of overweight and obesity to be 8.2 per cent. Overweight and obesity were more in urban (Males: 7.4% and Females: 16.9%) than rural areas (Males: 3% and Females: 6.6%) (Arifa *et al.*, 2018). In the second study from north with 720 adolescents (14-19 years) in Shimla district, 7.1 per cent were overweight while 1.3 per cent obese (Gupta *et al.*, 2014).

A larger number of studies reported the prevalence and associated factors for overnutrition from the Southern States of India. The study from Tirupati investigated the effects of social and environmental determinants on overweight and obesity prevalence among 2258 adolescent (12-16) children reported the prevalence of 21.5 per cent overweight and 9.6 per cent obesity. No significant differences were observed in the prevalence of

Table 3.1: National and regional prevalence of childhood overweight and obesity in India

Sl. No.	Author (year)	Zone	City	Age-group (y)	Sample size (n)	Prevalence(%) Overweight	Obesity	Combined
National Data on childhood overweight and obesity								
1.	MoHFW, 2019	India	Multiple states	0-<5	38081	1.8	0.2	—
				5-9	38366		1.3	5.3
				10-19	35869		1.1	4.8
2.	Ranjani *et al.*, 2016	India	16 states	1-18		19.3	19.3	19.3
Regional prevalence of overweight and obesity								
3.	Arifa *et al.*, 2018	North	Jammu	6-14	203	—	—	8.2
4.	Gupta *et al.*, 2014		Simla	14-19	720	7.1	1.3	8.4
5.	Shanmugam *et al.*, 2016	South	Coimbatore	5-15	890	8.32	4.72	13.04
6.	Anuradha *et al.*, 2015		Tirupati	12-16	2258	21.5	9.6	31.1
7.	Jagadesan *et al.*, 2014		Chennai	6-11	8025	—	—	42.9
				12-17	10930	—	—	55.5
8.	Prasanna *et al.*, 2012		Bangalore	12-15	761	10.0	5.0	15.0
9.	Daga *et al.*, 2020	West	Pune	3-16	1444	2.5	1.5	4.0
10.	Arora *et al.*, 2017		Pune	12-15	1652	6.1	4.8	10.9
11.	Iyer *et al.*, 2011		Vadodara	6-11	1067	14.4	5.9	20.3
12.	Saikia *et al.*, 2018	East	Assam	10-14	1200	20.9	10.2	31.1
13.	Panda *et al.*, 2017		Sambalpur	10-15	560	8.9	3.4	12.3
14.	Bhattacharya *et al.*, 2016		Guwahati	10-19	60	13.3	1.7	15.0
15.	Kar and Khandelwal, 2015		Gangtok	11-19	979	14.5	2.0	16.5
16.	Mondal *et al.*, 2015		Assam	5-11	1017	12.3	11.0	—
17.	Bagudai *et al.*, 2014		Odisha	10-16	5155	10.4	3.7	14.1

overnutrition across the age groups (Anuradha *et al.*, 2015). A study from Kerala that examined the prevalence of overweight and obesity in urban school children in different socio-economic strata. The prevalence of obesity and overweight significantly different among UIG, MIG and LIG boys was 5 per cent and 16 per cent, 3 per cent and 12 per cent, and 1 per cent and 2 per cent, respectively ($p<0.05$). The prevalence of obesity and overweight among girls of the UIG, MIG and LIG socio-economic groups was 10 per cent and 28 per cent, 4 per cent and 5 per cent, and 2 per cent and 3 per cent, respectively ($p<0.05$) (Cherian *et al.*, 2012). In their study from Chennai, Jagadesan *et al.* (2014) reported significantly higher prevalence of overweight/obesity in private compared to government schools using the International Obesity Task Force (IOTF) criteria (Private schools: 21.4%, Government schools: 3.6%, OR: 7.4, 95% CI: 6.3-8.6; $p<0.001$). Similar observations were reported using IAP growth standards (Private schools: 26.4%, Government schools: 4.6% OR: 6.9, 95% CI: 6.2-7.8; $p<0.001$). The differentials prevalence was attributed to the higher socio-economic status of children who attended private schools than government schools.

The Western Indian studies reported a combined prevalence of overweight and obesity between 4-20.3 per cent (Iyer *et al.*, 2017; Arora *et al.*; Daga *et al.* 2020). The higher prevalence was reported by Iyer *et al.* (2011) (20.3%) among 1067 subjects aged 6-12 years from Vadodara city assessed as per IOTF standards. Two studies from Pune reported different prevalence rates for combined overweight and obesity. Compared to the Arora *et al.* (2017), Daga *et al.* (2020), the study had a lower prevalence (4% vs. 10.9%). Among 1652 adolescents (12-15 years) residing in Pune city 6.1 per cent of students were overweight (i.e. 85th-95th percentile of BMI) and 4.78 per cent of students were obese (i.e. >95th percentile BMI) (Arora *et al.*, 2017). The Arora study focused primarily on the adolescent group while the Daga study focused on a mixed group of children including preschool, older children, and adolescents. A higher prevalence of overnutrition was observed in older children and adolescent group than the pre-school children or young Indian children (Arora *et al.*, 2017; Daga *et al.* 2020).

Studies from Eastern India primarily were on adolescent groups between 10-19 years old reported a combined prevalence of overweight and obesity between 12.3 per cent-31.1 per cent. Sakia *et al.* (2018) reported the highest prevalence of overweight and obesity among adolescents aged 10-14 years from Assam. The study participants attended schools located in Dibrugarh town and students were located on the urban side of the city. Bagudai *et al.* (2014) reported 10.4 per cent of students to be overweight and 3.7 per cent obese in a group of 5155 students (10-16 years, 3255 boys and 1900 girls) in Odisha. Among obese adolescents, 44.7 per cent were hypertensive. Another study from Gangtok reported the prevalence of obesity, overweight, and hypertension as 2.0 per cent, 14.5 per cent and 5.62 per cent, respectively among adolescents (Kar and Khandelwal, 2015). In their study in 560 adolescent school children (10-15 years) residing in urban Sambalpur, Odisha, Panda (2017) reported the prevalence was 8.9 per cent and 3.4 per cent for overweight and obesity, respectively.

Overall, studies from different regions of India showed a surge in the prevalence of overweight and obesity in children and adolescents. The Southern states reported a higher prevalence of overnutrition, followed by the Eastern states compared to other parts of India. Additionally, the smaller regional studies reported a higher prevalence of overweight and obesity in children compared to the national data from the recent CNSS (2016-18) data. The variations could be attributed to disparities in urban-rural residence or living, socio-economic status, differences in the adoption of sampling methods (i.e. smaller studies used convenient sampling that may overestimate the prevalence if private schools are selected), and smaller sample size of children or by chance. Regardless of the variations in the prevalence of overnutrition estimates from different parts of India, the mere fact that Indian children are gaining weight underscores the need for targeted intervention programmes based on the determinants of overnutrition. Hence, necessary steps to identify the modifiable determinants to improve them should be considered as priority.

Determinants of Overnutrition among Children

Aetiology of obesity remains complex and multifactorial. Several factors such as genetics, biological, social, behavioural and environmental cause either individually or collectively lead to obesity. A few of these factors are modifiable and could be negated through the maintenance of energy balance, balanced diet, and regular physical activity (Ebbeling *et al.*, 2002). The rising prevalence of obesity in genetically stable population groups indicates the roles of social and environmental or lifestyle determinants in the overweight and obesity epidemic in children (Hakala *et al.*, 1999). Understanding and identification of these determinants provide insights to develop evidence-based approaches in terms of interventions and policies to enable a reduction in the prevalence of childhood overweight and obesity. The present chapter explores the existing literature to identify socio-economic, demographic, and lifestyle determinants that contribute to the rising prevalence of childhood overnutrition. A few studies have investigated socio-economic and demographic determinants of childhood overnutrition for different communities. Studies from the last decade that explored the socio-economic and demographic factors are summarised (Table 3.2). Disparities exist in the distribution of these determinants across India, and regional variations in these determinants could be observed. Literature suggests the co-existence of under and overnutrition in communities. Often a life course-related evolution is observed with maternal and fetal undernutrition before, during or after gestation alludes to childhood or adult obesity in the offspring. Further, communities with high-risk for undernutrition from the high-risk Indian states report higher adult obesity prevalence in later years. A similar paradigm could be observed in urban and rural disparities, with the prevalence of childhood overnutrition significantly higher in children dwelling in urban areas than in rural villages. (Arifa *et al.*, 2018; MoHFW/UNICEF/Population Council, 2019).

The socio-economic status of the family was reported as a determinant of obesity in five Indian studies out of eight regardless of its regional allocations. A higher proportion of overnourished children was found in high socio-economic status families in all the four studies than low socio-economic families, indicating the significant association of family income with overweight or obesity (Iyer *et al.*, 2011; Cherian *et al.*, 2012; Jagadesan *et al.*, 2014; Anuradha *et al.*, 2015). In their study, Cherian *et al.* (2012) observed the impact of economic developments increased easy access to calorie-rich foods, especially for the higher socio-economic groups coupled with a lack of awareness in parents about childhood obesity.

The influence of gender was reported in two studies which indicated a higher risk of obesity in female children (Cherian *et al.*, 2012; Kar and Khandelwal, 2015). Also, Cherian, *et al.* (2012)

Table 3.2: Socio-economic and demographic determinants of overweight and obesity in Indian children

Sl. No.	*Author & Year*	*Place*	*Sample*	*Age group*	*Socio-economic-demographic determinants*
1.	Arifa *et al.*, 2018	Jammu	203	6-14 years	Urban setting (24.3%) vs. in rural setting(9.6%)
2.	Panda *et al.*, 2017	Sambalpur	560	10-15 years	Family history ($\chi2$=4.11, p=0.04)
3.	Bhattacharya *et al.*, 2016	Guwahati	60	10-19 years	% prevalence was low if mothers were housewives ($\chi2$=9.548, p=0.049)
4.	Anuradha *et al.*, 2015	Tirupati	2258	12-16 years	Mother's higher education (OR=1.57; 95% CI 1.048-2.35, p<0.05); High family income (OR=1.529; 95% CI 1.089-2.148, p<0.05)
5.	Kar and Khandelwal, 2015	Gangtok	979	11-19 years	Early adolescence ($\chi2$=11.8, p<0.0001); Female gender ($\chi2$=10.89, p<0.05); Pre-hypertensive ($\chi2$=56.3, p<0.0001); High socio-economic status ($\chi2$=101.5, p<0.0001)
6.	Mondal *et al.*, 2015	Assam	1017	5-11 years	Mothers lower education (≤10th standard) (OR=0.541 95% CI: (0.31-0.94), p<0.05); ≥7, Family size (OR=1.62; 95% CI: 1.10-2.36)
7.	Jagadesan *et al.*, 2014	Chennai	18955	6-17 years	High income (OR=7.4; 95% CI 6.3-8.6, p<0.001)
8.	Cherian *et al.*, 2012	Kerala	1634	6-15 years	High income (prevalence was 15% vs. 10% in low income, p<0.05); Female gender (prevalence was 17.4% vs. 13.2% in males, p=0.028)
9.	Iyer *et al.*, 2011	Vadodara	1067	6-12 years	High income ($\chi2$=11.52, p<0.01)

reported age-related trend in the percentages of obesity or overweight among girls, overweight increased with age. The percentage of obese and overweight girls were consistently higher along with all age groups than boys in the same age group. However, these studies have not adjusted for the potential developmental differences between female and male children that could precipitate a higher weight in female adolescents due to the onset of puberty and associated changes. The second growth spurt for female adolescents occurs at an earlier age (10-13 years) compared to their male peers (15-18 years) and physiological transformations that accompany this phase. On the other hand, a pooled meta-analysis of 21 Indian studies on both boys and girls, with 81,716 school children from 11 Indian states reported a higher burden of overnutrition in boys than girls (Jena and Jeena, 2018). The above study had adjusted for various confounders before the associations were examined.

A few parental or maternal factors were reported as determinants of childhood obesity such as the mother being a housewife reduced the risk of childhood obesity (Bhattacharya *et al.*, 2016). Also, family size ≥7 compared to <7 numbers increased the odds of overweight in 5-11 year old tribal Bodo children from Assam. Further, mothers' educational status was reported to influence the risk of overnutrition in their children; however, the results were mixed. Anuradha *et al.* (2015) reported a higher risk of childhood obesity among children of educated parents. Conversely, Mondal *et al.* (2015) reported a significantly lower risk (0.541 times) of overweight in children whose mothers were ≤10th standard educated ($p<0.05$), compared to their peers whose mothers had college or further education. Only one study reported the role of family history as a determinant of obesity in children with about 4.5 per cent obese children had a family history of overweight/obesity compared to that of non-obese children (7.3%) ($p<0.05$) (Panda, 2017). Collectively, studies indicated important determinants that should be considered while planning interventions and policies to address childhood obesity.

Lifestyle Determinants of Childhood Overweight and Obesity

Overnutrition is often considered as a manifestation of poor lifestyle choices that influence the life-course nutritional status.

The lifestyle factors include food-related, physical activity-related or behavioural or psychological, and in a majority of the population, these factors are amenable to behavioural changes. The present chapter summarizes modifiable lifestyle-related risk factors that potentially could reduce the prevalence of childhood overnutrition (Table 3.3). Evidence from Indian studies indicates that consumption of calorie-dense foods of low nutritional value (i.e. junk and fast foods) and low physical activity among Indian children as two important risk factors for childhood overweight/ obesity (Table 3.3). A surge in the consumption of junk and fast foods during childhood is reported from several studies in India, which often replace the major meals of the day. Increased use of such energy-laden foods adds significantly to the intake of energy. Excess calorie intake, consumption of fast foods, carbonated drinks, food from school canteens were significantly associated with overweight and obesity (Arifa *et al.*, 2018). In their Shimla study, Gupta *et al.* (2014) reported a significant positive association of overweight/obesity with frequent fast-food consumption (OR=4.45, 95% CI=2.42-8.18, $p<0.05$). Additionally, lower salt intake in their diet had lower odds of being overweight/obese (OR=0.47, 95% CI=0.25, 0.87, $p<0.05$). Panda *et al.* (2017) reported higher consumption of fast foods in obese children compared to that of non-obese children (65.2 *vs.* 34.6%) and a significant association between fast-food consumption and obesity ($p<0.05$). Many studies among school children reported increased access, availability of energy-dense foods, snacks, and carbonated beverages in school canteens (Sharma *et al.*, 2019). Additionally, working mothers or single-parent families, access to takeaway foods, increased frequency of eating out, and the addictive taste increase the higher use of fast and junk foods. The higher per capita income of family also increased the family's economic capacity and thus, the affordability of these foods. Therefore, to address childhood overweight and obesity, access, availability, and the use should be reduced and such foods need to be replaced by healthy foods.

Recent trends suggest increased physical inactivity among young children and adolescents due to their confinement to sedentary activities such as watching television and playing computer games and mobile usage. The Central Board of Secondary Education fact sheet (Global School-based health

Table 3.3: Lifestyle determinants of overweight and obesity in Indian children

Sl. No.	*Author & Year*	*Place*	*Sample size (n)*	*Age group (y)*	*Lifestyle determinants*
1.	Arifa *et al.*, 2018	Jammu	203	6-14 years	Excess calorie intake (OR=35.2; 95% CI 7.8-158.6, $p<0.001$); Fast food consumption (OR=6.1; 95% CI 2.2-16.9, $p<0.001$; Consumption of carbonated drinks (OR=5.2; 95% CI 1.89-14.32, $p<0.001$); Low physical activity (OR=6; 95% CI 2-18.13, $p<0.001$)
2.	Panda *et al.* 2017	Sambalpur	560	10-15 years	Fast food consumption ($\chi2=23.94$, $p<0.05$; Physical inactivity ($\chi2=11.83$, $p<0.05$)
3.	Bhattacharya *et al.*, 2016	Guwahati	60	10-19 years	Television watching >5 hours ($\chi2=18.63$, $p<0.001$); Playing video/computer games >5 hours ($\chi2=9.85$, $p<0.05$)
4.	Anuradha *et al.*, 2015	Tirupati	2258	12-16 years	<7 hours of sleep (OR=2.006; 95% CI 1.19-3.37, $p<0.001$)
5.	Kar and Khandelwal, 2015	Gangtok	979	11-19 years	Fast food consumption times per week (4.60 ± 1.8, $p<0.0001$); Screen time hours per day (16.86 ± 3.9, $p<0.0001$); Low outdoor activities hours per week (3.12 ± 1.2, $p<0.0001$)
6.	Gupta *et al.*, 2014	Shimla	720	14-19 years	Fast food consumption (OR=4.45; 95% CI 2.42-8.18, $p<0.05$); Low salt consumers were less obese (OR=0.47; 95% CI 0.25-0.87; $p<0.05$)
7.	Arora *et al.*, 2012	Delhi	1814	12-18 years	% Prevalence of obesity for daily vs. sometimes vs. never eating breakfast was 14.6 *vs.* 15.2 *vs.* 22.9 (F-test 3.25; p=0.039 for trend); Breakfast consumers had high physical activity (OR=2.9; 95% CI 1.9-4.4, $p<0.05$)

survey, 2007) reported that only 30 per cent of adolescents played regularly for at least 1 hour a day. A higher reliance on mechanized transportation, the use of labour-saving devices at home, and lesser inclination towards regular physical activities contribute to overweight and obesity in children (Global Strategy on Diet, Physical Activity and Health, 2002). Arora *et al.* (2017) reported a higher risk for childhood overweight and obesity with increased sedentary behaviours and physical inactivity. A higher prevalence of obesity and overweight was observed (11.68% and 10.9%, respectively) among children who were exposed to longer screen time such as watching television or using computers for a prolonged period as compared to the children with lesser sedentary activities. The results indicated that sedentary activity has a significant role in the development of obesity (Arora *et al.*, 2017). Also, physical inactivity among obese children was significantly higher than non-obese children (65.2% vs. 43.2%, $p<0.05$) (Panda *et al.*, 2017). Similar significant results were reported by the studies that explored the association between physical inactivity or sedentary behaviours or higher screen time use and overnutrition in children (Bhattacharya *et al.*, 2016; Kar and Khandelwal, 2015).

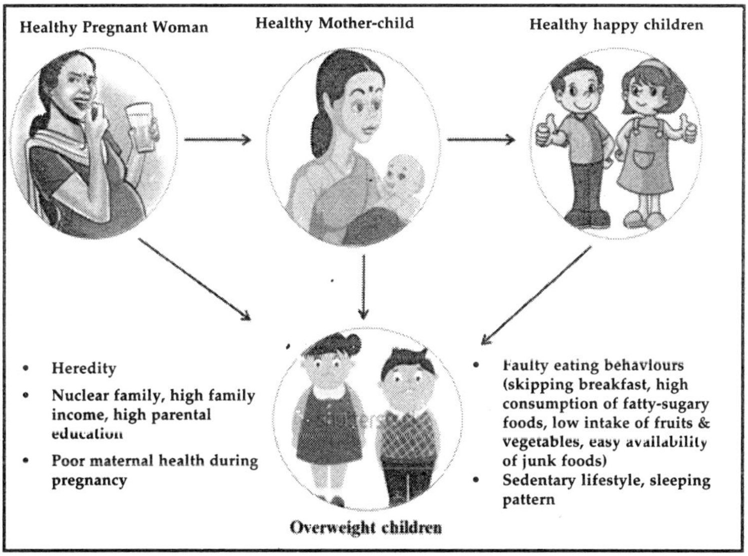

Fig. 3.1: Determinants of overweight and obesity in Indian children

Skipping breakfast was found to be associated with a higher risk of overweight and obesity in children. In a Delhi study among 1814 adolescents (12-18 years), it was observed that overall prevalence of overweight and obesity among adolescents who consumed breakfast daily (14.6%) was significantly lower against those who only sometimes (15.2%) or never (22.9%) consumed breakfast ($p<0.05$ for trend). However, this relationship was statistically significant for boys (15.4 % *vs.* 16.5% *vs.* 26.0; $p<0.05$ for trend) but not for girls. Children who consumed breakfast engaged in greater physical activity *versus* those who never consumed breakfast (Arora *et al.*, 2012). Additionally, child sleep duration <7 hrs per day increased the risk (OR=2.006; 95% CI: 1.194-3.371) for childhood overweight and obesity (Anuradha *et al.*, 2015). To sum up, evidence indicated relevant modifiable lifestyle determinants associated with childhood obesity (Fig. 3.1). These factors could be augmented in children through behaviour change strategies that could potentially prevent or decrease the prevalence of childhood overnutrition.

Conclusion

In India, a gradual increase in the prevalence of childhood overweight and obesity in tandem with the reduction of undernutrition is observed. Currently, the national prevalence of overweight and obesity remains less challenging as a young nation, however, the regional disparities warrant timely interventions. The research studies from the last decade have identified socio-economic, demographic and lifestyle factors that increased the risk of overnutrition in children. Multiple factors were identified, however, the interventions will need to be contextualized, and augmenting a few or more factors could improve the scenario. Behaviour change interventions in children could modify the lifestyle determinants such as developing healthy food habits and regular physical exercise among the vulnerable groups. Improving childhood nutrition practices requires effective and sustained multi-sectoral nutrition programming over the long term and an important step towards the same would be to achieve the World Health Association Target of no increase in childhood overweight.

REFERENCES

Anuradha, R., Sathyavathi, R., Reddy, M., Hemalatha, R., Sudhakar, G., Geetha, P. *et al.* 2015. "Effect of social and environmental determinants on overweight and obesity prevalence among adolescent school children." *IJEM,* **15**(2): 283-287.

Arifa, Q.A., Kumar, D., Rafiq, N., Nabi, T. 2018. "Association of overweight and obesity with dietary and physical activity behaviour among school-aged children in North India: a cross-sectional study." *International Journal of Community Medicine and Public Health,* **5**(7): 2944-2951.

Arora, M., Nazar, G., Gupta, V., Perry, C., Reddy, S., Stigler, M. 2012. "Association of breakfast intake with obesity, dietary and physical activity behavior among urban school-aged adolescents in Delhi, India: results of a cross-sectional study." *BMC Public Health,* **12**: 881-892.

Arora, M., Shinde, S., Patwardhan, R. 2017. "Prevalence of Overweight or Obesity in Adolescent School Children from Pune, India." *Imperial Journal of Interdisciplinary Research,* **3**(3): 1272-1276.

Bagudai, S., Nanda, P., Kodidala, S.R. 2014. "Prevelance of Obesity and Hypertension in adolescent school going children of Berhampur, Odisha, India." *International Journal of Physiotherapy and Research,* **2**(6): 777-780.

Bhattacharya, P.K., Gogoi, N., Roy, A. 2016. "Prevalence and awareness of obesity and its risk factors among adolescents in two schools in a northeast Indian city." *International Journal of Medical Science and Public Health,* **5**(6): 1111-1122.

Cherian, A., Cherian, S., Subbiah, S. 2012. "Prevalence of Obesity and Overweight in Urban School Children in Kerala, India." *Indian Pediatrics,* **49**: 475-477.

Daga, S., Mhatre, S., Kasbe, A., Dsouza, E. 2020. "Double burden of malnutrition among Indian school children and its measurement: a cross-sectional study in a single school." *BMJ Paediatr Open.* 2020; **4**(1):e000505. Published 2020 February 2. doi:10.1136/bmjpo-2019-000505

de Onis, M., Onyango, A.W., Borghi, E., Siyam, A., Nishida, C., Siekmann, J. 2007. "Development of a WHO growth reference for school-aged children and adolescents." *Bull World Health Organ.* 2007; **85**:660-7.

Ebbeling C., Pawlak, D., Ludwig, D. 2002. "Childhood obesity: Public health crisis, common sense cure." *Lancet,* **360**: 473-82.

Global School based health survey. 2007. Retrieved from http://www.who.int/chp/gshs/2007_India_CBSE_fact_sheet.pdf.

Global Strategy on Diet, Physical Activity and Health. 2002. Retrieved from http://www.who.int/dietphysicalactivity/childhood_why/en/index.html.

Gómez, M. 2013. "Post-green revolution food systems and the triple burden." *Food Policy,* **42**: 129-138.

Gupta, A., Sharma, D., Thakur, D., Thakur, A., Mazta, S.R. 2014. "Prevalence and predictors of the dual burden of malnutrition among adolescents in North India." *Saudi Journal of Obesity,* 2(2): 63-67.

Hakala, P., Rissanen, A., Koskenvuo, M., Kaprio, J., Ronnemaa, T. 1999. "Environmental factors in the development of obesity in identical twins." *Int J Obes Relat Metab Disord,* **23**: 746-753.

Hoddinott, J.B.Z. 2013. "Adult consequences of growth failure in early childhood." *Am J Clin Nutr,* **98**:1170-1178.

India State-Level Disease Burden Initiative Malnutrition Collaborators. 2019. "The burden of child and maternal malnutrition and trends in its indicators in the states of India: the Global Burden of Disease Study 1990-2017." *The Lancet. Child and adolescent health,* **3**(12): 855–870. https://doi.org/10.1016/S2352-4642(19)30273-1

International Institute for Population Sciences(IIPS).(1995). National Family Health Survey (MCH and Family Planning), (NFHS-1), India 1992-93. Bombay: IIPS.

International Institute for Population Sciences (IIPS) and ORC Macro. (2000). National Family Health Survey (NFHS-2), 1998-99: India. Mumbai

International Institute for Population Sciences. (2007). National Family Health Survey (NFHS-3), 2005-06: India. Mumbai, India: IIPS.

International Institute for Population Sciences. (2008). District Level Household and Facility Survey (DLHS-3), 2007-08. Mumbai: IIPS.

International Institute for Population Sciences (IIPS) and ICF. 2017. National Family Health Survey (NFHS-4), 2015-16: India. Mumbai: IIPS.

Iyer, U., Elayath, N., Akolkar, A. 2011. "Magnitude and Determinants of Overweight and Obesity in 6-12 year old school children of Vadodara City." *Current Pediatrics,* **15**(1): 105-109.

Jagadesan, S., Harish, R., Miranda, P., Unnikrishnan, R., Anjana, R.M., Mohan, V. 2014. "Prevalence of Overweight and Obesity Among School Children and Adolescents in Chennai." *Indian Pediatrics,* **15**: 544-549.

Jena, K.P., Jeena, P.B. 2018. "Overnutrition among school children in India: a review and meta-analysis." *Lancet Global Health,* 6: S25.

Kar, S., Khandelwal, B. 2015. "Fast foods and physical inactivity are risk factors for obesity and hypertension among adolescent school-children in east district of Sikkim, India." *J Nat Sci Biol Med,* **6**(2): 356–359.

Khadilkar, V., Yadav, S., Agrawal, K.K., Tamboli, S., Banerjee, M., Cherian, A., Goyal, J.P., Khadilkar, A., Kumaravel, V., Mohan, V., Narayanappa, D. 2015. "Revised IAP growth charts for height, weight and body mass index for 5 to 18-year-old Indian children." *Indian Paediatrics,* **52**(1): 47-55.

Meenakshi, J. 2016. "Trends and patterns in the triple burden of malnutrition in India." *Agricultural Economics* , **47**(S1): 115–134.

Ministry of Health and Family Welfare. 2014. Annual Health Survey: Clinical, anthropometric and biochemical (CAB). New Delhi, Ministry of Health and Family Welfare, Government of India. 2014.

Ministry of Health and Family Welfare (MoHFW), Government of India, UNICEF and Population Council. 2019. Comprehensive National Nutrition Survey (CNNS) National Report. New Delhi.https://www.popcouncil.org/uploads/pdfs/2019RH_CNNSreport.pdf accessed on June 21, 2020.

Ministry of Women and Child Development and UNICEF. (2014). Rapid survey on children (RSOC) 2013-14 National report. New Delhi, Ministry of Women and Child Development, India. 2013-14.

Mondal, N., Basumatary, B., Kropi, J., Bose, K. 2015. "Prevalence of double burden of malnutrition among urban school going Bodo children aged 5-11 years of Assam, Northeast India." *Epidemiology Biostatistics and Public Health,* **12**(4): e11497-1 to e11497-10.

Panda, S. C. (2017). "Overweight and obesity and lifestyle of urban adolescent school children of eastern state of India." *International Journal of Research in Medical Sciences,* **5**(11): 4770-75.

Prasanna, K.B., Bengalorkar, G.M., Deepthi, R., Muninarayan, C., and Ravishankar, S. (2012). "Prevalence of overweight and obesity among adolescent school going children (12-15 years) in urban area, South India." *Int J Cur Res Rev,* **4**(20): 99-105.

Ranjani, H., Mehreen, T.S., Pradeepa, R., Anjana, R.M., Garg, R. 2016. "Epidemiology of childhood overweight and obesity in India." *Indian J Med Res,* 143: 160-174.

Saikia, D., Ahmed, S.J., Saikia, H., Sarma, R. 2018. "Body mass index and body fat percentage in assessing obesity: An analytical study among the adolescents of Dibrugarh, Assam." *Indian Journal of Public Health,* **62**(4): 277-281. https://doi.org/10.4103/ijph.IJPH_24_18

Sharma, P., Yadav, S.S., Menon, K. 2019. "A Review of the Nutritional Quality of School Canteen Foods in South Asia." *International Journal of Public Health Research and Development,* **10**: 1600-06.

Shanmugam, K., Ravishankar, S.L., Kannappan, S., Thomas, V. Chacko, T.V. 2016. "Prevalence of overweight and obesity among children aged 5-15 years in a rural school in Coimbatore." *International Journal of Medical Science and Public Health,* **5**(10): 2186-89.

United Nations Children's Fund (UNICEF), World Health Organization, International Bank for Reconstruction and Development/The World Bank (2020). Levels and trends in child malnutrition: Key Findings of the 2020 Edition of the Joint Child Malnutrition Estimates. Geneva: World Health Organization; https://data.unicef.org/resources/jme-report-2020/ accessed on June 21, 2020.

WHO (2006). World Health Organization Child Growth Standards. https://www.who.int/growthref/en/ accessed on June 21, 2020.

4

Immunization Status of 0-59-month Children in India

Susmita Bharati, Manoranjan Pal and *Premananda Bharati*

Introduction

The proverb—"prevention is better than cure"—is very much applicable to children's diseases, because it affects the future of mankind. Prevention not only makes the children secure but also the future generation when children grow up healthy. Thus, the effectiveness of immunization of children is unquestionable. Globally, vaccine preventable diseases account for nearly 20 per cent of all deaths occurring annually among children under five years of age and immunization has a vital role to play in achieving the goals specified in the Millennium Declaration (WHO, 2012). It is also seen that during 2010, the mortality rate of children due to only measles was about 47 per cent (Simons *et al.*, 2012). India accounts for the highest number of under-five deaths in the world (WHO, UNCF, 2012). The average annual rate of decline in under-five mortality is 3.1 per cent during 1990-2009 and it was considered as insufficient to achieve the Fourth Millennium Development Goal (MDG) of minimizing under-five mortality to 39 per 1000 live births by 2015 (UNCF, 2010).

In India, Universal Immunization Programme (UIP) was launched in 1985 with much dynamism to attain the target to immunize all eligible children by 1990. Under (UIP), vaccines for six vaccine-preventable diseases such as tuberculosis, diphtheria, pertussis (whooping cough), tetanus, poliomyelitis, and measles are available for free of cost to all. Lot of energy and money have been spent on the UIP, but it does not reap the much-hyped outcome. Unmistakably, various survey results show the glaring gap between the target and achievement even after several years. So, to find out the prevalence of immunization and morbidity among children in India, the present objectives of the study are (i) to assess the immunization status of (0-5) year children and (ii) to assess the effectiveness of the socio-demographic factors on immunization.

Methodology

Data

The data has been accessed from the fourth round National Family Health Survey (NFHS-4) carried out during 2015-16. The survey was coordinated by International Institute for Population Sciences (IIPS) in collaboration with the Ministry of Health and Family Welfare. Data, relating to the children of age (0-59)-month, are taken in our study. The sample size for this study is 2,25,002. The child is considered as a fully immunized if the child has taken one dose for BCG, three doses for DPT and Polio each and single dose for measles. Data on immunization status are verified from vaccination cards and in case, where a vaccination card was not available or vaccination was not recorded on the card, the mother's recall of vaccination was accepted.

Places of residence are taken as "rural" and "urban". Sex of infants has also been considered. Mother's educational status are grouped into four categories such as illiterate (those who can neither read nor write), primary (literate up to class IV standard), secondary (class V to class X standard) and the fourth group is class XI and onwards (i.e. Higher Secondary, Graduate, Post graduate etc.). Birth order of the child, family size, awareness of mother through social media like TV, newspaper or magazine, gender of the household head and wealth index of the family have been considered as independent variables. Wealth index is a measure of the economic status of the household (Rutstein, 1999). Though it is an indicator of the level of the wealth in the household, it is consistent with expenditure and income measure. It is based on 33 household assets and housing characteristics, namely household electrification, type of windows, sources of drinking water, types of toilet facility, flooring, roofing, cooking fuel and house ownership, material of exterior walls, number of household members per sleeping room, ownership of a bank or post-office account, ownership of a mattress, a pressure cooker, a chair, a cot/ bed, a table, an electric fan, a radio/transistor, a black and white television, a colour television, a sewing machine, a mobile telephone, and any other telephone, a computer, a refrigerator, a watch or clock, a bicycle, a motorcycle or scooter, an animal-drawn cart, a car, a water pump, a thresher, and a tractor. Here each household asset was assigned a weight generated through principal component analysis and the resulting score was standardized in relation to a normal distribution and each household was assigned a score for each asset and the scores were summed for each household and individuals were ranked according to the score of the household and the scores were divided into five quintile groups starting from lower strata to higher strata like poorest, poorer, medium, richer and richest.

To see the relative and effective intervention, immunization status was regressed on socio-economic variables using categorical logistic regression analysis. Dependent variables are taken as binary. Children who have been immunized are coded as '1' and non-immunized children are coded as '0'. An estimated odd ratio of '1' indicates that the nature of dependent variable is not different from the reference category. If the estimated odd ratio is >1, the probability of becoming affected is more in this category compared to the reference category and if it is <1, then it is just opposite to that of '>1' case.

Results

Table 4.1 describes the immunization status of (0-59)-month children in India as well as its gender differences. It is seen that percentages of children who have taken BCG, triple doses of DPT, triple doses of Polio and measles vaccination are 88.6, 70.3, 64.8 and 68.7 respectively. The picture is more or less same for each sex. Table 4.2 shows the immunization status of (0-59) month

Table 4.1: Immunization status of (0-59)-month children in India and by gender

Type of vaccination	Total			Boys			Girls		
	N	Yes (%)	No (%)	N	Yes (%)	No (%)	N	Yes (%)	No (%)
BCG	225002 (100.0%)	88.6	11.4	116360 (100.0%)	88.9	11.1	108642 (100.0%)	88.3	11.7
DPT1	225002 (100.0%)	84.0	16.0	116360 (100.0%)	84.3	15.7	108642 (100.0%)	83.7	16.3
DPT2	225002 (100.0%)	78.5	21.5	116360 (100.0%)	78.8	21.2	108642 (100.0%)	78.2	21.8
DPT3	225002 (100.0%)	70.3	29.7	116360 (100.0%)	70.6	29.4	108642 (100.0%)	70.0	30.0
POLIO1	225002 (100.0%)	85.5	14.5	116360 (100.0%)	85.7	14.3	108642 (100.0%)	85.2	14.8
POLIO2	225002 (100.0%)	79.1	20.9	116360 (100.0%)	79.3	20.7	108642 (100.0%)	79.9	21.1
POLIO3	225002 (100.0%)	64.8	35.2	116360 (100.0%)	65.0	35.0	108642 (100.0%)	64.6	35.4
MEASLES	225002 (100.0%)	68.7	31.3	116360 (100.0%)	69.0	31.0	108642 (100.0%)	68.5	31.5
Complete immunized	225002 (100.0%)	64.8	35.2	116360 (100.0%)	65.0	35.0	108642 (100.0%)	64.5	35.5

Table 4.2: Immunization status of (0-59) month children in India and by age

Age groups (Months)	N	BCG	DPT1	DPT2	DPT3	Polio1	Polio2	Polio3	Measles	Comp. Immu-nization
0-11	41889	87.5	73.2	59.9	45.8	76.2	61.1	44.6	18.7	17.5
12-23	45289	91.0	88.8	84.9	77.8	89.9	85.2	73.2	79.6	75.5
24-35	45096	89.6	87.6	83.9	77.3	88.4	84.4	71.4	81.6	77.2
36-59	92728	87.4	84.8	81.2	74.4	86.0	81.7	66.6	79.8	74.9
0-59	225002	88.6	84.0	78.5	70.3	85.5	79.1	64.8	68.7	64.8

children in India and by age and through this table, it is seen that maximum immunization has been completed between 12 to 35 months of age. Table 4.3 describes the immunization status in relation to zones and states of India. It is seen that in India immunization status of BCG is 88.6 per cent. In case of DPT3, Polio3 and measles, immunization statuses are 70.3 per cent, 64.8 per cent and 68.7 per cent respectively and completely immunized children are 64.8 per cent only. The lowest immunized zone for BCG is north-east (78.0%) while the highest zone is south (94.2%). The

Table 4.3: Immunization status among (0-59) month children in different zones and states of India

Zones/States	*N*	*BCG*	*DPT3*	*Polio3*	*Measles*	*Complete Immunization*
North-east	**69.1**	**78.0**	**61.5**	**59.1**	**58.7**	**55.1**
Arunachal Pradesh	3851	63.6	43.3	46.7	45.5	39.8
Assam	8855	82.3	65.9	56.7	65.4	60.9
Manipur	5256	87.0	68.6	70.1	61.9	59.6
Meghalaya	3823	85.3	69.1	65.9	63.4	61.8
Mizoram	4309	70.3	59.2	57.0	56.6	54.6
Nagaland	3825	67.7	48.2	52.3	44.4	39.1
Sikkim	898	96.1	85.6	78.5	78.4	76.8
Tripura	1188	76.9	65.8	62.3	59.8	55.8
East	**47320**	**91.9**	**77.5**	**68.8**	**72.7**	**69.1**
Bihar	22275	90.2	74.5	64.4	69.9	65.3
Jharkhand	10507	93.5	76.2	68.9	73.1	68.6
Orissa	9728	92.1	82.5	73.8	76.1	74.6
West Bengal	4810	96.4	84.3	78.7	78.3	76.3
Central	**65967**	**88.1**	**63.8**	**61.0**	**65.7**	**61.0**
Madhya Pradesh	21272	89.8	65.5	55.4	70.0	64.8
Chhattisgarh	8230	96.9	77.9	69.8	75.1	72.3
Uttar Pradesh	36465	85.2	59.5	62.2	61.1	56.2
West	**15418**	**87.8**	**70.1**	**60.5**	**70.4**	**66.0**
Goa	378	97.9	89.2	86.0	85.7	83.1
Gujarat	6444	85.8	66.0	54.8	65.5	61.5
Maharashtra	7990	89.0	72.3	63.8	73.7	68.9
Dadra and NH	277	92.8	78.3	57.4	75.1	67.5
Daman and Diu	329	84.2	69.9	64.4	66.3	61.4
North	**42481**	**91.0**	**74.1**	**69.0**	**71.6**	**68.1**
Haryana	6875	90.3	72.0	67.0	69.8	65.4
Himachal Pradesh	2525	92.4	79.5	75.5	75.4	70.4
Jammu & Kashmir	7093	93.6	80.4	77.4	75.0	72.6
New Delhi	1145	94.4	81.3	75.8	79.4	74.1
Chandigarh	174	97.7	88.5	84.5	81.0	79.9
Uttarakhand	5007	91.2	75.0	65.3	70.6	66.3
Punjab	4746	98.2	89.7	88.9	81.1	80.4
Rajasthan	14916	87.1	65.2	59.0	66.8	62.8
South	**21811**	**94.2**	**80.2**	**70.9**	**77.4**	**74.0**
Andhra Pradesh	2599	95.9	81.0	59.2	77.3	74.4
Telangana	2029	95.6	78.3	63.9	76.3	71.5
Karnataka	6308	92.9	77.3	67.0	75.9	72.1
Kerala	2235	98.3	87.2	85.9	82.4	80.9
Tamil Nadu	6836	94.2	80.7	74.7	78.4	74.5
Poducherry	945	97.6	89.7	85.3	82.6	82.1
Lakshadweep	281	99.6	87.2	85.4	80.4	80.1
Andaman and NH	578	72.0	63.8	60.0	54.8	52.6
India	**225002**	**88.6**	**70.3**	**64.8**	**68.7**	**64.8**

highest immunized zone for the other three vaccination is south zone with 80.2 per cent, 70.9 per cent and 77.4 per cent immunization respectively for DPT3, Polio3 and Measles, while the lowest immunized zones for these three vaccinations is again north-east with 61.5 per cent, 59.1 per cent and 58.7 per cent immunization respectively. The highest complete immunized zone is south zone (74.0%) and lowest zone is north-east (55.1%). State-wise distribution for immunization of BCG, the lowest percentage is seen in Arunachal Pradesh (63.6%) and the highest percentage is in Lakshadweep (99.6 %) and then followed by Punjab (98.2%). The lowest immunized state for DPT3 is Arunachal Pradesh (43.3%) and the highest states are Punjab and Puducherry (89.7%). For Polio, the lowest immunized state is Arunachal Pradesh (46.7%) and the highest state is Punjab (88.9%). For measles, the lowest immunized state is Nagaland (44.4%) and then followed by Arunachal Pradesh (45.5%) and the highest percentage of immunization is seen in Goa (85.7%). For complete immunization, the highest occurrence is seen in Goa (83.1%) and the lowest occurrence is seen in Mizoram (39.1%) and then followed by Arunachal Pradesh (39.8%).

Table 4.4 shows the relationship between socio-demographic variables with immunization status of pre-school children in India. It is seen that socio-economic status has an impressive effect on immunization status, because it is significantly more in urban areas. Mother's education, mother's awareness through any media and wealth index of the family has positive impact on increasing the immunization rate among the pre-school children. Increment of birth order and family size has a negative impact on immunization and it is also seen that middle-aged mother, i.e. from (20-35)-year old mothers have the highest immunized children than early aged and late aged mothers. Practically sex of the children has no impact on the variation of immunization status in India.

Table 4.5 shows the impact of socio-demographic variables on immunization status among pre-school children in India through categorical logistic regression. Regression shows that education of mother, mother's age, awareness of mother and wealth index of the family have positive impact on the immunization status. Birth orders of the family and family size have negative impact on the immunization status because all these results are statistically significant at 1 per cent level of significance.

Table 4.4: Relationship between different socio-demographic variables and Immunization status of (0-59) month children in India

Independent variables	*N*	*BCG*	*DPT3*	*Polio3*	*Measles*	*Complete Immunization*
Residence						
Rural	171519	87.8	69.1	63.8	67.8	63.7
Urban	53483	91.2	74.3	68.1	71.8	68.2
Mother's education						
Illiterate	68978	82.5	61.1	57.1	62.3	57.8
Primary	32835	87.6	68.4	63.3	67.8	63.7
Secondary	102191	91.7	75.1	68.8	71.9	68.3
Higher	20998	95.2	80.3	73.0	75.7	72.5
Mother's age						
15-19	5452	87.1	55.8	51.7	45.4	42.7
20-35	197043	89.3	71.2	65.5	69.5	65.6
36+	22507	82.7	66.1	62.0	67.9	63.5
Birth order						
1st	83046	91.4	74.7	68.2	72.0	68.3
2nd	69784	90.1	72.3	66.1	70.4	66.6
3rd-4th	54265	86.0	65.9	61.0	65.6	61.3
5th and above	17907	77.0	55.6	55.3	56.9	52.5
Family size						
<6	95043	89.6	72.8	67.1	71.2	67.3
6 and above	129959	87.9	68.5	63.1	66.9	62.9
Awareness through						
TV- No	71557	83.0	61.4	57.7	61.9	57.2
Yes	153445	91.2	74.5	68.1	71.9	68.3
Newspaper- No	154290	86.7	67.1	62.2	66.2	62.0
Yes	70712	92.9	77.5	70.5	74.3	70.8
Magazine- No	192699	88.4	69.9	64.5	68.4	64.5
Yes	32303	89.7	72.6	66.8	70.6	66.5
Gender of the Household Head						
Female	197992	88.5	70.2	64.7	68.7	64.8
Male	27010	89.3	71.1	65.4	68.7	64.7
Wealth index						
Poorest or poorer	111492	85.0	64.3	59.7	64.2	59.8
Middle	45136	90.3	73.0	67.3	70.7	67.0
Richer or Richest	68374	93.4	78.3	71.5	74.9	71.5

Table 4.5 Categorical logistic regression between different socio demographic variables and Immunization status of (0-59) month children in India

Residence	*BCG*	*DPT3*	*Polio3*	*Measles*	*Complete Immunization*
Rural ®	1.00	1.00	1.00	1.00	1.00
Urban	0.903**	0.902**	0.920**	0.919**	0.925**
Mother's education					
Illiterate®	1.00	1.00	1.00	1.00	1.00
Primary	1.128**	1.186**	1.172**	1.125**	1.130**
Secondary	1.522**	1.372**	1.312**	1.164**	1.176**
Higher	2.190**	1.487**	1.373**	1.142**	1.168**
Mother's age					
15-19®	1.00	1.00	1.00	1.00	1.00
20-35	1.377**	2.180**	1.879**	3.007**	2.790**
36+	1.185**	2.491**	2.031**	3.875**	3.495**
Birth order					
1st®	1.00	1.00	1.00	1.00	1.00
2nd	0.921**	0.888**	0.916**	0.892**	0.900**
3rd-4th	0.772**	0.969**	0.840**	0.781**	0.788**
5th and above	0.577**	0.578**	0.766**	0.572**	0.592**
Family size					
<6®	1.00	1.00	1.00	1.00	1.00
6 and above	0.951**	0.873**	0.867**	0.869**	0.875**
Awareness through					
TV- No®	1.00	1.00	1.00	1.00	1.00
Yes	1.407**	1.319**	1.206**	1.249**	1.278**
Newspaper- No®	1.00	1.00	1.00	1.00	1.00
Yes	1.059**	1.079**	1.033**	1.106**	1.107**
Magazine- No®	1.00	1.00	1.00	1.00	1.00
Yes	0.912**	0.962**	0.985**	0.976	0.953**
Gender of the household					
Female®	1.00	1.00	1.00	1.00	1.00
Male	0.894**	0.949**	0.966**	1.000	0.999
Wealth index					
Poorest or poorer®	1.00	1.00	1.00	1.00	1.00
Middle	1.176**	1.170**	1.176**	1.122**	1.128**
Richer or Richest	1.480**	1.369**	1.320**	1.270**	1.264**

** $p > 0.05$

Discussion

In respect of immunization status, India's motto was to be immunized all children and pregnant mothers by 1990 (Banerjee, D., 1990). From our study, it is seen that during 2015-16, among pre-school children in India, 88.6 per cent, 68.7 per cent, 70.3 per cent and 64.8 per cent are immunized by BCG, measles, DPT (triple dose) and Polio (triple doses) respectively. About 64.8 per cent are completely immunized during 2015-16. The highest percentages of immunized children are seen in south zone and the lowest percentage is seen in north-east zone. In state-wise distribution, the highest percentage of immunized children are found in Puducherry, Punjab, Lakshadweep, Goa and the lowest immunized states are mainly Arunachal Pradesh, Nagaland or Mizoram. It is also interesting to note that there has been no gender discrimination on immunization status of the children. But, still now in India, 35 per cent children have incomplete immunization.

Socio-demographic factor has a very significant relationship with the immunization status. Mainly, children of higher educated mother have the highest percentage of complete immunization. Similar findings show a positive correlation between mother's education and complete immunization (Mathews, 2012). Furthermore, birth order, mother's awareness and wealth index of the family have strong positive effect on the status of immunization. Thus, it appears that unless mothers become educated and income of the families are increased, it is difficult to improve the immunization status of children. So, it is necessary to spread the awareness among mothers. Thus, we can say that strengthening of health education activities and proper motivation specially among mothers by health workers can definitely improve the awareness and thereby improve the immunization coverage and mainly female education alone can solve this purpose.

Besides this, one of the strong arguments for low immunization coverage is the failure of the 'demand' and 'supply' sides (Pande *et al.*, 2003). The demand failure includes the knowledge gap about the benefits of immunization, possibly due to lack of immunization campaigns and families not being adequately informed (Phukan, 2009). However, supply or system failure includes failure of the health worker to arrive on time or be regular, inadequate supplies and so on. Besides this, immunization is also very much dependent upon the state health infrastructure, because immunization programme has become fruitful through public programme only and not by private programme. So, it is suggested to strengthen the programme, revitalize and strengthen routine immunization services with particular reference to illiterate mothers, inaccessible and tribal areas and low performing states.

REFERENCES

Banerjee, Debabar. 1986. "Technocratic Approach to Health: Western Response to Alma Ata." *Economic and Political Weekly,* **28**(12): 1233-1234.

Brown, K.E., Black, R.E. and Becker, S. 1982. "Seasonal changes in nutritional status and the prevalence of malnutrition in a longitudinal study of young children in rural Bangladesh." *American Journal of Clinical Nutrition,* **36**: 303-13.

Chen, L.C., Chowdhury, K.M.A., and Huffman, S.L. 1980. "Anthropometric assessment of energy-protein malnutrition and subsequent risk of mortality among preschool aged children." *American Journal of Clinical Nutrition,* **33**: 1836-45.

International Institute for Population Sciences (IIPS) and ORC Macro. 2007. National Family Health Survey (NFHS-3), 2005-06, Vol.1: India, Mumbai; IIPS.

Mathew, J.L. "Inequity in Childhood Immunization in India: A Systematic Review." *Indian Pediatr,* 2012; **49**: 203-22.

Pande, R.P. and Yazbeck, A.S. 2003. "What's in a country average? Wealth, gender, and regional inequalities in immunization in India." *Social Science and Medicine,* **57**: 2075-88.

Phukan, R.K., Barman, M.P. and Mahanta, J. 2009. "Factors Associated with Immunization Coverage of Children in Assam, India: Over the First Year of Life." *Journal of Tropical Pediatrics,* **55**: 249-252.

Rutstein, S. 1999. Wealth *versus* expenditure: Comparison between the DHS wealth index and household expenditures in your departments of Guatemala. Calverton, Maryland: ORCMacro.

Ruzicka, L.T. and Kane, P. 1985. "Nutrition and child survival in south Asia." In K. Srinivasan and S. Mukerji, eds. *Dynamics of Population and Family Welfare,* pp. 333-57. Bombay: Himalaya Publishing House.

Santhanakrishnan, B.R. and Ramalingam, R. 1987. "Risk factors of mortality in children with diarrhoeal disease in Madras, India." *Journal of Diarrhoeal Disease Research,* **5**: 36–9.

Simons, E., Ferrari, M., Fricks, J., Wannemuehler, K., Burton, A. and Strebel, A. 2012. "Assessment of the 2010 global measles mortality reduction goal: results from amodel of surveillance data." *The Lancet,* **379**: 2173–2178.

Singh, K.P. 1989. "Green revolution and child survival in the state of Punjab." In *International Population Conference, New Delhi: Proceedings,* Vol. 1, pp. 379-88. Liege, Belgium: International Union for the Scientific Study of Population (IUSSP).

Sommer, A. and Loewenstein, M.S. 1975. "Nutritional status and mortality: A prospective validation of the QUAC stick." *American Journal of Clinical Nutrition,* **28**: 287-92.

Sommerfelt, A.E. and Stewart, M.K. 1994. *Children's nutritional status.* DHS Comparative Studies, No. 12. Calverton, Maryland: Macro International, Demographic and Health Surveys.

United Nations Children's Fund (2010). Levels and Trends in Child Mortality. Estimates Developed by the UN Inter-agency Group for Child Mortality Estimation. New York, USA.

Vella, V., Tomkins, A., Borghesi, A., Migliori, G.B., Adriko, B.C. and Crevatin, E. 1992a. "Determinants of child nutrition and mortality in north-west Uganda." *Bulletin of the World Health Organization,* **705**: 637-43.

World Bank Organization. 2006. News and Broadcast—Urgent action needed to overcome persistent malnutrition in India, say 'World Bank Report' web. Worldbank.org. May 11.

World Health Organization. 1995. Physical Status: The Use and Interpretation of Anthropometry. *WHO Technical Report Series No. 854.* Geneva: WHO.

World Health Organization. 2012. *Millennium Development Goals: Immunization's contribution to reaching the Millennium Development Goal on child survival.* World Health Organization, Geneva.

5

Socio-economic and Demographic Determinants of Undernutrition among the Nyishi Women

Nitamoni Bharali, Nitish Mondal and Kh. Narendra Singh

Introduction

There were 821 million undernourished people living in the world in 2018 (10.8% of the total population). It was estimated that another billion people had a lack of vitamins and minerals. In 2015, protein-energy malnutrition (PEM) was estimated to have resulted in 3,23,000 deaths—down from 5,10,000 deaths in 1990. In 2010, malnutrition was the cause of 1.4 per cent of all disability adjusted life years (Murray *et al.*, 2012). In 2010, it was estimated to have contributed to about 1.5 million deaths in women though some estimate the number may be greater than 3 million (Lim *et al.*, 2012). From the day of beginning undernutrition is more common in developing countries including India. Certain groups have higher rates of undernutrition, including women, in particular while pregnant or breastfeeding mothers. In adults, undernutrition becomes more common due to physical, psychological, and socio-economic factors (Ronnie *et al.*, 2011) therefore, undernutrition or Chronic Energy Deficiency (CED) causes several ill-health condition, mortality, morbidity and generate a poor reproductive outcome among women, and therefore, it is considered to be the major public health issues in developing countries. Due to its immense population size, socio-economic disparities, illiteracy and inadequate access to health care facilities, the Indian population are found to be undernourished and underprivileged. Several research studies have reported the similar prevalence of undernourishment among different Indian population (Khongsdier, 2002; Gogoi and Sengupta, 2002; Mungreipy and Kapoor, 2010; Mahanta *et al.*, 2012; Bharali *et al.*, 2017; Tigga *et al.*, 2018). Moreover, the prevalence of undernutrition or CED among adults will reduce the physical activity, productivity and reproductive performance in the population (Mahanta *et al.*, 2012; Bharali *et al.*, 2017; Tigga *et al.*, 2018). A large number of studies also have explored the relation between BMI and mortality in adults (Seidell and Flegal, 1997; Dudeja *et al.*, 2001; Shukla *et al.*, 2002; Musaad *et al.*, 2013) and results apparent that underweight was associated with an increased risk of pre-mature mortality and increased risks of morbidity in adults (WHO Expert Consultation, 1995; 2004).

Prevalence of undernutrition among adult women in India is among the highest in the world. About 36 per cent of adult women (15-49 years) in India had chronic energy deficiency (CED), i.e. body mass index (BMI) below 18.5 kg/m^2 in 2005-06 (Jose, 2014). This is much higher than the prevalence in most countries of Sub-Saharan Africa (for which comparable data exist). Mainly, the global cut-off used to measure undernutrition, such as BMI below 18.5, overestimates its prevalence among Indian adults, because Indians as an ethnic group have something genetically specific to them which endow them with a relatively low BMI (WHO, 1995). Therefore, it is evident from the above discussion that the individual belonging to the above-mentioned vulnerable segments, residing in the rural regions are found to be nutritionally more susceptible than the individual residing in the urban regions in India. Therefore, the objectives of the present study are as follows:

1. To assess the prevalence of different grade of Undernutrition or CED (e.g. mild/moderate and severe) among adult Nyishi tribal women belonging to reproductive ages (15-44 years) of Arunachal Pradesh.
2. To determine the effect of socio-economic and demographic variables with different grades of undernutrition or CED status (e.g., mild/moderate and severe) among tribal women.

Material and Methods

The present community based cross-sectional study was conducted among 600 Nyishi tribal women aged 15-44 years residing in rural areas of Kemin and Kakoi Block (latitude 26°55'N and 28°40' and longitude between 92°40' and 94°21') of Papung Pare district of Arunachal Pradesh. It is estimated that the total population of 1,76,385 individuals, (males: 90,447 females: 85,938) Literacy Rate 82.14 per cent, Sex Ratio 975:1000) Arunachal Pradesh, India. The data of the present study was covered homogenous 14 villages of the studied area. The community block consists of predominant tribal ethnic communities like Nyishi, Hill Miri and Adi ethnic populations. Initially subjects were identified in the present study are belonging to the major dominant ethnic groups of this region include Nyishi tribal ethnic population. Ethnically, they are belonging to Sino-Tibetian family and showing close ethnic affinity with quasi-Tibetian origin. Age of the subjects was collected from the birth certificates and relevant official records issued by the local government officials. All the subjects were free from any physical deformities, systematic diseases, nutritional deficiencies apperently health and previous histories related to medical and surgical episodes. An informed consent was obtained by local village level authorities, and research precipitants prior to the data collection. The participation of the subject in this study is completely voluntary in nature, and the study was conducted in accordance with the ethical guidelines for human experiments as laid down in the Helsinki Declaration (Touitou *et al.*, 2004).

Collection of Socio-economic and Demographic Data

Demographic data including monthly family income, sanitation facility, dependent children, and parental education and occupation were recorded for each household before the collection of anthropometric data. Further, necessary information on dependent children, house type, water sources, consumption of alcohol, chewing of tobacco and smoking habits were also obtained. A structured schedule was completed by house visits and interviewing the subjects. The socio-economic status (SES) was evaluated using a modified version of Kuppuswamy's scale proposed by (Kumar *et al.*, 2007). The scale determines the SES based on a score calculated from education, occupation and monthly income. It was subsequently observed that all selected women belonged to a lower SES group.

Anthropometric Measurements

Anthropometric measurements were obtained from the women using the standard procedure (Hall *et al.*, 2007). The height was collected using the standard anthropometer rod nearest to 0.01 cm head oriented in Frankfort horizontal plan. The weight of the subjects, wearing minimum clothing and with bare feet was taken using a portable weighing scale (Libra, Edryl-India, Tiswadi, Goa) to the nearest 100 gm. The differences in anthropometric measurements were calculated for testing the co-efficient of reliability [R={1–(TEM) 2/SD2}, the SD= standard deviation of all measurements] using the technical error measurement {TEM=√(ΣD2/2N), D=difference between the measurements, N= number of individuals measured} following the method of Ulijaszek and Kerr (1999). Very high values of R (>0.98) were obtained for height and weight using TEM analysis and values were found within the cut-off values (0.95) as suggested by Ulijaszek and Kerr (1999).

Assessment of Nutritional Status

The nutritional status of adult Nyishi women was assessed using the BMI. BMI was calculated using standard equation of the WHO (1995, 2004): **BMI (kg/m²) = Weight (kg)/ Height² (m²).** Nutritional status has been assessed using the internationally accepted BMI guidelines as suggested by the WHO (WHO, 1995, 2004). For the screening of undernutrition, different CED grades of BMI were used. Studies have indicated the BMI values <18.50 kg/m² as the cut-off point to determine the nutritional status of different target populations, both in India and abroad (Khongsdier, 2001; 2005; Bose *et al.*, 2006; 2007; Subramanian *et al.*, 2007). Where the individuals with the BMI 16.99-18.49, <16.00 kg/m² was considered to be mild/moderate and severe undernutrition or CED, respectively. The BMI cut-off points as specified by WHO (1995, 2004) for Asian populations was used to assess the nutritional status of the adult Nyishi married individual. The utilized cut-off values are given in Table 5.1.

Table 5.1. Cut-off values of different Grade of Undernutrition or CED in Adults

Cut-off Points (BMI kg/m²)	*CED/Undernutrition Grade*
>18.50	Normal
17.0-18.49	Mild CED (Grade I)
16.0-16.99	Moderate CED (Grade II)
<16.00	Severe CED (Grade III)

Statistical Analysis

The data were compiled in MS Excel and Binary Logistics Regression (BLR) analysis done using Statistical Package for Social Sciences (SPSS, Inc., Chicago, IL; version 16.0). Binary logistic regression (BLR) analysis was undertaken to estimate the odds ratios (ORs), minimum of 95 per cent confidence intervals (CIs) and to assess possible differences in risk factors associated with those individuals being undernourished (BMI<18.50 kg/m^2), mild to moderate undernourished (BMI<16.00 -18.50 kg/m^2) and severely undernourished (BMI<16.00 kg/m^2), separately. In the BLR analysis, the different socio-economic, demographic and lifestyle predictor variables were used as univariate independent regression model analyses. To create the dichotomous individuals who were undernourished (BMI<18.50 kg/m^2) were coded as '1' in the respective BLR model. Similarly, individuals who happen to be mild-moderate and severely undernourished were also coded as '1' in the respective BLR model. Individuals who exhibited normal BMI were coded as '0' in the BLR models. These different regression models were utilized to identify possible risk factor(s) associated with undernutrition. The BLR analysis allows the creation of categorical depended variables and odds ratios were obtained by comparing with the reference categories. The predictor variables were entered in the regression equation and the results were obtained by comparing them with the reference categories. A p-value of less than 0.05 and 0.01 were considered to be statistically significant.

Results

Assessment of Nutritional Status among Nyishi Women

The prevalence of different grades of malnutrition status among adult Nyishi tribal women was evaluated using proposed BMI classification for Asia-specific population (WHO, 1995, 2004) and the results are presented in Table 5.2. The overall prevalence of undernutrition or CED (BMI<18.50 kg/m^2) and normal nutritional status was observed to be 26.33 per cent and 74.66 per cent, respectively. The overall prevalence of Mild undernutrition/CED (BMI 17.0-18.49 kg/m^2), Moderate undernutrition/CED (BMI 16.0-16.99 kg/m^2) and Severe undernutrition/CED (BMI <16.0 kg/m^2) was observed to be 8.33 per cent, 2.50 per cent and 15.00 per cent among tribal women, it was also depicted in Figure 5.1 also respectively.

Table 5.2: Nutritional status among the Nyishi tribal women

Category	*BMI (kg/m²)**	*Frequency*	*Percentages*
Mild Undernutrition (CED)	17.00-18.49	50	8.33%
Moderate Undernutrition (CED)	16.00-16.99	18	2.50%
Severe Undernutrition (CED)	<16.00	90	15.00%
Total Undernutrition(CED)	<16.00-18.49	158	26.33%

*WHO (1995).

The BLR model was fitted to find out the odds for the socio-economic, demographic, lifestyle related variables for being undernutrition (BMI<18.50 kg/m^2) in Nyishi women was depicted in Table 5.3. The results of the BLR analysis further showed significant effects to being undernourished was associated with having 3 and more dependent children (Odds: 0.620), which have a non-bricked house (Odds: 14.61), using the water source by river (Odds: 0.427) and supply water from river (Odds: 0.392) ($p<0.05$) and found highly associated with the education of the head who were illiterate (Odds: 31.11), studies till class 5 (Odds: 14.28) and till class 10th (Odds: 36.51), occupation of head doing cultivation (Odds: 35.54), monthly income is less (Rs. 2000-5000) (Odds: 10.76), non-sanitary toilet facility (Odds: 3.83), and the women consume alcohol (Odds: 4.23), chew tobacco (Odds:14.66) and do smoke

(Odds: 0.30) ($p<0.01$). On the other hand the occupation of women like housewife and service was not found any significant association with the prevalence of undernutrition among Nyishi women.

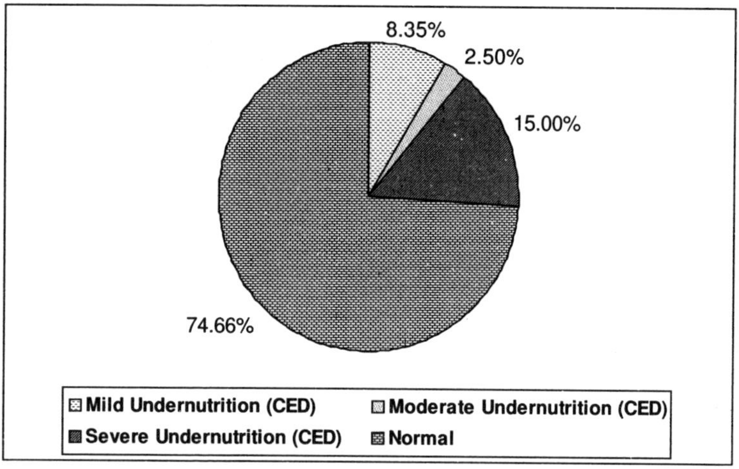

Figure 5.1: Prevelance of different grades of Undernutritional level among the Nyishi tribal women.

The BLR model was fitted to find out the odds for the socio-economic, demographic, lifestyle related variables for being Mild/ Moderate undernutrition (BMI 16.99 to <18.50 kg/m^2) in Nyishi women was depicted in Table 5.4. The results of the BLR analysis further showed significant effects to being undernourished was associated with having 3 and more dependent children (Odds: 0.46), using non-sanitary toilet facility (Odds: 3.52) ($p<0.05$) and found highly associated with the education of the head who studies till class 10th (Odds: 0.01), monthly income is less (Rs. 2000-5000) (Odds: 8.90) and the women consumes alcohol (Odds: 2.87), chew tobacco (Odds: 4.89) and do smoke (Odds: 0.28) ($p<0.01$). On the other hand, the occupation of women like housewife and service, occupation of the head, house type and used water source were not found any significant association with the prevalence of undernutrition among Nyishi women.

The BLR model was fitted to find out the odds for the socio-economic, demographic, lifestyle related variables for being Severe undernutrition (CED; BMI<16.00 kg/m^2) in Nyishi women was

Table 5.3: Binary logistic regression (BLR) analysis and association of socio-economic, demographic and lifestyle determinants of undernutrition (BMI <18.50 kg/m^2) among the Nyishi women

Variables	*Category*	*Wald*	*Odds*	*95%CI*	*p-value*
Education of the Head	Illiterate	51.132	31.114	12.127-79.831	0.000**
	Class 1-5th	75.371	14.286	7.837-26.039	0.000**
	Class 10th	27.323	6.513	3.226-13.151	0.000**
	>12th ®	1			
Education of Mother	Illiterate	0.162	1.219	0.465-3.195	0.687
	Class 1-5th	1.363	0.543	0.195-1.513	0.243
	Class 10th	28.677	0.010	0.002-0.055	0.000**
	>12th ®	1			
Occupation of Head	Daily wage	0.000	5.186	0.000	0.997
	Cultivation	33.860	35.548	49.163-2.570	0.000**
	Service	1			
Occupation of Mother	House Wife	0.000	8.508	0.000	0.990
	Service	1			
Monthly income of family	1000-1999	0.000	0.000	0.000	0.998
	2000-5000	11.891	10.763	7.022-16.496	0.000**
	5000< ®	1			
Dependent children	1-2 child ®	1			
	3< child	5.946	0.620	0.422-0.910	0.015*
House type	Bricked House	0.865	2.633	0.342-20.250	0.352
	Non-bricked house	6.739	14.615	1.929-110.718	0.009*
	Semi-bricked House®	1			
Toilet facility	Non-sanitary	26.967	3.839	2.310-6.378	0.000**
	Sanitary ®	1			
Water source	River	6.237	0.427	0.219-0.833	0.013*
	Supply	9.077	0.393	0.214-0.721	0.003*
	Well	1			
Alcohol consumption	No ®	1			
	Yes	6.431	4.235	4.235-9.765	0.000**
Tobacco chew	No ®	1			
	Yes	14.560	14.665	9.481-22.683	0.000**
Smoking habit	No ®	1			
	Yes	31.538	0.320	0.215-0.477	0.000**

® Reference category.
* $p < 0.05$; ** $p < 0.01$

Table 5.4: Binary logistic regression (BLR) analysis and socio-economic, demographic and lifestyle determinants of mild and moderate (BMI 16.99 to <18.50 kg/m^2) undernutrition among the Nyishi women

Variables	*Category*	*Wald*	*Odds*	*95%CI*	*p-value*
Education of the Head	Illiterate	0.094	0.834	0.262-2.653	0.759
	Class 1-5th	0.262	0.726	0.213-2.477	0.609
	Class 10th	1.151	0.014	0.002-0.138	0.000**
	>12th ®	1			
Education of Mother	Illiterate	0.094	0.834	0.262-2.653	0.75
	Class 1-5th	0.262	0.726	0.213-2.477	0.609
	Class 10th	13.564	0.014	0.002-0.138	0.000**
	>12th ®	1			
Occupation of Head	Daily wage	0.000	1.000	0.000	1.000
	Cultivation	0.000	5.874	0.000	0.993
	Service	1			
Occupation of Mother	House Wife	0.000	2.167	0.000	0.998
	Service	1			
Monthly Income of family	1000-1999	0.000	0.000	0.000	0.998
	2000-5000	48.221	8.909	4.805-16.516	0.000**
	5000< ®	1			
Dependent children	1-2 child ®	1			
	3< child	6.787	0.465	0.262-0.827	0.009*
House type	Bricked House	0.013	1.125	0.142-8.915	0.911
	Non-bricked house	1.914	4.204	0.550-32.137	0.166
	Semi-bricked House ®	1			
Toilet facility	Non-sanitary	10.546	3.522	1.647-7.530	0.001*
	Sanitary ®	1			
Water source	River	1.197	2.333	0.511-10.646	0.274
	Supply	2.957	3.552	0.838-15.066	0.086
	Well	1			
Alcohol consumption	No ®	1			
	Yes	14.889	2.875	1.681-4.916	0.000**
Tobacco chew	No ®	1			
	Yes	34.128	4.893	2.872-8.336	0.000**
Smoking habit	No ®	1			
	Yes	17.122	0.283	0.156-0.515	0.000**

® Reference category.
* $p < 0.05$; ** $p < 0.01$

depicted in Table 5.5. The results of the BLR analysis further showed significant effects to being undernourished was associated with using the water source by river (Odds: 0.29) and having a smoking habit (Odds: 0.45) ($p<0.05$) and found highly associated with the education of the head who were illiterate (Odds: 18.69), studies till class 5 (Odds: 6.04), occupation of head doing cultivation (Odds: 11.20), monthly income is less (Rs. 2000-5000) (Odds: 5.87), using a non-sanitary toilet facility (Odds: 12.43), using the water source supply water from river (Odds: 0.18) and the women consume alcohol (Odds: 8.07) and chew tobacco (Odds: 14.58) ($p<0.01$). On the other hand, the occupation of women like housewife and service, dependent children and house types were not found any significant association with the prevalence of undernutrition among Nyishi women.

Discussion

The prevalence of undernutrition (i.e., CED) is considered to be a serious public health problem among the adult population of North-east India. Present study was also showing a greater proportion of undernutrition or CED (i.e., 26.33%) prevalence in Nyishi women of Arunachal Predesh, North-east India. Khongsider, (2001) using the data from 12 populations of 18-60 years of North-east India reported that the prevalence of CED was found to be significantly lower in the tribal (19.00%) than in the Hinduized (49.00%) and caste (52.00%) populations. The prevalence of CED was found to be 21.43% among Dibongiya Deoris of Assam (Gogoi and Sengupta, 2002). When the population-specific comparison of prevalence of undernutrition (e.g. CED) was taken into consideration, the data showed a significantly ($p<0.01$) lower prevalence was observed than the other Indian tribal populations (47.40%) (Kshatriya *et al.*, 2016), Dhimal (47.20) (Banik *et al.*, 2007), Indian women (45.00%) (Griffiths and Bentley, 2001), Oraon tribe (62.50%) (Dutta Banik, 2011), Sarak women (46.36%) (Table 5.6). The prevalence of CED was reported to be higher in the Hinduized Mongoloid groups like Ahom (52.00%), Koch (50.00%) and Rajbanshi (42.00%) (Khongsider, 2002). Therefore, appropriate nutritional intervention programmes are necessary to improve the actual magnitude of undernutrition in the target population.

Table 5.5: Binary logistic regression (BLR) analysis and association of socio-economic, demographic and lifestyle determinants of severe (CED; BMI<16.00 kg/m^2) undernutrition among the Nyishi women

Variables	*Category*	*Wald*	*Odds*	*95%CI*	*p-value*
Education of the Head	Illiterate	38.294	18.69	7.394-47259	0.000**
	Class 1-5th	30.667	6.04	3.197-11.426	0.000**
	Class 10th	2.209	1.95	0.808-4.739	0.137
	>12th ®				
Education of Mother	Illiterate	0.496	1.509	0.480-4.742	0.481
	Class 1-5th	0.989	0.529	0.151-1.856	0.320
	Class 10th	13.564	0.014	0.002-0.138	0.000**
	>12th ®	1			
Occupation of Head	Daily wage	0.000	5.186	0.000	0.997
	Cultivation	21.760	11.20	15.432-814.284	0.000**
	Service	1			
Occupation of Mother	House Wife	0.000	2.998	0.000	0.998
	Service				
Monthly Income of family	1000-1999	0.000	0.000	0.000	0.000
	2000-5000	49.076	5.874	3.579-9.639	0.000**
	5000< ®	1			
Dependent children	1-2 child ®	1			
	3< child	0.442	0.854	0.537-1.359	0.506
House type	Bricked House	0.000	1.138	0.000	0.998
	Non-bricked house	0.000	5.490	0.000	0.998
	Semi-bricked House®	1			
Toilet facility	Non-sanitary	0.000	12.436	1.662-5.921	0.000**
	Sanitary ®	1			
Water source	River	11.579	0.292	0.144-0.594	0.001*
	Supply	26.505	0.181	0.095-0.347	0.000**
	Well	1			
Alcohol consumption	No ®	1			
	Yes	49.420	8.077	4.511-14.461	0.000**
Tobacco chew	No ®	1			
	Yes	85.831	14.585	8.273-25.713	0.000**
Smoking habit	No ®	1			
	Yes	10.173	0.459	0.284-0.741	0.001*

® Reference category.
* $p < 0.05$; ** $p < 0.01$

The association of socio-economic variables with undernutrition (Mild/Moderate and Severe) was earlier reported by various studies (Subramanium and Smith, 2006; Subramanium *et al.*, 2007; Pal *et al.*, 2017). Similarly, the results of the present investigation explained that the women belong to lower educational status (Class 10th), lower education of the head of the family (Illiterate, Class 1-5th, Class 10th), lower monthly income (Rs.2000-5000), lower occupation of the head of the family (cultivation) and non-sanitary toilets were significantly exhibited 0.01, 31.11, 14.28, 6.51, 35.54, 10.76 times and 3.89 times higher odds ($p<0.05$, $p<0.01$) to being undernutrition or CED (Mild/ Moderate and Severe), respectively (Tables 5.3, 5.4 and 5.5). Some similar studies also reported on this issue (Subramanium and Smith, 2006; Subramanian *et al.*, 2007; Sen *et al.*, 2013; Islam *et al.*, 2016; Pal *et al.*, 2017; Ravaoarisoa *et al.*, 2018). The more consumption of alcohol, tabbacco chew and habits of smoking can lead to have higher (Odds: 4.25, 14.66, 0.32) undernutrition status (Tables 5.3, 5.4 and 5.5). It was also observed that by a study smoking is linked with a poorer BMI and termination of smoking may increase adiposity and waist circumference among populations (Koster *et al.*, 2008, Rengma *et al.*, 2015).

Conclusion

The prevalence of undernutrition or CED (Mild, Moderate and Severe) within a population is considered a risk factor for various ill-health conditions, abnormalities, deficiencies and communicable diseases. Furthermore, lower socio-economic condition, lack of proper nutritional intake and consumption of various qualities of harmful products (e.g. alcohol, tobacco, smoking), poor quality of living condition may increase the prevalence of undernutrition or CED. There arises a need to address the challenges of establishing measures that would reduce the future ill-effects of undernutrition related morbidity. The results of the present study suggested that education, occupation and lower income have significantly contributed immense effects on different grades of undernutrition or CED (CED: Mild-Grade I, Moderate-Grade II and Severe-Grade III) prevalence in Nyishi women. Suitable health care strategies and intervention programmes are needed for combating such prevalence in

Table 5.6: Comparison of undernutrition or CED prevalence among studies done in Indian women and the present study

Population	*Area*	*Sample*	*Age (years)*	*Undernutrition Prevalence (%)*	*Source*
Indian Women	Andhra Pradesh	4032	15-49	45.00	Griffiths and Bentley, 2001
Tangkhul Naga	Manipur	346	20-70	16.20	Mungreipy and Kapoor, 2010
Indian	26 Indian states	81712	15-49	31.20	Bharati et al., 2007
Punjabi Women	Jalandhar, Punjab	65	17-80	18.50	Singh and Kirchengast, 2011
Indian Women	India	77220	15-49	32.10	Subramanium and Smith, 2006
Orang Women	Jharkhand	216	39-60	62.50	Dutta Banik, 2011
Sarak Women	Jharkhand	110	39-60	46.36	Dutta Banik, 2011
Indian Tribes	India	1090	20-60	47.40	Kshatriya *et al.,* 2016
Dhimal	West Bengal	146	≥18	46.20	Banik et al., 2007
Kora-Mudi	West Bengal	250	18-65	56.40	Bose et al., 2006
Savar	Orissa	300	≥18	49.00	Bose et al., 2006
Rural Women	Assam	285	≥18	48.00	Mahanta et al., 2012
Bathudi	Orissa	183	≥18	64.50	Bose and Chakraborty, 2005
Nyshi Women	Arunachal Pradesh	543	15-49	10.50	Bharali et al., 2017
Nyishi Tribal Women	**Papum-pere, Arunachal Pradesh**	**600**	**15-44**	**26.33**	**Present Study**

population. Finally, the results are important for effective implementation of any public health programme and appropriate intervention strategies to reduce the prevalence and associated risks of Undernutrition or CED.

REFERENCES

Banik, S.D., Bose, K., Bisai, S., Bhattacharya, M., Das, S., Jana, A., Purkait, P. 2007. "Undernutrition among adult Dhimals of Naxalbari, West Bengal: comparison with other tribes of eastern India." *Food Nutr Bull*, **28**: 348-352.

Bharali, N., Mondal, N., Singh, K.N. 2017. "Prevalence of Undernutrition, Overweight and Obesity among Nyishi tribal Women of Arunachal Pradesh, Northeast India." *Hum Biol Rev*, **6**:63-78.

Bose, K., Bisai, S., Das, P., Dikshit, S., Pradhan, S. 2007. "Interrelationships of income, chronic energy deficiency, morbidity and hospitalization among adult male slum dwellers of Midnapore, West Bengal, India." *J Biosoc Sci*, **39**: 779-786.

Bose, K., Chakraborty, F., Mitra, K., Bisai, S. 2006. "Nutritional status of adult Santal men in Keonjhar District, Orissa, India." *Food Nutr Bull*, **27**: 353-356.

Datta Banik, S. 2011. "Nutritional status adiposity and body composition of Oraon and Sarak females in Ranchi District, India—a comparison." *Ecol Food Nutr*, **50**: 43-62.

Dudeja, V., Misra, A., Pandey, R.M., Devina, G., Kumar, G., Vikram, N.K. 2001. "BMI does not accurately predict overweight in Asian Indians in northern India." *Br J Nutr*, **86**: 105-112.

Gogoi, G., Sengupta, S. 2002. "Body Mass Index among the Dibongiya Deoris of Assam, India." *J Hum Ecol*, **13**: 271-273.

Griffiths, P.L., Bentley, M.E. 2001. "The nutrition transition is underway in India." *Nutr*, **131**: 2692-2700.

Hall, J.G., Allanson, J.E., Gripp, K.W., Slavotinek, A.M. 2007. *Handbook of Physical Measurements.* Oxford, UK: Oxford University Press.

Islam, A., Islam, N., Bharati, P., Aik, S., Hossain, G. 2016. "Socio-economic and demographic factors influencing nutritional status among early childbearing young mothers in Bangladesh." *BMC Women's Health*, **16**.

Jose, S. 2014. "Adult Undernutrition in India—Poverty or Ethnicity?" *Economic and Political Weekly*. **49**: 72-74.

Khongsdier R. 2002. "Body mass index and morbidity in adult males of the War Khasi in North-east India." *Eur J Clin Nutr*, **56**: 484-489.

Khongsdier R. 2001. "Body mass index of adult males in 12 populations of north-east India." *Ann Hum Biol*, **28**: 374-383.

Khongsdier R. 2005. "BMI and morbidity in relation to body composition: a cross-sectional study of a rural community in North-East India." *Br J Nutr*, **93**: 101-107.

Koster, A., Leitzmann, M.F., Schatzkin, A., Adams, K.F., Jacques, Th.M. van Eijk, Hollenbeck, A.R., Harris, T.B. 2008. "The combined relations of adiposity and smoking on mortality." *Am J Clin Nutr,* **88**: 1206-1212.

Kshatriya, G.K., Acharya, S.K. 2016. "Gender Disparities in the Prevalence of Undernutrition and the Higher Risk among the Young Women of Indian Tribes." PLoS One **11**:e0158308.

Kumar, N., Shekhar, C., Kumar, P., Kundu, A.S. 2007. "Kuppuswamy's socio-economic status scale-updating for 2007." *Indian J Pediatr,* **74**: 1131-1132.

Lim, S.S., Vos, T., Flaxman, A.D., *et al.* 2012. "A comparative risk assessment of burden of disease and injury attributable to 67 risk factors and risk factor clusters in 21 regions, 1990-2010: a systematic analysis for the Global Burden of Disease Study 2010". *Lancet.* **380**: 2224–60.

Mahanta, L.B., Roy, T.D., Dutta, R.G., Devi, A. 2012. "Nutritional status and the impact of socio-economic factors on pregnant women in Kamrup district of Assam." *Ecol Food Nutr,* **51**: 463-480.

Mungreiphy, N.K., Kapoor, S. 2010. "Socio-economic changes as covariates of overweight and obesity among Tangkhul Naga tribal women of Manipur, north-east India." *J Biosoc Sci,* **42**: 289-305.

Murray C. 2012. "Disability-adjusted life years (DALYs) for 291 diseases and injuries in 21 regions, 1990–2010: a systematic analysis for the Global Burden of Disease Study 2010." *Lancet,* **380**: 2197–223.

Pal, A., Pari, A.K., Sinha, A., Dhara, P.C. 2017. "Prevalence of undernutrition and associated factors: "A cross-sectional study among rural adolescents in West Bengal, India." *Int J Pediatr Adolescent Med,* **4**:9e18.

Ravaoarisoa, L., Randriamanantsaina, L., Rakotonirina, J., Rakotomanga, J.D.M., Donnen, P., Dramaix, M.W. 2018. "Socio-economic determinants of malnutrition among mothers in the Amoron'I Mania region of Madagascar: a cross-sectional study." *BMC Nutr,* **4**: 6.

Rengma, M.S., Sen, J., Mondal, N. 2015. "Socio-Economic, Demographic and Lifestyle Determinants of Overweight and Obesity among Adults of Northeast India." *Ethiop J Health Sci,* **25**: 199-208.

Ronnie A. Rosenthal, Michael E. Zenilman, Mark R. Katlic. 2011. *Principles and practice of geriatric surgery* (2nd ed.). Berlin: Springer. p. 78.

Seidell, J.C., Flegal, K.M. 1997. "Assessing obesity: classification and epidemiology." *Br Med Bull,* **53**: 238-252.

Sen, J., Mondal, N., Dutta, S. 2013. "Factors affecting overweight and obesity among urban adults: across-sectional study." *Epidemiol Biostat Public Health,* **10**: e8741–1-8.

Shukla, R. 2002. *Solvent Extraction of Metal with Potassium dihydro-bispyrazolyl-borate,* **57**: 633-639.

Subramanian, S.V., Kawachi, I., Smith, G.D. 2007. "Income inequality and the double burden of under- and overnutrition in India." *J Epidemiol Community Health,* **61**: 802-809.

Subramanian, S.V., Smith, G.D. 2006. "Patterns, distribution, and determinants of under- and overnutrition: a population-based study of women in India." *Am J Clin Nutr,* **84**: 633-40.

Tigga, P.L., Debnath, S., Das, M., Mondal, N., Sen, J. 2018. "Prevalence of undernutrition and overweight or obesity among the Bengali Muslim population of West Bengal, India." *Anthropol Open J*, **3**: 1-10.

Touitou, Y., Portaluppi, F., Smolensky, M.H., Rensing, L. 2004. "Ethical principles and standards for the conduct of human and animal biological rhythm research." *Chronobiol Int*, **21**: 61-70.

Ulijaszek, S.J., Kerr, D.A. 1999. "Anthropometric measurement error and the assessment of nutritional status." *Br J Nutr*, **82**: 165-177.

WHO Expert Consultation. 2004. "Appropriate body-mass index for Asian populations and its implications for policy and intervention strategies." *Lancet* **363**: 157-163.

World Health Organization. 1995. Physical status: The use and interpretation of Anthropometry. Report of a WHO expert committee. World Health Organization, Geneva.

SECTION-II

Maternal Health Status, Child Mortality and Human Rights Issues

6

Maternal Health Upgradation
Impact of Knowledge, Attitude and Practice

Debidas Ghosh, Sujata Bhowmick (Ganguly) and *Dibya Pal*

Introduction

Health care is a big, complex industry having a simple definition: get healthy and stay healthy. It is a field where maintenance, improvement or restoration of the mental health as well as physical health is maintained through diagnosis, treatment and prevention. Health care is delivered by health professionals in allied health fields. Socio-economic condition and health policies largely influence the access to health care across the countries, communities and individuals. Geographic barriers like transportation, personal limitations like poor ability to communicate with health care providers, insufficient health literacy also influence the health care. Health care may be primary, secondary, tertiary as well as public health.

Primary level health care (PHC) means primary medical care by health professionals at grassroots level of health services. It forms an integral part of country's health system. PHC encompasses primary care, disease prevention, health promotion, population health, and community development within a holistic framework, with the aim of providing essential community-focused health care (Shoultz and Hatcher, 1997). The five underlying principles are—equitable distribution, community involvement, focuses on prevention, appropriate technology, and multi-sectoral approach (Walt and Vaughan, 1982). This is provided by sub-centre, primary health centre which are collectively known as primary tier of health care services delivery system.

Secondary level health care deals with more complex health problems of the community which are resolved at secondary level care through community health centres and district hospitals. Tertiary level health care is the highest level of health care available to the community for dealing with their most complex health problems, which cannot be solved at the primary and secondary levels. The institutions involved in providing the requisite facilities and cares include Medical College Hospitals, All India Medical Institutes, Regional Hospitals, Specialized Health Centres etc.

Current National Scenario of Maternal Health

WHO commends India for its groundbreaking progress in recent years in reducing the maternal mortality ratio (MMR) by 77 per cent, from 556 per 1,00,000 live births in 1990 to 130 per 1,00,000 live births in 2016. Sample registration system (SRS) studies showed that MMR (Maternal Mortality Rate) is declined up to 26.9 per cent. Assam has pointed as the highest MMR (229/ per lakh births) while Kerala pointed as lowest one (42/per lakh births). Last year WHO proclaimed India's progress in reducing the rate of MMR to achieve sustainable development goal (SDG) in 2030 (WHO, 2018). In India, haemorrhage (25.6%) ranked first as the cause of maternal death followed by sepsis (13%), toxemia (11.9%), abortion (8%), obstructed labour (6.2%) and other (35.3%).

1. Maternal Mortality and Morbidity

1.1. Maternal mortality: The death of a woman while pregnant or within 42 days of the termination of pregnancy, irrespective of the duration and site of pregnancy, from any cause related to or aggravated by the pregnancy or its management but not from accidental or incidental causes is known as maternal mortality.

1.2. Late maternal mortality: A maternal death resulting from direct or indirect obstetric causes more than 42 days but less than one year after termination of pregnancy.

1.3. Pregnancy-related mortality: A maternal death occurring during pregnancy or within 42 days of termination of pregnancy, irrespective of cause.

1.4. Maternal mortality ratio (MMR or MMRatio): The number of maternal deaths per 1,00,000 live births in a given time period. The MMR expresses obstetric risk, or a woman's chances of dying from a given pregnancy. This is the most commonly used indicator of maternal health.

$$\text{MMR} = \frac{\text{Number of maternal deaths}}{\text{Per 1,00,000 live births in a given time period}}$$

1.5. Maternal mortality rate: The number of maternal deaths per 1,000 women of reproductive age (usually 15-49 years).This is an indicator of the risk of maternal death among women of reproductive age and provides an indication of the burden of maternal deaths in the adult female population.

$$\text{MMR} = \frac{\text{Number of maternal deaths}}{\text{Per 1000 women of reproducti ve age (15 - 49 years)}}$$

1.6. Lifetime risk of maternal mortality: The annual maternal mortality rate multiplied by the length of the reproductive period (usually 35 years). This measure reflects the cumulative risk of becoming pregnant and dying as a result of pregnancy in a woman's lifetime.

1.7. Reproductive morbidity: Illness that includes conditions of physical ill-health related to the concepts of "successful childbearing" and of "freedom from gynaecological disease and risk". According to this definition, reproductive morbidities can be classified as follows:

(i) *Obstetric morbidity*: Maternal illness during pregnancy, delivery, and the postpartum period.

(ii) *Gynaecological morbidity*: Illness of the female reproductive tract not associated with a particular pregnancy, such as reproductive tract infections, cervical cell changes, prolapse, and infertility.

2. Risk of Maternal Health

A large proportion of women die due to mainly pregnancy related anaemia including postpartum haemorrhage, unsafe abortion, pregnancy induced hypertension, obstructed labour and sepsis (Vora *et al.*, 2009). In fact, an estimated 5,85,000 women die each year, 20 million women develop chronic illness as a result of pregnancy related complications. Out of these maternal deaths, an estimated 94 per cent takes place in low and lower middle-income countries. Young adolescents (ages 10-14) face a higher risk of complications and death as a result of pregnancy than other women (WHO, 2019).

(a) Pregnancy related anaemia: Anaemia is most commonly encountered medical disorders during pregnancy where iron deficiency anaemia is more predominant. Preterm deliveries, intrauterine growth retardation, intrauterine death increases due to anaemia (Maka *et al.*, 2017). In India, more than 50 per cent women in rural and more than 45 per cent in urban areas are anaemic (**NFHS-4**). Early diagnosis and treatment can improve both maternal and neonatal outcome. Anaemia is defined as a reduction in either the percentage of red blood cells (hematocrit), or a reduction in the concentration of haemoglobin in a sample of venous blood when compared with reference values. The normal value of haemoglobin in women is 11 gm/dl. In case of pregnant women, ICMR categorizes different level of anaemia as follows:

Category	*Hb level (gm/dl)*
Non-anaemia	11 or higher
Mild anaemia	10-10.9
Moderate anaemia	7-10
Severe anaemia	<7

Source: Indian Council of Medical Research Criteria (ICMR).

(b) Pregnancy induced hypertension: Pregnancy induced hypertension (PIH) is hypertension that occurs after 20 weeks of gestation in women with previously normal blood pressure, when the **systolic** blood pressure is ≥140 mmHg or diastolic blood pressure is ≥90 mmHg or both. The broad classification of pregnancy induced hypertension during pregnancy is gestational hypertension, pre-eclampsia and eclampsia. Severe pre-eclampsia in pregnancy is a systolic blood pressure ≥160 mmHg or diastolic blood pressure ≥110 mmHg or both. Eclampsia is a severe type of pregnancy induced hypertension, and it happens in about one in 1,600 pregnancies and develops near the end of pregnancy (Tesfaye and Tilahun, 2019).

(c) Puerperal sepsis: It is an infective condition in the mother following childbirth. It is the third most common cause of maternal death worldwide as a result of childbirth after haemorrhage and abortion. According to World Health Organization (WHO), puerperal sepsis accounts for 15 per cent of the 5,00,000 maternal deaths annually. In low and middle income countries puerperal infections are the sixth leading cause of disease burden in women during their reproductive years. The debilitating sequelae of this untreated pregnancy complications can be both short term and long term. Puerperal sepsis was defined as infection of the genital tract occurring at any time between the onset of rupture of membranes or labour, and the 42nd day postpartum in which two or more of the following are present:

(i) Fever (oral temperature 38.5°C/101.3°F or higher on any occasion).
(ii) Pelvic pain.
(iii) Abnormal vaginal discharge, e.g. presence of pus.
(iv) Abnormal smell/foul odour of discharge.
(v) Delay in the rate of reduction of the size of the uterus (involution) (Shamshad *et al.*, 2010).

(d) Pregnancy linked undernutrition: Maternal undernutrition in the low and middle-income countries is an underliying cause for a 3.5 million mother's deaths and disabilities due to physical and mental effects of poor dietary intake in the earliest months of life. Undernourished pregnant women suffer from a combination of chronic energy deficiency that leads them to have a low birth weight (LBW), preterm and unsuccessful birth outcomes (Dadi *et al.*, 2019). So, the nutritional statuses of the mother at conception affect growth and development of foetus. Any stimulus or insult during embryonic development would have a permanent effect on the structure and physiology of the human body.

So, nutrient reduction, deprivation or imbalance could result poor pregnancy outcomes like obstructed labour, premature or low-birth-weight babies and postpartum haemorrhage. Evidence also shows that nutrient imbalance before implantation may result in endocrine and metabolic dysfunctions in post-natal life. In addition, the maternal malnutrition could exert a suppressive effect on the maternal and foetal immune response. It could also affect both the proliferation of myogenic precursors reducing the number of muscle fibers and the future reproductive maturation with possible consequent impaired fertility and quality of gametes (Castrogiovanni *et al.*, 2017).

3. Maternal Health Care

According to Alma Ata declaration, maternal health is an important part of primary health care. Women's health during prepartum and postpartum period are more crucial to stay healthy in later part of life and have better birth outcomes, influencing infancy, childhood as well as adulthood. Not only is that, for the development of healthy future, maternal health care is one of the important pillars in this concern. Therefore, the health and well-being of women matter to every person, society and country and are essential for the achievement of the Sustainable Development Goals (SDGs). Nutrition and health service delivery are the two most important determinants of maternal health (WHO, 2017).

3.1. Essential maternal health care coverage

(a) Antenatal care (ANC) which is also known as prenatal care. It is a type of preventive routine health care. Its goal is to provide regular check-ups that allow doctors or midwives to treat and prevent potential health problems throughout the course of the pregnancy and to promote healthy lifestyles that benefit both mother and child.

The components of ANC include:

(i) Risk identification;
(ii) Prevention and management of pregnancy-related or concurrent diseases; and
(iii) Health education and health promotion (WHO, 2002).

(b) Post-natal care (PNC) is the care given to the mother and her newborn baby immediately after the birth and for the first six weeks of life. First 42 days after delivery is vulnerable for both the mother and newborn. The main purpose of providing optimal post-natal care is to avert both maternal and neonatal death, as well as long-term complications (WHO, 2002).

Now, in addition to post-natal care with two full assessments on the first day, three additional visits are recommended: day 3 (48–72 hours), between days 7– 14 and 6 weeks after birth. Actions are necessary across sectors and settings to eliminate avoidable maternal and perinatal mortality and morbidity.

Before pregnancy, the overall health and lifestyle choices of parents can affect fertility, maternal health and their infants' probability of developing chronic conditions later in life. People contemplating pregnancy should be screened for health problems, which need to be identified and managed.

During pregnancy, high-quality antenatal care is essential to ensure not only a healthy pregnancy for mother and baby but also an effective transition to positive labour and childbirth. Services should include the provision of education and basic information on health care for expectant parents.

During delivery, high-quality, evidence-based obstetric and neonatal care are one of the highest priorities to reduce illness and death in mothers and their newborn babies.

- In the postpartum period, it is critical to monitor maternal and newborn health as the risk of death is higher during the first week postpartum for both. Timely detection and management of symptoms reduce the risk of mortality and complications.

4. Relationship among Knowledge-Attitude-Practice (KAP)

Knowledge, attitude and practice are important pillars for health development. Links among knowledge, attitude and practices have been derived internationally in relation to health issues. Good level of knowledge helps to generate positive/innovative attitude. Again positive or innovative attitude provoke a person to be in good practice. While an individual is benefited by good practice, his or her desire towards healthy lifestyle is increased which again helps or encourages to gain new knowledge in other field of life. So it is a cyclic process (Fig. 6.1).

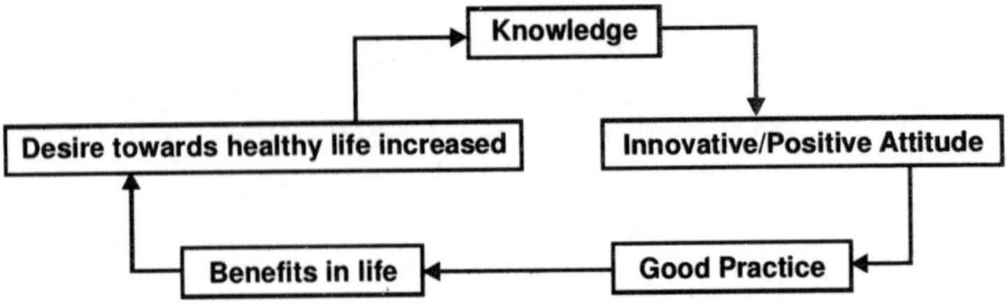

Fig. 6.1: Vicious cycle among knowledge, attitude and practice.

Importance of KAP for Betterment of Maternal Health

Maternal and child health are important indicators for describing mortality conditions, health progress and the overall social and economic well-being of a country. Pregnancy is a natural process and every woman have the right to access to appropriate health care services that will enable her to plan and go safely through pregnancy and childbirth. Pregnancy and childbirth related complications are the leading causes of maternal mortality. The health of women is a crucial factor for the health of children. The maternal and neonatal deaths can be appropriately addressed with antenatal, intranatal and post-natal care. A sound knowledge, correct attitude and proper practice of antenatal, intranatal and post-natal care and early detection of danger signs and seeking medical help from appropriate centres could lower the mortality and morbidity (Shirin, 2011). Despite international and government efforts to increase the provision of a basic package of essential maternal health services, the majority of women in developing countries are still not able to access these potentially life-saving services. In poor countries, shortages of skilled health workers and equipped facilities, and the often-unequal distribution of existing health resources, create barriers to care for large segments of the population. Women's use of care tends to be further restricted by educational, social, cultural, and financial factors. Low level of awareness among mothers can lead to unsuccessful results in terms of care giving due to deep-rooted cultural and traditional beliefs as well as ignorance among caregivers. Therefore, to increase the practices, improving overall knowledge status of mothers covering proper health education to them regarding care of newborn and discouraging the unhealthy traditional beliefs are very important. Implementation of the guidelines outlined in the Maternal and Child Health Handbook is highly recommended in this regard. Measures should be taken to provide mother targeted education consists of nutritional education, personal hygiene, childrearing and immunization of newborn at birth. To deal with that, parents of the children as well as grandparents or other caretakers need to be included in any training sessions or education process (Majumder *et al.*, 2018).

4.1. *Knowledge*

Knowledge defines familiarity, awareness, or realization of specific domain (such as facts, information, descriptions, or skills) obtained through experience or education. Characteristics of knowledge are:

(i) Knowledge can change the attitude.
(ii) Mentioned both theoretical and practical understanding of a subject.
(iii) Can be implicit (as with practical skill or expertise) or explicit (as with the theoretical understanding).
(iv) Can be more or less formal or systematic.
(v) Involves complex cognitive processes: perception, communication, and reasoning.

(a) Nutritional Knowledge for Maternal Health

The word "Nutrition" is often paired with the word "Food" as these two go together. Nutrition is science of food, the nutrient and other substances their in, their action, interaction and balance in relationship to health and diseases. The process by which the organism ingests, digests, absorbs, transport and utilizes nutrient and disposes of their end products refer as nutrition. Not only that, nutrition is also related with social, economic, cultural and physiological involvement of food and eating.

So, nutrition is a broad and very essential spectrum in everyday life. It helps us to know:

1. About health and how good health is maintained.
2. About the nutrients—macronutrients as well as micronutrients with their functions and sources.

3. Different pathological states of undernutrition, overnutrition, imbalance, specific deficiencies, extreme deficiency/excess of essential nutrients.
4. Nutritional requirements for special physiological condition—such as pregnancy, lactation, sick individual, pre-operative and post-operative conditions.
5. Proper idea for meal planning considering the different food groups, funding news, economic status, time and energy, individuals' likes and dislikes variety, satiety, religion, tradition and customs.
6. The idea regarding the role of microorganism (moulds, yeasts and bacteria) in food spoilage, their effect on body (both detrimental and beneficial) as well as the way to preserve food.

Mothers play a key role for maintaining the health in family. Mother's limited knowledge about food choice, feeding and health care seeking practices contributing significantly to negative nutrition outcomes for children in most developing countries. Independent and positive associations are found with mother's knowledge and nutritional status (stunting, wasting) of children. Research evidence showing that nutrition education has significantly impact on dietary habit of pregnant women and on maternal and birth outcome of pregnancy. WHO recommended that health care provided need to give adequate, specific and acceptable nutrition related advice to pregnant women during every visit of antenatal care (ANC) (Zelalem *et al.*, 2017). School education (informal) is suggested by many researchers to incorporate the information on nutrition which is more practical (Fadare *et al.*, 2019). It has been seen that poor nutritional knowledge leads to high rate of malnutrition both in mother and children. A well resourced, targeted and coordinated nutrition education can improve maternal nutritional knowledge, health care seeking behaviours and practices significantly. Nutrition education have been promoting proper child care practices and management of childhood illnesses such as diarrhoea, health and nutrition messages are usually targeted to mothers specially whom have not received formal education. These types of women are usually patronize health services at primary health care centres. So, effective utilization of nutritional knowledge will help to gain health and nutrition education which is, therefore, expected to improve the health and nutritional status of mother as well as children through selection of healthy food habit, participation in maternal and child health care programmes. Thus, attention should be given to promote nutrition education for every woman.

(b) Reproductive Knowledge for Maternal Health

Reproductive knowledge is a crucial factor for the maintenance of maternal health as near about 2.5 million deaths are reported every year globally that may be due to the lack of knowledge among the mothers. Knowledge regarding menstrual hygiene, conception, appropriate age of marriage as well as the childrearing age, contraception, sexually transmitted diseases, considering the same. In India, sex education is not offered in school. Generally, adolescent gets the information about their reproductive health from peer group or mother but not all the information is accurate enough as some of them are biased with local taboos. So, proper knowledge about reproductive health is necessary for a safe motherhood.

Importance of reproductive knowledge:

- (i) Reproductive knowledge among mothers helps to protect them from unwanted pregnancies and unsafe abortion.
- (ii) Serious complications such as ectopic pregnancy, pelvic inflammatory disease, miscarriage, congenital infection, preterm labour, come from STIs/RTIs. These serious complications may lead to some severe chronic conditions such as infertility, genital cancer and death. To reduce the jaws of death from RTIs/STIs, reproductive knowledge is very much essential among them.

(c) Hygiene and Sanitation Knowledge for Maternal Health

Hygiene refers to condition and practice that helps to maintain health and prevent the spreading of disease. Whereas sanitation refers to the provision of safe drinking water and adequate sewage disposal. Both sanitation and hygiene are related and effective tools for maternal health. More broadly sanitation also included the safe management of solid waste and animal waste. Inadequate sanitation is a major cause of infectious diseases such as cholera, typhoid and dysentery world-wide. Maternal health is highly related to WASH (water, sanitation and hygiene) condition and practice. Its help to maintain better health of the mother and prevent infection from harmful microorganisms. Sanitation and hygiene reduce maternal and new born morbidity and mortality rate. There is a close relationship among sanitation, hygiene and maternal health. Poor sanitation and unhygienic condition may influence the risk of infection such as sepsis, diarrhoea, tetanus, pneumonia which increases the chances of maternal and neonatal death rate. During pregnancy, childbirth, and postpartum period, maternal health is very sensitive to disease and infection.

Importance

(i) *Ascaris lumbricoides and hook worm infection* are the major causes of anaemia in mothers due to poor sanitation which may lead to listeria. In that case, the chances of infection in pregnant women increase more than 17 times and ultimately cause of spontaneous abortion and preterm birth.

(ii) Drinking water which is a vital thing in our day-to-day life. If it is unsafe or polluted with high amount of arsenic or fluoride, it may cause still birth and increases the rate of spontaneous abortion.

Determinants of Hygiene and Sanitation

(i) *Low socio-economic status:* Maintenance of hygienic condition among low socio-economic group is a bigger challenge due to their financial condition. As they give more importance to secure the daily food of their family rather than hygiene and sanitation.

(ii) *Education:* Education can change the behaviour of the people towards a standard and healthy lifestyle by using proper hygienic and sanitary conditions and practices (Akpakli *et al.*, 2018).

4.1.1. Source of knowledge for maternal health upgradation

There are different sources for information regarding health especially maternal health. But education is the main thing that encourages us to distinguish between right and wrong. So, education is the passage to progress in any field.

(a) **Formal education**: A process of acquiring knowledge through study or imparting the knowledge by way of instructions or some other practical procedure usually takes place in the premises of educational institutions like schools or colleges. Here planned education of different subjects having proper syllabus are acquired by attending the institution. It is hierarchically structured and having chronological grading system.
Thus, education improves health, while health improves learning potential. Education and health complement enhance and support each other; together, they serve as the foundation for a better world. So, educated women have better health status and higher rate of health care access by taking correct decision on family planning (chances of unwanted and unplanned pregnancies are less) to immunization. Formal education also helps to acquire life skills like problem solving, critical thinking, communication, self-assessment which helps to adopt healthy lifestyle (Luthra, 2007). Women's education level modulated the effects of total fertility rate (TFR), birth order, delivery by skilled attendants, clean water, and sanitary sewer access. In the fully adjusted model, for every additional year of maternal education, there was a corresponding decrease in the MMR (Koch *et al.*, 2012).

(b) **Informal education**: A more natural process of acquiring knowledge outside the educational institutional premises without the involvement of conscious efforts. It is neither pre-planned nor deliberate. Informal education does not require fixed curriculum and timetable rather it consists of experiences and actually living in the family or community. Different sources of informal education are— mass media, periodicals and campaign.

Mass media

The term 'mass' in mass media means that we can reach large number of people at a time through the means of communications and techniques by which specialized groups employ technological devices to disseminate symbolic content to large heterogeneous and widely dispersed audience. Television, radio, audio-visual aids like films and documentaries, newspapers, magazines, booklets, leaflets, exhibitions with models, posters, charts are used as mass media.

Advantages of mass media

(i) Provides quick method to reach huge audience even to illiterate.
(ii) Makes good use of scarce manpower.
(iii) Helps to motivate and teach people.
(iv) Inexpensive in comparison with the cost to reach individual.

Periodicals

Periodical is a primary source of informal information. Primary sources of information are the first published records of original research and development or description of new application or new interpretation of an old theme or idea. These are original documents representing original ideas and constitute the latest available information. Researchers produce new information can make it available to the community through the primary sources. Periodical article is the main medium of communication for the exchange of scientific information. Periodical is a publication in the form of magazines, journals, newspapers and newsletters. These are called periodicals because they are published at periodic intervals, i.e., daily, weekly, fortnightly, monthly, quarterly, or yearly. They are extremely important sources of information (Rao and Reddy, 2018) to the general community where more technical information are expressed in common and understanding level.

Campaign

It is another media to promote public health by making new health interventions available. Public health campaigns involve a broad set of communication strategies and activities that specialists in health promotion engage into disseminate relevant and persuasive health information to groups of people who need such information to lead healthy lives. Typically, these campaigns are designed to raise public consciousness about important health issues by educating specific groups (i.e. target audiences) about imminent health threats and risky behaviours that might harm them. Health campaigns are generally designed to increase awareness of health threats and to move target audiences to take necessary action in favour of public health. These behaviours can include adopting healthy lifestyles that include exercise, nutrition, and stress-reduction; avoiding dangerous substances such as poisons, carcinogens, or other toxic materials; seeking opportunities for early screening and diagnosis for serious health problems; and availing themselves of the best available health care services, which can be adopted easily to minimize harm.

Outreach services

It means the act of reaching out; an effort to build connections from one person or group to another. Community outreach programme empowering health care professionals effectively to improve knowledge and behaviours of women about maternal health in women. Dramatic increase has seen in the institutional delivery all-over world (Bang *et al.*, 2018). Health outreach programmes play a critical role in improving and extending the reach of health care through activities such as health education, case management, basic health screening, and facilitating access to services. These activities can directly and indirectly improve health outcomes of individuals and communities. Outreach programmes can show that they take initiatives to improve health outcomes by using evidence-based measures, or measures that have been shown to indicate health status. Community Health Workers and Popular Educators are two outreach models that are powerful in improving health outcomes. Activities stemming from these models include:

(i) Sharing culturally appropriate health education.
(ii) Providing informal counselling and social support.
(iii) Acting as advocates and connecting people to services.
(iv) Supporting ongoing disease self-management skills.
(v) Facilitating community organizing and community empowerment (this can be done by bringing community members together in order to identify their health issues and to develop plans addressing those issues).

(c) **Non-formal education:** Apart from organization, the knowledge which is gathered from home, nature, own experiences, observation in daily life is called non-formal education. Generally, the purpose of this education is to enhance the skill as well as the aptitude of the people to live in society.

Characteristics

(i) More flexible.
(ii) No time bound.
(iii) No age limit.
(iv) Learner centric.

4.1.2. Strategies for knowledge dissemination to maternal community:

Dissemination of knowledge to maternal community is another important factor. Face-to-face or interpersonal communication among the women involving direct interaction between the source and receiver. In this method voice is the main organ of communication, but the use of other support materials (printed, visual, and audio-visual) are highly recommended. These supportive material reinforce the oral communication between the educator and the target audience. Interpersonal communication is a very effective way of studying maternal health problems and for adapting the necessary messages.

Interpersonal communication are of two kinds, they are:

One-to-one communication: This takes place when the caregivers or mother visits the doctor, health worker or Anganwadi Worker. These functionaries can listen to the mothers problems and help find solution to her problems. The advantages of face-to-face communication over mass media are that it creates opportunities for questions, discussion, participation and feedback.

Group discussions: This involves face-to-face interaction with a group of people. Sometimes, it is desirable to work with groups of people not only to save time and money but also to benefit from group dynamics. Examples of face-to-face group discussion are—lecture, demonstration, meetings, community events etc.

At rural sectors, two strategies are very much fruitful for knowledge dissemination. They are—

Women to women strategy: Educated women or health aware women who have knowledge regarding maternal health issues may transfer or circulate their knowledge to other women who are in dark about health issues. In this strategy Accredited Social Health Activist (ASHA) and Anganwadi Worker are the key women, plays an important role to circulate health related information including family planning to immunization. The advantages of this type of communication are:

(i) Generally women are more sympathetic to other women health issues and try to solve the situation utmost.
(ii) Feel free while discussing.
(iii) Women can easily rely on other women.

Child to women strategy: School going children are getting primary health related knowledge or information from formal education system which is conveyed to parents specially mothers. Thus, women are also enlightened to health issues.

Feedback responses to resources: The key women communicate to the resource person at a regular interval to depict the real health status of a particular region. According to the information, health care services are simplified if needed and packages are modulated based on the regional need. Again the key women deliver the modulated package to the target women for improving health status.

4.2. Attitude

According to Winston Churchill, "attitude is a little thing that makes a big difference". Thurstone said, "An attitude denotes the sum total of man's inclinations and feelings, prejudice or bias, preconceived notions, ideas, fears, threats, and other any specific topic." As a whole attitudes refer the mental setup or viewpoint to accept or reject or indifferent of anything or events or actions.

Characteristics of Attitude:

- (i) Knowledge can change the attitude.
- (ii) Complex combination of personality, beliefs, values, behaviours and motivations.
- (iii) A continuum from very favourable to very unfavourable.
- (iv) Can be explicit (consciously aware) and implicit (unconscious, but have an effect on behaviour).
- (v) Component of attitude—(1) cognitive component, (2) affective component, and (3) behavioural component.

Attitude can be influenced by different factors such as—social factors, family, media, direct instruction, prejudices, educational and religious institutions, personal experience, physical factors, economic status and occupations etc.

4.2.1. Types of Attitude

There are four types of attitude—(a) Innovative attitude, (b) Negative attitude, (c) Indifferent attitude, and (d) Positive attitude.

(a) Innovative attitude: This is an excellent attitude and individuals having such attitude not only follow the positive and healthy guidelines but also influence the other's community members in this concern.

(b) Positive attitude: A state of mind that visualize and expects favourable results, recognize opportunities and made positive thinking. It is essential for the progression of life favourably in all areas. People having positive attitudes accept and handle challenges with confidence as confidence is the basic thing of positive attitudes. So positive attitude brings strength, energy, motivation and initiative.

(c) Negative attitude: A negative attitude is something that every person should avoid. Generally, people with negative attitude ignore the good things in life and only think about whether they will fail. They often find a way out of tough situations by running away from it. They often compare themselves with other persons and find the bad in them only. In short, he is exactly the opposite of the one with a positive mindset. There are certain bad effects that a person with a negative mindset has to face. Anger, doubt, frustration are very common expression of negative attitude.

(d) Indifferent attitude: In this case mindset is neutral. There is neither hope nor doubt. The people generally tend to ignore the problems in life. They wait for some other individuals to take care of their problems. They generally have a lazy life and they are often unemotional. However, indifferent attitude may change to only positive attitude.

4.2.2. Process for changing attitude: from negative to positive

Attitude change occurs anytime. Thus, changes occur when a person goes from being negative to positive, from slightly positive to very positive, or from having no attitude to having one. Because of the functional value of attitudes, the processes that change them have been a major focus throughout the history of social psychology. For better health and quality of life negative to positive or very positive attitude is desirable. Positive attitude can be obtained by positive stimulus. The another ways are—

(i) Experiences sharing of them who are benefited by accessing health care services.
(ii) Increasing the exposure to the mass media either by health awareness presentation or group discussion.
(iii) Individual counselling.
(iv) Explaining the bad/worse/harmful aspects of negative attitude on health care.
(v) Repeated exposure to the fact.

4.3. Practice/Behaviour

Practice defines behaviour under the guidance of attitude. Recurring patterns of human activities mediated by socially shared knowledge objects that are grounded in tradition and shared by a particular professional knowledge community. Colloquially, practice is associated with the terms such as—traditions, rules, norms, habits, mentalities and so on.

4.3.1. Healthy Behaviour

Healthy behaviour is the activity undertaken by individuals for the purpose of maintaining or enhancing their health, preventing health problems, or achieving a positive body image. It is not limited to healthy people trying to stay healthy, but also includes the physically handicapped and persons with chronic diseases who seek to control, minimize, or contain their affliction through positive forms of health behaviour, such as diet, exercise, and avoiding smoking (Cockerham, 2014).

4.3.2. Process for Changing Behaviour: from Unhealthy to Healthy

Habit can not be changed in one day but through a long duration with positive attitude habit can be changed. Like the letter sequence of the word 'Habit' is less lasting. If 'H' is omitted from the word 'a bit' exists, further more omitting 'a' letter from the word 'bit' exists and by omitting the letter 'b' from the word 'it' exists until/ unless the word is demolished completely. Experts who study behaviour change agree that long lasting change is most likely when it is self-motivated and rooted in positive thinking (positive attitude). On the other hand, aroused fear or regret of an individual may affect the person attempting to make change in behaviour. Unhealthy behaviour for maternal health such as improper food intake (not maintaining the basic requirements), irregular hand washing, alcohol intake or smoking, not using contraceptive or family planning methods, preferring home delivery by untrained birth attendant rather institutional delivery, not accepting anti-natal services, using water/fruit juices feeding instead of colostrums and breast milk, avoiding immunization for mother and children, not maintaining personal sanitation and hygiene, not using sanitary toilets etc. All these unhealthy behaviour depend on several factors. By the following key processes healthy behaviour can be achieved:

(i) Deal with real problem.
(ii) Repeated encouragement for accepting healthy habits specially food habit, work habit and hygienic practices.
(iii) Reducing the frequencies of unhealthy habits and incorporating healthy habits gradually.

4.4. Attitude and Behavior for Maternal Health

High maternal mortality and morbidity persist, in large part due to inadequate access to timely and quality health care. Several factors—cultural norms, gender discrimination and lack of a right's based approach which emphasizes human dignity and attention to the needs of women in planning and delivering health services, inadequate knowledge of sign and symptoms of illness and services available, cost of services, lack of transport options and poor quality of care. Attitudes and behaviours of maternal health care influence health seeking and quality of care. Negative attitude and behaviour could undermine the quality of care and the effectiveness of maternal and infant health promotion efforts (WHO, 2014).

It has seen that risk of poor maternal and newborn health outcomes are the effect of reluctance to attend antenatal care and other health services. Attitude towards pregnancy significantly influence health seeking behaviour among women. Women's freedom of movement had a significant influence on their health seeking behavior. Proportion of women having positive attitude towards pregnancy among attendees of ANC is higher than among the non-attendees of ANC (Akhtar *et al.*, 2018; Gopalakrishnan *et al.*, 2019). WHO recommends that all women must have access to high quality care before, during and after childbirth to optimized maternal health. Women's attitude towards ANC is crucial to her ability to access the requisite care. More sensitization is required to change the attitude of pregnant women towards antenatal and intrapartum care (WHO, 2018). Pregnancy and childbirth are holistic experience that is profoundly affected by women's attitude and the care received (Ogu and Alegbeleye, 2018).

Different phases of KAP modification

Enrichment in KAP is performed through following process—

(a) Precontemplation phase:

This is the initial phase when information, message, literature etc. are involved for awareness upgradation. Even formal, informal, non-formal educations are also involved here. So, in this step knowledge upgradation is mainly emphasized.

(a) Contemplation

In this phase, mental conflict starts between existing knowledge and present inputted knowledge. The candidates try to select out of these two on the basis of analysis. This is transitional stage between knowledge and attitude.

(b) Preparation

After analysis an output of the 2nd phase, the candidate accept the better one as prepare own self to follow it. This is initial stage of attitude development.

(c) Action

On the basis of 3rd phase, the action is started where attitude is shifted to practice.

(d) Maintenance

In this phase, the candidate follows up the new action and stabilizes the practice and habit.

(e) Relapse

If there is sliding from the maintenance phase due to lack of seriousness, casual activities, then it would be restarted from preparation or action.

REFERENCES

Akhtar, S., Hussain, M., Majeed, I. and Afzal, M. 2018. "Knowledge attitude and practice regarding antenatal care among pregnant women in rural area of Lahore." *Int J Soc Sc Manage.* **5**:155-162.

Akpakli, D.E., Manyeh, A.K., Akpakli, J.K., Kukula, V., Gyapong, M. 2018. "Determinants of access to improved sanitation facilities in rural districts of southern Ghana: Evidenced from dodowa health and demographic surveillance site." *BMS Res Notes.* **11**: 473-480.

Bang, K.S., Chae, S.M., Lee, I., Yu, J. and Kim, J. 2018. "Effects of a community outreach program for maternal health and family planning in Tigray, Ethiopia." *Asn Nur Res.* **12**:223-230.

Castrogiovanni, P. and Imbesi, R. 2017. "The role of malnutrition during pregnancy and its effects on brain and skeletal muscle, post-natal development." *J. Funct. Morphol. Kinesiol.* **2**:1-10.

Cockerham, W.C. 2014. *Health behavior.* The Wily Blackwel Encyl Health, Illness, Behavior Society.

Dadi, A.F. and Desyibelew, H.D. 2019. "Undernutrition and its associated factors among pregnant mothers in Gondar town, North-west Ethiopia." *Pols One.* **4**:1-11.

Fadare, O., Amare, M., Mavrotas, G. and Akerel, D. 2019. "Mother's nutrition-related knowledge and child nutrition outcomes:empirical evidence from Nigeria." *PLoS One.* **4**:1-17.

Gopalakrishnan, S., Eashwar, V.M.A. and Mithulakshmi, M. 2019. "Health seeking behavior among antenatal and post-natal rural women in Kanchipuram District of Tamil Nadu: A cross-sectional study." *J Family Med Prim Care.* **8**:1035-1042.

ICMR, 1989. "Evaluation of the National Nutritional Anemia Prophylaxis Programme." An ICMR Task Force Study. New Delhi ICMR.

Koch, E., Throp, J., Bravo, M., Gatica, S., Romero, C.X., Aguilera, H. and Ahlers, I. 2012. "Women's education level, maternal health facilities, abortion legislation and maternal deaths: a natural experiment in Chile from 1957 to 2007." *PLOSOne.* **7**:1-16.

Majumder, S., Najnin, Z., Ahmed, S. and Bhuiyan, S.U. 2018. "Knowledge and attitude of essential newborn care among post-natal mothers in Bangladesh." *J H Res.* **5**:1 11.

Maka, S.S., Tandare, S.B. and Tandare, M.B. 2017. "Study of impact of anemia on pregnancy." *Int J Reprod Contracept Obstet Gynecol.* **6**:4847-4850.

National Family Health Survey 4 (NFHS 4). 2016. West Bengal. International Institute for Population Sciences. Deonar, Mumbai.

Ogu, R.N. and Alegbele 2018. "Improving maternal health: women's attitude to antenatal care ultilization is crucial." *Clin Obstet Reprod Med.* **4**:1-3.

Rao P.M., and Reddy V.P. 2018. "Importance of periodical literature in research." *Int I Library Information Studies.* **8**:256-260.

Shamshad, Shamsher, S. and Rauf, B. 2010. "Puerperial sepsis—still a major threat for parturient." *J.Ayub Med Coll Abbottabad.* **23**:18-22.

Shirin, S. 2011. "Knowledge, attitude and practice of maternal health care amongst the married women in a rural area of Bangladesh." *Ibrahim Med. Coll. J.* **5**: 13-16.

Shoultz, J. and Hatcher, P. 1997. "Looking beyond primary care to primary health care: An approach to community-based action." *Nursing Outlook.* **45**:23-26.

Smith, E., Murray, S.F., Yousafzai, A.K. and Kasonka, L. 2004. "Barriers to accessing safe motherhood and reproductive health services: the situation of women with disabilities in Luska, Zambia." *J. Disablity Rehabilitation.* **26**:121-127.

Tesfaye, A.B. and Tilahun, M.R. 2019. "Pregnancy induced hypertension and associated factors among women attending delivery service at Mizan-Tepi University Teaching Hospital, Tepi General Hospital and Gebretsadik Shawo Hospital, Southwest, Ethiopia." *Ethiop J Health Sci.* **29**: 831-841.

Vora, K.S., Mavalankar, D., Ramani, K.V., Upadhyaya, M., Sharma, B., Iyengar, S., Gupta, V. and Iyengar, K. 2009. "Maternal health situation in India: A case study." *J Health Popul Nutr.* **27**:184-201.

Walt, G. and Vaughan, P. 1982. "Primary health care: what does it mean?" *Trop Doct.* **12**:99-100.

World Health Organization. 2002. "Essential antenatal, perinatal and postpartum care." Regional Office for Europe: WHO.

World Health Organization. 2008. "Standards for maternal and neonatal care." Geneva: WHO.

World Health Organization. 2016. "Sexual and reproductive health: New guidelines on antenatal care for a positive pregnancy experience." Geneva: WHO.

World Health Organization. 2017. "Maternal and newborn health." Copenhagen: WHO.

World Health Organization. 2019. "Maternal mortality: Fact sheet." Geneva: WHO.

Zelealem, A., Endeshaw, M., Ayenew M., Shiferaw, S. and Yirgu, R. 2017. "Effect of nutrition education on pregnancy specific nutrition knowledge and healthy dietary practice among pregnant women in Addis Ababa." *Clinics Mother Child Health.* **14**:1-10.

7

Maternal and Child Health Status in North East India

Thangjam Chitralekha Devi, Subal Das and *Huidrom Suraj Singh*

Introduction

Maternal health is defined as the health of women during pregnancy, childbirth, and the postpartum period (WHO, 2016). The health of women is of particular concern because women's health matter not only to themselves but it is also crucial to the health of the children they will bear. Investing in the health of women and children will help to take necessary actions for the reduction of infant mortality rate and for the development of the child. Further improving maternal, reproductive and child health reduces poverty and stimulates economic growth of the society (WHO, 2010). The reproductive health embraces mother and child care in order to improve quality of life of the family. Reproductive health profile of mothers is affected particularly with the shortcomings in the health care services like poor coverage and quality of antenatal care, unsafe deliveries, lack of emergency obstetric care and poor referral services also contributed to high maternal deaths (WHO, 2018). Maternal health is also influenced by several factors. Some of the study shows that age, family size, as well as type of family, relation with family etc. will have an effect on the mother's health status (Rao *et al.*, 1998). Moreover, lack of knowledge and ignorant about dietary pattern during pregnancy is another promising risk factor affecting on maternal health. On the other hand, shortage of qualified and trained midwives is one of the primary factors behind poor maternal health status particularly in rural areas. Therefore, maternal health care has become a major concern that reflects the status of women in the society and empowerment level and also appalling the basic health care facilities in a particular region (Gogoi, 2014). Thus, empowering women with knowledge and awareness about health from the time of conception till childbirth is fundamental to achieve global health. The utilization of maternal health services with special reference to antenatal check-up, nutrition, financial assistance are intended for pregnant women in order to screen and detect early signs of risk factors for diseases followed by timely intervention, originally with the objective of reducing maternal and prenatal mortality and morbidity (WHO, 2016). In order to minimize the rate of maternal and child morbidity as well as mortality, the Government of India has initiated financial assistance to the mothers for a safe motherhood by promoting institutional deliveries under Janani Suraksha Yojana (JSY) launched by National Rural Health Mission (2005). The JSY scheme is implemented across the country and provides cash assistance to the poorest and the marginalized sections of the societies.

The term child health refers the physical, mental, emotional, spiritual, and social well-being of the children. As the First Five Year Plan in India stated, "Health is a positive state of well-being in which harmonious development of mental and physical capacities of the individual lead to the enjoyment of a rich and full life." It suggests that lack of health whether physical, mental or emotional is a bad sign for the nation while also being harmful for the children. The lack of maternal health often affects a child's health in adverse ways. Poor health condition also deprives them from school attendance. Thus, the quality of children's life depends on the implementation of the child development scheme as well as proper dissemination of information to parents and guardians in different regions. Health status of the children largely depends on the status of the mother, socio-economic status, education, awareness level, health practices during pregnancy, periodical immunization of the child, fertility records, antenatal care etc. Sandiford *et al.* (1995) show that mother's education is the key factor that leads to changes in a woman's values, beliefs, power or knowledge which in turn leads to lower child mortality either through better domestic child care or more effective use of health services.

The World Health Organization (WHO) estimates that, of 5,36,000 maternal deaths occurring globally each year, 1,36,000 takes place in India. Moreover, 45,000 women died from preventable pregnancy-related complications in India (WHO, 2015). India alone contributes more than 25 per cent of the global disability due to maternal conditions (WHO, 2011). Therefore, the present chapter seeks to examine the status of maternal and child health care in the north-eastern region (NER) of India, which is one of the most remote and backward regions of the country; wherein about 81.6 per cent of population lives in the rural hilly areas (Census, 2011). The main objectives of the present review chapter is to understand the present situation of maternal and child health particularly on antenatal check-up, mode of delivery, health-care facilities, immunization and vaccination, and health status in North East (NE) states. Attempts were also made to assess the impact of national maternal and child health programmes in the NE states.

Methodology

The present chapter is a review of data on North East states of India comparing reports of National Family Health Survey-3 (2005-06) and National Family Health Survey-4 (2015-16). It examines data on health indicators of mother and child, i.e. total fertility rate, age at marriage, antenatal check up, mode of delivery, health care facilities, immunization and vaccination, and health status in NE states and compares with all-India average levels. All two rounds of NFHS data are nationally representative because it has covered more than 99 per cent of both the general population as well as child population in India. Apart from the NFHS data, the chapter also reviews and compares with available literatures on maternal and child health in India.

Results and Discussion

(i) Literacy and Early Marriage and Pregnancy

Educational status of the mother is considered as an important social determinant of health for children. Therefore, rate of literacy was examined to understand the health conditions of both mother and children of NE states. Literacy rate in most of the NE states is above the national average level (68.4%) except in Arunachal Pradesh (65.6%). But, there is significant difference in rural and urban populations. The highest literacy rate in NE states is recorded from Mizoram (93.5%). States like Meghalaya and Sikkim show significantly increase in literacy rate from NFHS-3 to NFHS-4. However, literacy rate has increased to a certain extent in Assam, Manipur, Nagaland and Sikkim in the last decade (Table 7.1).

Age at marriage and rate of early pregnancy was also examined to understand its effects on maternal and child health status. The overall rate of women age 20-24 years married before 18 years of age decreases in NFHS-4 as compared to NFHS-3. Prevalence of early marriage before attending 18 years of age is observed to be significantly higher among the rural populations compared with urban population of NE states except in Sikkim. The highest rate of early marriage is reported from Assam (38.6%) followed by Tripura (33.1%) and Arunachal Pradesh (23.5%) in the entire NE states whereas, the least frequency is observed in Mizoram (10.8%). According to NFHS-3 report, NE states showed high incidence of women age 15-19 years who are already mothers or pregnant. However, the incidence rate is extensively decreased in the last decade in most of the NE states according to NFHS-4 reports. Moreover, the entire rural population of NE states reports extensively high frequency of early pregnancy than the respective urban population. Tripura shows slightly increased rate with 13.3 per cent in urban and 20.7 per cent in rural population than the other NE states while Sikkim shows the least frequency of 2.8 per cent (Table 7.1).

(ii) Antenatal Care during Pregnancy Period

Overall antenatal check-up during the first trimester keeps increasing rate from the last ten years in the entire NE states except Nagaland. However, majority of the states still not able to reach the national average level that is 58.6 per cent. Situation is more pronounced when we look into the rural areas of the NE states comparing to the urban population.

State-wise, Manipur records the highest rate (77.0%) of antenatal check-up in the first trimester and the least frequency is

Table 7.1: Literacy, Early marriage and Women who were pregnant or already mother at the age of 15-19 years

	India	*Arunachal Pradesh*	*Assam*	*Manipur*	*Meghalaya*	*Mizoram*	*Nagaland*	*Sikkim*	*Tripura*
Literacy									
Urban	81.4	80.9	87.0	89.9	93.4	98.6	89.9	89.5	88.4
Rural	61.5	60.1	69.2	81.7	79.6	85.4	75.1	85.2	77.0
Total	68.4	65.6	71.8	85.0	82.8	93.5	81.0	86.6	80.4
NFHS-3 (2005-06)	56.1	52.7	63.0	72.6	69.5	94.0	75.2	72.3	68.5
Women age 20-24 years married before age 18 years (%)									
Urban	17.5	18.7	24.3	12.1	8.5	7.1	9.3	16.4	26.5
Rural	31.5	25.5	31.9	14.7	19.7	17.0	15.8	14.1	35.7
Total	26.8	23.5	30.8	13.7	16.9	10.8	13.3	15.0	33.1
NFHS 3 (2005-06)	47.4	42.0	38.6	12.9	24.6	20.6	21.4	30.1	41.6
Women age 15-19 years who were already mothers or pregnant at the time of the survey									
Urban	5.0	9.8	8.1	6.1	3.4	6.2	2.8	2.4	13.3
Rural	9.2	10.8	14.4	8.2	10.1	8.9	7.9	3.0	20.7
Total	7.9	10.5	13.6	7.4	8.6	7.2	5.7	2.8	18.6
NFHS-3 (2005-06)	16.0	15.4	16.4	7.3	8.3	10.1	7.5	12.0	18.5

Source: Based on authors' computation from National Family Health Survey-4 (NFHS-4), 2015–16.

reported from the Nagaland (24.9%). According to the NFHS-4 report, the rates of mothers who had at least 4 antenatal care visits are considerably greater than the NFHS-3 report. Some of the NE states show more or less equal prevalence as that of the national average level (57.6%). However, Nagaland reports to have an incredibly least rate (15.0%) in the entire NE states as well as both in urban (28.7%) and rural (9.2%) population. Sikkim records the overall highest rate (74.7%) followed by Manipur (69.0%) in the NE states. But, the rate of at least 4 antenatal care visits by mothers were reported to be highest in Manipur (81.7%) followed by Mizoram (77.5%), and Tripura (77.0%).

In India, the overall national rate of mother who consumed iron folic acid shows considerably increase from NFHS-3 (15.2%) to NFHS-4 (30.3%). Moreover, the rates of iron folic acid consumption in some NE states are higher than the national average level (30.3%) except in Arunachal Pradesh (8.3%), Nagaland (4.4%) and Tripura (13.4%). These three states are very poor in terms of rates of iron folic acid consumption by mothers during pregnancy periods in both rural and urban areas as compared to other states of NE Region. In NE states, prevalence of full antenatal care is significantly increased from the past 10 years except in Arunachal Pradesh where it decreases from 4.9 per cent to 3.6 per cent. Sikkim reported highest frequency of antenatal care in rural population (40.2%) than urban population (36.7%). On the other hand, other remaining NE states show highest frequency in urban populations. Particularly three states Arunachal Pradesh, Nagaland and Tripura had very poor prevalence rate of full antenatal care received by less than 10 per cent of mothers in both rural and urban areas (Table 7.2).

(iii) Institutional Birth and Caesarean Section Delivery

In the last 10 years (NFHS-3 to NFHS-4), the total rate of institutional births show tremendously increased to certain extent in most of the NE states. The increased rate is significantly higher in Sikkim from 47.2% to 94.7%. The rate is, however, greater in urban population than the rural in all NE states. Sikkim records the highest institutional births (94.7%) from the rest of the NE states followed by Mizoram (80.1%) and the least frequency is reported from Nagaland (32.8%). Moreover, an increasing trend of institutional births in public facility over the last decades was also

Table 7.2: Antenatal care and consumption of iron folic acid by Mothers during pregnancy period

	India	*Arunachal Pradesh*	*Assam*	*Manipur*	*Meghalaya*	*Mizoram*	*Nagaland*	*Sikkim*	*Tripura*
Mothers who had antenatal Check-up in the First Trimester									
Urban	69.1	39.2	68.5	84.9	68.3	77.0	36.7	77.2	77.1
Rural	54.2	36.3	53.5	72.6	50.7	52.1	19.8	75.7	62.7
Total	58.6	37.0	55.1	77.0	53.3	65.7	24.9	76.2	66.4
NFHS-3 (2005-06)	43.9	24.2	40.0	64.5	32.6	42.9	29.2	57.9	47.2
Mothers who had at least 4 antenatal care visits									
Urban	66.4	37.3	60.4	81.7	71.3	77.5	28.7	75.6	77.0
Rural	54.2	23.6	44.8	62.0	46.3	42.5	9.2	74.2	59.9
Total	57.6	26.8	46.5	69.0	50.0	61.7	15.0	74.7	64.3
NFHS-3 (2005-06)	43.9	22.4	23.5	54.1	42.8	45.6	12.1	56.2	50.6
Mothers who consumed iron folic acid for 100 days or more during pregnancy									
Urban	40.8	11.1	44.0	50.9	53.8	59.3	7.7	48.7	16.3
Rural	25.9	7.5	30.5	32.7	33.2	47.2	3.0	54.9	12.4
Total	30.3	8.3	32.0	39.2	36.2	53.8	4.4	52.8	13.4
NFHS-3 (2005-06)	15.2	7.3	10.3	6.8	5.9	17.8	1.2	26.3	11.5
Mother who had full antenatal care									
Urban	31.1	3.9	30.4	45.1	38.4	47.9	4.9	36.7	9.8
Rural	16.7	3.5	16.6	27.8	20.9	27.0	1.3	40.2	6.8
Total	21.0	3.6	18.1	33.9	23.5	38.5	2.4	39.0	7.6
NFHS-3 (2005-06)	11.6	4.9	6.7	5.8	4.2	11.8	0.6	22.4	7.4

Source: Based on authors' computation from National Family Health Survey-4 (NFHS-4), 2015–16.

observed. Unlike, from the rest of the states, Sikkim and Tripura show higher frequencies of having institutional births in rural than the urban population.

However, there is lesser rate of occurrence below the national average level (52.1%) in Arunachal Pradesh (42.7%), Manipur (45.7%), Meghalaya (39.4%), and Nagaland (25.1%) (Table 7.3). According to NFHS-4 Report overall caesarean section delivery status in some of the NE states is more or less equal to the national average level (17.2%). The rate of caesarean section delivery increased double times over the last decade in most of the NE states. However, Tripura records highest rates among the urban population (45.8%) followed by Assam (36.9%) and Manipur (33.0%). Most of the rural population shows lower prevalence of caesarean section delivery at an average below 10.0 per cent in NE states (Table 7.3).

The rates of caesarean section deliveries were compared between the Private and Public Health sectors, the caesarean delivery at Private Health sectors is significantly higher than the Public health sectors in all the NE states. Moreover, urban populations show significantly higher frequencies of delivery by caesarean section in private sectors than the rural populations in the entire NE states. Tripura records the highest caesarean section delivery in NE states with 87.1 per cent in urban and 57.6 per cent in rural. However, the least incidence is recorded from Mizoram (30.0%). On the other hand, overall rate of caesarean section delivery in public health facility considerably decreased from the last 10 years. However, there is increase in the rate of using public health facility in urban population. Meghalaya is the only state that shows least frequency (9.8%) while the other states show higher frequency than the national average level. Similar trend of caesarean section delivery is also observed in Tripura (18.1%) and Manipur (22.6%) (Table 7.3).

(iv) Fertility and Infant Mortality Rate

There is a gradual reduce in the total fertility rate in NFHS-4 reports as compared to NFHS-3 reports. Further, the rural populations show higher prevalence of total fertility rate than the urban population in the entire NE states. Three states, namely Arunachal Pradesh (2.1), Tripura (1.7) and Sikkim (1.2) reports fertility rate below the national average level (2.2). Sikkim records the lowest

Table 7.3: Institutional birth and delivery by Caesarean Section in Private and Public Health Facility Centres

	India	Arunachal Pradesh	Assam	Manipur	Meghalaya	Mizoram	Nagaland	Sikkim	Tripura
Institutional Births									
Urban	38.7	81.5	92.9	86.3	88.1	97.2	56.3	95.3	92.6
Rural	75.1	44.2	68.2	60.5	45.7	61.0	24.0	94.4	75.7
Total	78.9	52.3	70.6	69.1	51.4	80.1	32.8	94.7	79.9
NFHS-3 (2005-06)	38.7	28.5	22.4	45.9	29.0	59.8	11.6	47.2	46.9
Institutional Births in Public Facility									
Urban	46.2	59.5	61.7	55.3	53.1	70.2	40.2	77.5	68.9
Rural	54.4	38.0	59.8	40.9	37.3	56.6	19.5	85.2	69.2
Total	52.1	42.7	60.0	45.7	39.4	63.8	25.1	82.7	69.1
NFHS-3 (2005-06)	18.0	19.5	13.0	36.1	19.7	51.6	7.3	44.5	43.0
Birth Delivered by Caesarean Section									
Urban	28.3	20.1	36.9	33.0	20.5	19.0	12.4	28.8	45.8
Rural	12.9	5.8	10.8	15.2	5.6	5.7	3.4	17.1	12.2
Total	17.2	8.9	13.4	21.1	7.6	12.7	5.8	20.9	20.5
NFHS-3 (2005-06)	8.5	2.9	5.3	9.0	4.1	6.2	2.0	12.3	12.9
Births in a Private Health Facility Delivered by Caesarean Section									
Urban	44.8	42.2	65.6	52.8	34.5	31.4	35.7	(48.3)	87.1
Rural	37.8	32.8	48.3	40.9	29.3	20.2	25.8	50.1	57.6
Total	40.9	37.5	53.3	46.2	31.4	30.0	31.4	49.3	73.7
NFHS-3 (2005-06)	27.7	9.9	26.7	26.7	26.7	19.5	18.5	*	(69.5)
Births in a Public Health Facility Delivered by Caesarean Section									
Urban	19.9	18.2	26.6	30.0	16.0	15.1	16.5	26.0	36.4
Rural	9.3	10.0	11.4	17.6	8.5	8.6	11.2	14.7	12.1
Total	11.9	12.5	12.9	22.6	9.8	12.3	13.5	18.1	18.1
NFHS-3 (2005-06)	15.2	10.5	21.0	17.6	8.3	8.9	15.8	25.0	23.7

Source: Based on authors' computation from National Family Health Survey-4 (NFHS-4), 2015–16.
( )-Based on 25-49 unweighted cases.
*Percentage not shown; based on fewer than 25 unweighted cases

total fertility rate both in rural and urban populations (Table 7.4). Rural populations show significantly higher frequencies of Infant Mortality Rate (IMR) than the urban population in the entire NE states. Assam records the highest IMR in the NE states with 48 per 1000 live births and the least frequency is reported from Manipur with 22 per 1000 live births. In general, IMR is reducing from the last decade as observed from NFHS reports except Mizoram. A similar trend is also observed for under-five Mortality rate (U5MR) where rural populations are more hazardous than the urban population. Assam records the highest U5MR with 57 per 1000 live births and the least U5MR is reported from Manipur with 26 per 1000 live births. Assam is the only state in NE (57 per 1000 live births) that records above the national average level of U5MR (50 per 1000 live births). Moreover, the level of U5MR in Assam is much higher in both rural (58 per 1000 live births) and urban population (40 per 1000 live births) when compared with other NE states and it even exceeds the national average levels (Table 7.4).

(v) Immunization and Vaccination of Children

The rates of immunization show extensively improved in all NE states from the last 10 years to a certain extent. Manipur (65.8%) and Sikkim (83.0%) reported higher frequency of children at age 12-23 months fully immunized which is above the national average level (62.0%). Yet, Nagaland and Arunachal Pradesh show the least frequencies of immunization rates with 35.7 per cent and 38.2 per cent respectively. Most of the urban populations of NE states exceed the rate of immunization while compared with rural populations except in Mizoram and Sikkim. Such difference in rate of immunization level among rural and urban children age 12-33 months is observed to be significantly varied in Assam and Meghalaya (Table 7.5).

Regarding overall rate of vaccination in public health facility is significantly higher in the rural children than urban children populations. Moreover, the rates of vaccination in rural children of NE states are more or less equal to the national average level (94.2%) except Meghalaya reporting 91.7 per cent. Tripura shows the highest frequency in both rural (99.2%) and urban children populations (92.6%). Vaccination received by urban children populations of two states, namely Assam (77.3%) and Meghalaya

Table 7.4: Fertility and Infant Mortality Rate

	India	Arunachal Pradesh	Assam	Manipur	Meghalaya	Mizoram	Nagaland	Sikkim	Tripura
Women age 20-24 years married before age 18 years (%)									
Urban	17.5	18.7	24.3	12.1	8.5	7.1	9.3	16.4	26.5
Rural	31.5	25.5	31.9	14.7	19.7	17.0	15.8	14.1	35.7
Total	26.8	23.5	30.8	13.7	16.9	10.8	13.3	15.0	33.1
NFHS-3 (2005-06)	47.4	42.0	38.6	12.9	24.6	20.6	21.4	30.1	41.6
Women age 15-19 years who were already mothers or pregnant at the time of the survey									
Urban	5.0	9.8	8.1	6.1	3.4	6.2	2.8	2.4	13.3
Rural	9.2	10.8	14.4	8.2	10.1	8.9	7.9	3.0	20.7
Total	7.9	10.5	13.6	7.4	8.6	7.2	5.7	2.8	18.6
NFHS-3 (2005-06)	16.0	15.4	16.4	7.3	8.3	10.1	7.5	12.0	18.5
Total Fertility Rate (Children per Women)									
Urban	1.8	1.7	1.5	2.1	1.7	2.0	1.8	1.1	1.4
Rural	2.4	2.3	2.3	2.9	3.5	2.7	3.4	1.2	1.8
Total	2.2	2.1	2.2	2.6	3.0	2.3	2.7	1.2	1.7
NFHS-3 (2005-06)	2.7	3.0	2.4	2.8	3.6	2.9	3.7	2.0	2.2
Infant Mortality Rate (IMR)									
Urban	29	19	28	16	16	31	21	(13)	(12)
Rural	46	24	50	25	32	50	33	38	32
Total	41	23	48	22	30	40	29	30	27
NFHS-3 (2005-06)	57	61	66	30	45	34	36	34	51
Under five Mortality Rate (U5MR)									
Urban	34	25	40	18	20	35	25	(18)	(21)
Rural	56	35	58	30	43	58	42	39	36
Total	50	33	57	26	40	46	37	32	33
NFHS-3 (2005-06)	74	86	85	42	70	53	65	40	59

Source: Based on authors' computation from National Family Health Survey-4 (NFHS-4), 2015–16.
( ) - Based on 25-49 unweighted cases.

(81.1%) reports below the National average level of urban children population (82.1%). On the other hand, the rates of receiving vaccinations in private health facility are drastically decreased in most of the NE states from the last decades. However, the urban children populations show significantly increase rate of receiving vaccinations from the private health facility while compared to rural children population according to NFHS-4 reports. Though, six out of eight NE states, namely Arunachal Pradesh (8.7%), Manipur (7.0%), Mizoram (13.1%), Nagaland (15.4%), Sikkim (8.1%) and Tripura (7.4%) received vaccination by the urban children population below the national average level (16.7%). It is evidence from the available reports that majority of the rural NE children received vaccinations from Public Health facility centres while urban children received from Private Health facility centres (Table 7.5).

Adequate diet received by children of NE states was also assessed from NFHS reports. There is overall increase rates in receiving adequate diet in most of the NE states than the national average level (9.6%) among the children age 6-23 months. However, Assam and Tripura reports lowest prevalence of this rate in both rural and urban children population. Urban populations in NE states like Manipur, Meghalaya, Mizoram, and Nagaland show higher frequencies to certain extent (Table 7.5).

The rate of severely wasting (weight-for-height) in all NE states are below the national average level showing improvement particularly weight for height (NFHS-4). The prevalence increases from the last 10 years in Arunachal Pradesh (from 6.1% to 8.0%), Assam (4.0% to 6.2%), and Sikkim (from 3.3% to 5.9%). Though, children of Meghalaya show rapid decrease in severely wasted children in the last 10 years (from 19.9% to 6.5%). The urban and rural children of all the NE states did not show any significant difference with respect to distribution of severely wasted level except for Arunachal Pradesh. Since, the rate of severely wasted children particularly in rural and total population of Arunachal Pradesh is above the national average level (Table 7.5).

(vi) Biochemical and Physiological Variables

Overall anaemic status of pregnant women (15-49 years) as well as children age 6-59 months in all the NE states slightly decreases

Table 7.5: Immunization and Vaccinations of the Children in Private and Public Health Facility Centres

	India	Arunachal Pradesh	Assam	Manipur	Meghalaya	Mizoram	Nagaland	Sikkim	Tripura
Children (age 12-33 months) fully immunized									
Urban	63.9	44.2	70.9	74.3	81.4	49.8	41.6	(81.4)	64.2
Rural	61.3	36.4	44.4	61.7	45.7	51.3	33.4	83.7	51.2
Total	62.0	38.2	47.1	65.8	51.4	50.5	35.7	83.0	54.5
NFHS-3 (2005-06)	43.5	28.4	31.4	46.8	29.0	46.5	21.0	69.6	49.7
Children who Received Vaccinations in Public Health Facility									
Urban	82.1	90.3	77.3	92.8	81.1	86.8	84.6	(91.9)	92.6
Rural	94.2	95.1	95.3	92.9	94.3	98.3	94.7	95.1	99.2
Total	90.7	93.9	93.3	92.9	92.4	92.2	91.7	94.1	97.4
NFHS-3 (2005-06)	82.0	95.4	87.0	92.7	87.0	93.7	93.1	98.6	87.2
Children who Received Vaccinations in Private Health Facility									
Urban	16.7	8.7	21.8	7.0	18.9	13.1	15.4	(8.1)	7.4
Rural	3.4	4.5	3.3	5.6	2.5	0.6	4.5	4.9	0.0
Total	7.2	5.5	5.3	6.1	4.9	7.2	7.8	5.9	2.0
NFHS-3 (2005-06)	10.5	3.2	7.3	3.3	8.9	5.7	6.1	0.4	1.7
Children receiving an adequate Diet									
Urban	11.6	11.1	11.8	22.1	26.6	16.0	19.4	20.7	7.2
Rural	8.8	14.8	8.5	17.3	23.1	13.2	16.9	24.4	5.5
Total	9.6	13.9	8.9	18.8	23.6	14.6	17.5	23.1	5.9
NFHS-3 (2005-06)	-	-	-	-	-	-	-	-	-
Children under 5 years who are severely wasted									
Urban	4.1	4.5	1.8	6.5	1.2	3.9	5.7	5.3	7.5
Rural	3.9	6.4	2.4	6.5	3.4	4.3	6.0	6.7	7.4
Total	3.0	6.2	2.2	6.5	2.3	4.2	5.9	6.3	7.5
NFHS-3 (2005-06)	6.1	4.0	2.1	19.9	3.6	5.2	3.3	8.6	6.4

Source: Based on authors' computation from National Family Health Survey-4 (NFHS-4), 2015–16.
( ) - Based on 25-49 unweighted cases.

from the past 10 years according to NFHS-3 and NFHS-4 reports. However, Tripura (54.4%) still exceeds over the national average level (50.3%) with respect to anaemic status of pregnant women. The highest frequencies are reported from Tripura (54.7%) followed by Meghalaya (49.5%), and Assam (44.8%). On the other hand, states like Arunachal Pradesh (35.7%), Manipur (28.5%), Nagaland (29.1%), Sikkim (33.6%) and Tripura (49.8%) reports more anaemic status among the urban pregnant women while compared with the rural populations. Sikkim records the least frequency particularly in rural (19.6%) and total population (23.6%) among the NE states (Table 7.6). Among the children of age 6-59 months, the overall anaemic status in some of NE states is more or less equal to the national average level (58.5%). Sikkim reported to be the highest in anaemic status (55.1%) followed by Arunachal Pradesh (50.7%), and the least frequency is reported from Mizoram (19.1%). More frequency is reported from the rural population rather than urban, however, the opposite trend is seen in states like Manipur and Sikkim where urban children are more anaemic than the rural children (Table 7.6).

Frequencies of high blood sugar level (>160 mg/dl) among the women of 15-49 years in most of the NE states is above the national average level (2.8%) for example, Tripura (4.0%), Mizoram (3.9%), Manipur (3.0%), and Sikkim (2.9%). It is more evidence when we observe for urban populations. All the NE states reported to be higher in frequencies of high sugar level in urban than the rural population except in Nagaland (Table 7.6).

The prevalence of very high systolic (≥180 mm of Hg) and or diastolic pressure (≥110 mm of Hg) is more than the national average level in most of the NE states. The highest frequencies are observed from the Nagaland (4.7%) followed by Arunachal Pradesh (2.2%). The lowest frequencies are reported from Tripura (0.2%) and Mizoram (0.6%). More or less equal frequencies were observed between rural and urban populations.

(vii) Delivery: Expenditure and Financial Assistance, Violence

Overall rate of women experienced violence during their pregnancy by NE women is less than the national average level (3.3%) except Manipur (3.4%). In general, urban women population experienced significantly higher frequencies of violence during

Table 7.6: Anaemia, Blood Sugar and Blood Pressure levels among the NE children and women population

	India	Arunachal Pradesh	Assam	Manipur	Meghalaya	Mizoram	Nagaland	Sikkim	Tripura
Pregnant Women age 15-49 who are anaemic (<11.0g/dl)									
Urban	45.7	35.7	37.9	28.5	38.6	24.1	29.1	(33.6)	(49.8)
Rural	52.1	33.4	45.7	23.7	51.3	29.9	28.8	19.6	55.8
Total	50.3	33.8	44.8	25.2	49.5	26.6	28.9	23.6	54.4
NFHS-3 (2005-2006)	57.9	51.8	72.0	36.3	58.1	48.3	*	62.1	57.6
Children age 6-59 months who are anaemic									
Urban	55.9	49.7	27.6	24.5	33.6	14.1	17.6	59.7	45.7
Rural	59.4	51.0	36.5	22.0	41.8	24.5	23.1	52.7	49.2
Total	58.5	50.7	35.7	22.8	40.7	19.1	21.6	55.1	48.3
NFHS-3 (2005-2006)	69.4	56.9	69.4	41.1	63.8	43.8	*	58.1	62.9
Blood Sugar Level 15-49									
Urban	3.6	2.1	4.1	3.7	2.5	4.6	2.7	3.5	5.8
Rural	2.3	1.7	2.1	2.6	1.6	2.9	2.9	2.6	3.2
Total	2.8	1.8	2.4	3.0	1.8	3.9	2.8	2.9	4.0
NFHS-3 (2005-2006)	NA	NA	NA	NA	NA	NA	NA	NA	NA
Very High Blood Pressure 15-49									
Urban	0.7	2.1	1.3	1.2	0.9	0.5	5.7	1.9	0.0
Rural	0.7	2.3	1.6	0.8	1.0	0.8	4.0	1.6	0.2
Total	0.7	2.2	1.5	1.0	1.0	0.6	4.7	1.7	0.2
NFHS-3 (2005-2006)	NA	NA	NA	NA	NA	NA	NA	NA	NA

Source: Based on authors' computation from National Family Health Survey-4 (NFHS-4), 2015–2016).

* Percentage not shown, based on fewer than 25 unweighted cases.

NA - Not available

( ) - Based on 25-49 unweighted cases.

pregnancy than rural populations. But, Assam (2.1%), Nagaland (2.3%), Sikkim (0.6%) and Tripura (2.5%) records higher frequencies than their respective urban population. Such domestic violence related with pregnancy was reported to be lowest in Meghalaya and Sikkim with 0.4 per cent each.

In general, the rates of pocket expenditure per delivery in Public Health Facility in all NE states are above the national average level (3198/-) suggesting spending of more expenditure in delivery. The highest frequency is reported from Manipur which cost up to 10,348/- and the lowest expenditure from Meghalaya with 3324/-. Most of the urban populations of NE states spend more expenditure on delivery while compared with rural population. Expenditure on delivery spends from own pocket ranges from 3281/- to 9886/- in rural population and 4032/- to 11007/- in urban population (Table 7.7).

In NE, the overall rate of mothers who received financial assistance under JSY was observed to be significantly higher among the rural population as compared to urban population. Assam (66.1%) and Mizoram (47.5%) received highest financial assistance which crosses even from the national average level. Arunachal Pradesh (20.5%) received the lowest assistance followed by Manipur (26.2%) (Table 7.7).

Literacy rate is one of the important keys to measure socio-economic progress as well as living healthily. As per 2011 Census, the literacy rate of women in India is 64.8 per cent. However, the literacy rate in the latest NFHS-4 reports reveals 68.4 per cent of which the urban population shows 81.4 per cent. It suggests significant difference in literacy rate between urban and rural population. Situation becomes worse when we look into rural women population. It holds true when we compared between rural and urban women population of NE states.

In a society, age at marriage is a key indicator of the maternal health status. Global data released by UNICEF shows that in South Asia, the child marriage (below 18 years of age) rate has dropped by more than a third from 50 per cent to 30 per cent. This could be due to decline on early marriage prevalence rates in India, which has registered a drop from 47.4 per cent in 2005-06 to 26.8 per cent 2015-16. Same decreasing trend in early marriage is also observed in most of the NE states. However, its prevalence is still high in most of the rural populations as compared with the urban population. It is further evidenced from the NRHM (2013)

Table 7.7: Delivery Expenditure, Financial Assistance and Domestic violence experienced by NE women

	India	*Arunachal Pradesh*	*Assam*	*Manipur*	*Meghalaya*	*Mizoram*	*Nagaland*	*Sikkim*	*Tripura*
Average out of Pocket expenditure per delivery in Public Health Facility (D)									
Urban	3913	9640	5244	11007	2915	5019	6448	4032	5449
Rural	2947	5028	3645	9886	3414	3281	5401	3975	4571
Total	3198	6474	3821	10348	3324	4327	5834	3993	4784
Mother who received financial assistance under JSY									
Urban	21.4	12.9	42.4	21.2	26.2	44.9	27.5	11.9	21.3
Rural	43.8	24.5	69.9	30.0	28.6	52.5	31.8	38.3	37.3
Total	36.4	20.5	66.1	26.2	28.0	47.5	29.7	29.4	32.6
Ever Married Women who have experienced violence during any pregnancy									
Urban	2.9	2.6	1.8	4.1	0.5	2.8	0.4	0.0	1.5
Rural	3.5	1.2	2.1	3.0	0.4	1.1	2.3	0.6	2.5
Total	3.3	1.5	2.1	3.4	0.4	2.1	1.5	0.4	2.2

Source: Based on authors' computation from National Family Health Survey-4 (NFHS-4), 2015–2016.
Note: No records available for NFHS-3 on expenditure on delivery, financial assistance under JSY and violence during pregnancy.

reports indicating high percentage (38 %) of rural Khasi girls of Ri Bhoi who were married below the legal age at marriage. Approximately 10 million girls aged 15 to 19 years give birth each year in developing regions (UNFPA, 2015). However, the global adolescent birth rate has been declined from 65 births per 1000 women in 1990 to 47 births per 1000 women in 2015 (UN DESA, 2015). Most of the NE states also decline birth rate of women age 15-19 years who are mothers or pregnant.

Limited studies are conducted for antenatal check-up among the North-east region. According to Purkayastha and Singh (2017), the antenatal check-up is more common among younger women age below 35 years than the older rural Khasi women of Ri Bhoi, district Meghalaya. It further reveals that mothers who did not have any antenatal check-ups felt that antenatal care (ANC) are not necessary during pregnancy. Hence, the institutional delivery was reported very low among the studied population constituting only about 6.9 per cent. Studies among the four regions of Andhra Pradesh for the utilization of antenatal care revealed regional variation in reception of adequate ANC ranging from 27.9 per cent to 42.4 per cent. Moreover, utilization of private health facilities for ANC is high in the studied urban populations (Ponna *et al.* 2018). Literatures on the utilization of antenatal care of NER of India are very limited. In North East region, 42.6 per cent of women got full ANC as reported from urban area of Imphal East, Manipur (Laishram *et al.*, 2013). According to NFHS-4 reports, the full ANC has increased in urban population of Manipur (45.1%) which is even higher compared with the national average level (31.1%). Further, majority of the women consume iron folic acid tablets (94%), though only 45.3 per cent of them completed the required 100 tablets (Laishram *et al.*, 2013). These findings are even lower while compared with other studies (Singh *et al.*, 2000). First visit during first trimester by pregnant mothers is very low in most of the NE states. It is supported by other studies reporting lower frequency (50.41%) of first trimester visit among the Aimol tribe of Manipur (Aimol and Phukan, 2014). According to the findings, 56 per cent of child-birth had institutional deliveries and only few 11 per cent had undergone caesarean section delivery among Aimol tribe of Manipur. Rural-urban differentials existed with regard to place of delivery and the person attending the home delivery across the states/union territories. In rural areas, institutional deliveries ranged from 24.3 per cent in Nagaland to

100 per cent each in Kerala and Goa. In contrast, the percentage of institutional deliveries in urban areas ranged from 60.0 per cent in Nagaland to 99.7 per cent each in Kerala and Goa (MHFW, 2009).

The trend of caesarean delivery is increasing throughout the country with regional variations. Nambiar and Singh (2017) reports the current scenario of caesarean section delivery across the districts of NE states of India. According to the study, the institutional delivery has high-high spatial 94 association at West and South districts of Sikkim, Dhemaji district of Assam and Champhai, Aizawl, Serchhip districts of Mizoram whereas low-low spatial association in Phek, Zunheboto, Wokha, Kiphire and Tuensang districts of Nagaland. The percentage observed was highest in Imphal East and Imphal West districts of Manipur; Morigaon, Dibrugarh, Kamrup districts of Assam; and West Tripura district, whereas, the rate of caesarean section in Nagaland is very low as compared to the other NE states.

According to the United Nations Population Division, a total fertility rate (TFR), i.e., the number of children born per woman is 2.1, is called Replacement-level fertility, which if maintained for few decades, will lead to a stable population. So, as per the reports from NFHS-4, the TFR levels in the NE states are more or less equal to replacement-level fertility.

In India, the coverage levels for immunization programme varied across the country. Its frequency is relatively lower in some of the states like Bihar, Rajasthan, Uttar Pradesh, Madhya Pradesh and entire NE states (Singh and Yadav, 2000a). It is further supported by many other studies reporting less per cent of immunization rate in different population groups located in different parts of the country such as North India (25%), Rajasthan (50%), Lucknow (44.1%), Agra (30%), and Delhi (17.8%) (Mathew *et al.*, 2002; Manjunath and Pareek, 2003; Nath *et al.*, 2007; Saxena *et al.*, 2008; Kumar *et al.*, 2010). On the other hand, the full immunization coverage among the children of Assam reaches up to 62.2 per cent which is also comparable with other studies conducted in different parts of the country like Kerala (77.5%), Maharashtra (64.28%), and Madhya Pradesh (60.8%) (Nair *et al.*, 1994; Yadav and Singh, 2004; Phukan *et al.*, 2008; Wadgave and Pore, 2012). Variations in child immunization rate are further evidenced from the study of Singh (2013). According to the coverage across different six geographical regions of India, children residing in rural areas and girls remained disadvantaged (Mathew *et al.*, 2002; Yadav and Singh, 2004). Moreover, the low coverage of immunization was mainly affected by maternal education and place of delivery. Deliveries in the hospital were more likely to be fully immunized. In a hospital based study, 61.9 per cent of children born in hospitals were completely immunized. It is in accordance with the findings of NFHS-4 (62%). However, some of the NE states still show least frequency of immunization in states like Nagaland (35.7%) and Arunachal Pradesh (38.2%).

There is limited number of studies conducted in NER of India particularly about the vaccination status. Studies reveal that children who utilize private care are almost twice as likely to receive preventive care from private sources, but the majority of the population in India still obtains preventive care from public providers (Howard and Roy, 2004). However, according to NFHS-4 report, vaccination in public health facility is considerably higher in rural populations (94.2%) than urban (82.1%). Most of the children in urban populations receive preventive care from the private health facility (16.7%) comparing to rural populations (3.4 %).

The nutritional status of reproductive age women is very much important in both maternal and child health status. Particularly, the rural women were reported to have high prevalence of underweight in most of the NE states. It is supported by the study of Baidya *et al.* (2016) reporting 28.10 per cent of the reproductive age women were underweight in Tripura. The study further shows that women of 15-29 years of age were significantly more underweight compared to women between 45 to 49 years of age.

Tripathi *et al.* (2017) reported that the pocket expenditure on hospitalization for childbirth in private sector led to a significantly higher prevalence of catastrophic expenditure than hospitalization in a public sector (7%). Most of the public sector health facilities were observed to be used by rural populations as evidence from the pocket expenditure due to hospitalization for childbirth.

Conclusion

The overall maternal and child health status in North East India has improved over the last decades. However, the overall vaccination rate, institutional births, antenatal care, fertility rate, and financial assistance under JSY—irrespective of rural and urban sectors—are still very low in most of the NE states as compared to other neighbouring states of mainland India. Whereas, frequencies of caesarean section delivery, severely wasted children, early marriage and pregnancy, infant mortality rate and U5MR, pocket expenditure against delivery, and domestic violence during pregnancy are comparatively very high. There is still a significant gap between rural and urban population in terms of maternal and child health status in most of the variables considered in the present study. Most of the NE states require full attention and regular monitoring particularly on vaccination programmes launched by the government as well as the antenatal check-up as the rate of vaccination and antenatal care in these states are very low while compared with national average level. Moreover, in-depth research works are very much essential to identify the potential risk factors for low fertility rate as well as high incidence of caesarean section delivery in NE states. The complex non-communicable diseases like diabetes, obesity and high blood pressure are found to be increased particularly among the urban population. Therefore, mass public awareness should be given on such increasing trends of lifestyle associated diseases in order to educate the people. Health facilities and other schemes provided by government should also reach to remote areas to improve maternal and child health. Moreover, active participation of the people and taking full responsibilities in any family welfare programmes and activities equally by both male and female is very much important to achieve the development goals.

REFERENCES

Aimol, K.R., Phukan, M. 2014. "Cultural beliefs associated with pregnancy and childbirth among Aimol tribe of Manipur." *Asian Journal of Home Science*, **9**(1): 11-16.

Baidya, S., Das, R., Deb, D. 2016. "Undernutrition among Reproductive Age Women: A Persistent Public Health Problem in a North-Eastern State of India." *Indian Journal of Nutrition* **3**(2): 136.

Gogoi, M. 2014. "Women Empowerment and Maternal Health Care Utilisation in North-East India." *Journal of North East India Studies*, **4**(2): 69-80.

Government of India. 2011. Census of India 2011: Population Enumeration. Office of the Registrar General and Census Commissioner, India. (http://www.censusindia.gov.in/2011census/population_enumeration.html)

Howard, D.H., Roy, K. 2004. "Private Care and Public Health: Do Vaccination and Prenatal Care Rates Differ between Users of Private *versus* Public Sector Care in India?" *Human Health Services Research,* **39**(6): 2013-26.

Kumar, D., Aggarwal, A., Gomber, S. 2010. "Immunization Status of Children Admitted to a Tertiary-care Hospital of North India: Reasons for Partial Immunization or Non-immunization." *Health Population Nutrition,* **28**(3): 300-304.

Laishram, J., Thounaojam, U.D., Panmei, J., Mukhia, S., Devi, H.S. 2013. "Knowledge and Practice of Ante-natal Care in an Urban Area." *Indian Medical Gazette.* 101-106.

Manjunath, U., Pareek, R.P. 2003. "Maternal Knowledge and Perceptions about the Routine Immunization Programme—a study in a semiurban area in Rajasthan. *Indian Journal of Medical Science,* **57**: 158-63.

Mathew, J.L., Babber, H., Yadav, S. 2002. "Reasons for nonimmunization of children in an urban, low income group in North India." *Trop Doct,* **32**:135-38.

Ministry of Health and Family Welfare (MHFW). Coverage Evaluation Survey, All India Report. 2009.

Nair, T.N.P., Varughese, E. 1994. "Immunization coverage of infants-Rural-Urban difference in Kerala." *Indian Paediatrics,* **31**: 139-43.

Nambiar, A., Singh, K.J. 2017. "A Spatial Analysis of Caesarean birth in Northeast States, India." *Demography India,* 90-97.

Nath, B., Singh, J.V., Awasthi, S., Bhushan, V., Kumar, V., Singh, S.K. 2007. "A study on determinants of immunization coverage among 12-23 months old children in urban slums of Lucknow district, India." *Indian Journal of Medical Science,* **61**: 598-606.

National Family Health Survey (NFHS) India, 2005-06. International Institute for Population Science. Ministry of Health and Family Welfare, New Delhi, 2007.

National Family Health Survey (NFHS) India, 2015-16. International Institute for Population Science, Ministry of Health and Family Welfare, New Delhi, 2017.

National Rural Health Mission (NRHM). District Level Household and Facility Survey 2012-13, Meghalaya. Ministry of Health and Family Welfare. 2013.

National Rural Health Mission (NRHM). Janani Suraksha Yojana (JSY). Ministry of Health and Family Welfare, Government of India. 2005.

Phukan, R.K., Barman, M.P., Mahanta, J. 2008. "Factors associated with immunization coverage of children in Assam, India: Over the First Year of life." *Journal of Tropical Paediatrics,* **55**(4): 249-52.

Ponna, S.N., Upadrasta, V.P., Babu Geddam, J.J., Dudala, S.R., Sadasivuni, R., Bathina, H. 2017. "Regional variation in utilization of Antenatal care services in the state of Andhra Pradesh." *Journal of Family Medicine and Primary Care,* **6**: 231-39.

Purkayastha, P., Singh, K.N. 2017. "Fertility preferences and antenatal check-ups among the rural Khasi women of Ri Bhoi district, Meghalaya, India." *International Journal of Recent Scientific Research* **8**(8): 19423-19427.

Rao, K.V., Mishra, V.K., Retherford, R.D. 1998. "Effects of expo-sure to mass media on knowledge and use of oral rehydration therapy for childhood diarrhea in India. National Family Health Survey Subject Report No.10. Mumbai: International Institute for Population Sciences and Honolulu: East West Center Program on Population."

Sandiford, P., Cassel, J., Montenegro, M., Sanchez, G. 1995. "The Impact of Women's Literacy on Child Health and its Interaction with Access to Health Services." *Population Studies*, **49**(1): 5-17.

Saxena, P., Prakash, D., Saxena, V., Kansal, S. 2008. "Assessment of routine immunization in urban slum of Agra district." *Indian Journal Prev Soc Med*, **39**: 60-2.

Singh, P., Yadav, R.J. 2000A. "Immunization status of children of India." *Indian Pediatrics*, **37**(11): 1194-1199. .

Singh, P.K. 2013. "Trends in Child Immunization across Geographical Regions in India: Focus on Urban-Rural and Gender Differentials." *PLOSONE*, **8**(9): 2013.

Tripathy, J.P., Shewade, H.D., Mishra, S., Kumar, A.M.V., Harries, A.D. 2017. "Cost of hospitalization for childbirth in India: how equitable it is in the post-NRHM era?" *BioMed Central Research Notes*, **10**: 409.

United Nations Department of Economics and Social Affairs (UN DESA). 2015. Population Division, World Population Prospects, The 2015 Revision (DVD edition). New York: UNDESA, Population Division.

United Nations Department of Economics and Social Affairs (UN DESA), Population Division. World Population Prospects: The 2017 Revision, DVD Edition. New York: UN DESA; 2017.

United Nations Population Fund (UNFPA). Girlhood, not motherhood: Preventing adolescent pregnancy. New York: UNFPA; 2015.

Wadgave, H.V., Pore P.D. 2012. "Missed opportunities of immunization in under-fives in adopted area of Urban Health Centre." *Ann Trop Med Public Health*, **5**: 436-40.

World Health Organization (WHO). Maternal Health http://www.who.int/maternal-health/en/. 2016.

World Health Organization (WHO). Maternal mortality. Fact sheet No. 348 http://www.who.int/mediacentre /factsheets/fs348/en/. Updated November 2015.

World Health Organization (WHO). Maternal Mortality. http://www.who.int/news-room/fact-sheets/detail/maternal-mortality, 2018.

World Health Organization (WHO). The Global strategy for women's and children's health. Geneva: World Health Organization; 2010: 7 (http://www.who.int/pmnch/topics/maternal /20100914_gswch_en.pdf

World Health Organization (WHO). World Report on Disability. http://www.who.int/ disabilities/world_ report/2011/report.pdf, 2011.

Yadav, R.J., Singh, P. 2004. "Immunization status of children and mothers in the state of Madhya Pradesh." *Indian Journal of Community Medicine*, **29**: 147-8.

8

Malaria Infection and Malnutrition during Pregnancy

Sanghamitra Pati and *Rajeshwari Sinha*

Introduction

Malaria and malnutrition are two very important health problems that have been impacting global public health since long. In case of pregnant women, both malarial infection and inadequate nutrition are known to severely impact maternal and fetal health. One of the most common infectious diseases today, malaria is caused largely by the parasite *Plasmodium falciparum,* although the infection may also be caused by other parasites such as *P. vivax, P. ovale, P. malariae,* and *P. knowlesi.* In 2017, there were an estimated 219 million cases and 4,35,000 related deaths due to malaria (World Health Organization, 2018). About 15 countries in the sub-Saharan African region and India carried almost 80 per cent of the global malaria burden. Given equal exposure, adult men and women are equally vulnerable to malarial infection. The rate of infection is, however, still higher in pregnant women. Another key barrier in successful pregnancy is malnutrition. Maternal macronutrient as well as micronutrient undernutrition will also substantially impact pregnancy outcomes and neonatal health. Anaemia, which is often used as a proxy indicator for iron deficiency in pregnant women, affected 35.3 million pregnant women in 2016, contributing to a global prevalence of 40.1 per cent worldwide (Development Initiatives, 2018). Presently, there is a growing evidence base that suggests that malaria and malnutrition in pregnant women together interact to worsen pregnancy outcomes. However, a molecular level understanding of the dual effects these two during pregnancy and its impact on maternal health is not very adequately available. The chapter explores the biological basis and linkages between these malaria and malnutrition during pregnancy. Additionally, it also aims to capture available understanding on the mechanism of action that could lead to unfavourable outcomes in pregnant women. In view of improved maternal and child health, an understanding of the interplay between malarial infection and malnutrition in pregnant women would be pertinent, and also aid the design of well integrated and impactful interventions. The chapter focuses on malarial infection largely caused by *P. falciparum*, and both macro- and micro-nutrient undernutrition.

Malaria and Pregnancy

Malaria in Pregnancy (MiP) is known to pose significant risk for both the pregnant mother and unborn foetus. Malarial infection among pregnant women leads to reduced immune response in the mother, as a result of which the infection can spread easily and have severe implications. Pregnant women are said to be more vulnerable and at a higher risk of contracting malarial infection compared to non-pregnant women. This could be because pregnancy compromises a woman's immunity to malaria. In addition to this, female mosquitoes are also attracted to people based on an array of sensory information such as carbon dioxide exhaled, body odour, heat, moisture etc. A study conducted in Gambia found that women at advanced stage of pregnancy exhaled greater volume of carbon dioxide than non-pregnant women (Dobson, 2000). Moreover, pregnant women were also observed to release more volatile substances from the surface of their skin, owing to their bodies being comparatively warmer than women who were not pregnant. Hence, there is greater attraction for mosquitoes by pregnant women.

Upon infection by the *P. falciparum*, erythrocytes infected with the parasite accumulate on the maternal placental vascular space, where parasites replicate. *P. falciparum* parasites export a protein VAR2CSE to the erythrocytes that facilitates its binding to specific ligands in the placenta especially chondroitin sulphate A. The accumulation of infected erythrocytes is at a much higher density as compared to that in the peripheral blood and is often found to sequester the placenta (a phenomenon termed as placental sequestration). This is also followed by number of histological changes such as infiltration of mononuclear cells, deposition of malaria pigment, release of pro-inflammatory mediators etc.

Complications of malaria in pregnancy can be manifested through abortions, premature delivery, low birth weight (LBW), congenial infection, fetal and perinatal death, acute pulmonary edema, still-births, and anaemia (Uneke, 2012; Bauserman *et al.*, 2019). In malaria endemic areas, where infection transmission is high, and women have acquired substantially high levels of immunity, the nature of *P. falciparum* infection during pregnancy is asymptomatic, implying that symptoms of malaria are not readily observed. In this case, the parasites may continue to be present in the placenta and contribute to maternal anaemia in pregnant women even in the absence of a clinical sign of the disease (World Health Organization, 2017). In low-transmission settings, where women of reproductive age have relatively little acquired immunity to malaria, MiP is associated with anaemia, severe malaria, spontaneous abortion, still-birth, prematurity and LBW (World Health Organization, 2017).

Additionally, malaria is also an important contributor to anaemia during pregnancy which leads to LBW (White, 2018). Several mechanisms are thought to be involved in the production of anaemia during malaria, and these include direct hemolysis, accelerated removal of red blood cells in the spleen and retardation of erythropoiesis. In India, 50.3 per cent of pregnant women were found to be anaemic (National Family Health Survey-4, 2015-16).

Malnutrition and Pregnancy

Maternal macronutrient and micronutrients play an important role in maternal and child health. Pregnant women are required to meet their own nutritional needs and at the same time supply nutrients to the growing foetus. The association between maternal dietary patterns and pregnancy and infant outcomes have been studied across many prospective pregnancy and birth cohort population studies. It has been found that women with high intake of vegetables, plant foods, and vegetable oils were at lesser risk of preeclampsia, whereas women with high intake of processed meat, sweet drinks, and salty snacks were at an increased risk (Cetin and Laoreti, 2015). Inadequacies in maternal nutrition during pregnancy, therefore, increase the risk of gestational anaemia, hypertension, miscarriages and fetal deaths, pre-term delivery and maternal mortality (Ramachandran, 2002). Maternal undernutrition also leads to a reduced nutrient supply, due to poor placental formation. As a result, normal blood flow to the placenta is restricted and nutrient supply is decreased.

Malaria-malnutrition Linkages in Pregnancy

There have been few studies that document the relationship between malaria and malnutrition during pregnancy. However, those that are available indicate that the nutritional status of the mother having malaria infection is linked to the low birth weight of fetus (Das *et al.*, 2018; Unger *et al.*, 2016). It is well-accepted that living conditions of populations who reside in malaria-endemic areas, often contribute to poor nutritional status. In addition, various articles shed light on the intricate bidirectional relationship between infection and malnutrition (Katona and Katona-Apte, 2008; Macallan, 2009; Farhadi and Ovchinnikov, 2018).

Nutritional deficiency (due to reduced dietary intake) is associated with poor immune response and impaired body resistance to infection. As a result, a person's susceptibility to infection increases. In addition to immune system dysregulation, inadequate nutrient intake also leads to weight loss, mucosal damage, pathogen invasion, and impaired growth and development. The symptoms can be further aggravated in a sick person, such as diarrhea, loss of appetite, nutrient losses, damage to body's defence mechanisms. In pregnant women with malaria, undernutrition may worsen the already increased susceptibility to the infection and further impair development of protective immunity to malaria. On the other hand, infection can also contribute to malnutrition. Inflammation and sequestration in the placenta due to MiP, as discussed earlier, has been linked to impaired trans-placental transport of nutrients such as glucose, amino acids etc., thus leading to nutritional depletion (Boeuf *et al.*, 2013).

Schaible and Kaufmann (2007), along similar lines, discuss the linkages between protein energy malnutrition (PEM) with compromised immunity, infection and disease, ultimately leading to loss of productivity, unstable socio-economic status and inadequate nutrition. An early publication of the WHO entitled *Interactions of Nutrition and Infection,* outlines that the high prevalence of an infectious disease may affect the nutritional status of a population (Scrimshaw *et al.,* 1968). This is because that the ability of many from the population to produce or earn food supply will be reduced. On the other hand, deficiencies in nutrition will tend to lower the capacity of the host to resist the consequences of an infection. It states that *"when infection aggravates malnutrition or malnutrition lowers resistance to infection, the relationship between the two can be classified as synergistic."*

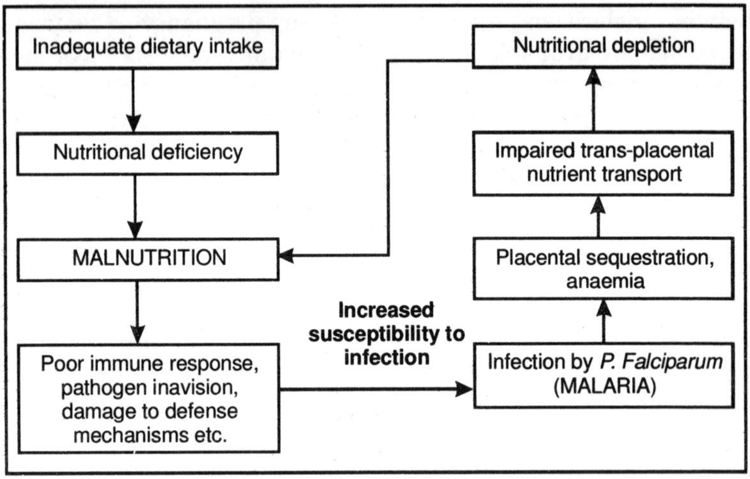

Fig 8.1: Possible linkages between malnutrition and malaria.

A prospective ultrasound study in Democratic Republic of Congo examined the impact of maternal malaria and under-nutrition on intrauterine growth restriction (IUGR). It was found that the risk of IUGR associated with malaria was 2-8 times higher among women with evidence of undernutrition (Landis *et al.,* 2009). Similarly, macronutrient undernutrition and anaemia was found to increase the risk of fetal growth restriction in a malaria-endemic area in Papua New Guinea (Unger *et al.,* 2015). The Maternal Malaria and Malnutrition (M3) initiative attempted to understand the relationship between maternal malaria and malnutrition and their relationship with birth weight. As part of this study, 14,633 singlet on live pregnancies from women participating in 13 studies from 1996-2015 in multiple low and middle income countries were investigated (Cates *et al.*, 2017). The study indicated that pregnant women who were both infected with malaria and malnourished were at a greater risk of babies with low birth weight and reduced mean birth weight of babies, as compared to their counterparts who were well nourished and not infected by malaria infection. However, unlike the WHO view of the infection-nutrition relationship being synergistic, the study under the M3 initiative found it difficult to establish a synergistic linkage between maternal malaria and malnutrition. It mentioned that these two largely acted independently to influence fetal and gestational growth. Micronutrient deficiencies examined among pregnant women with *Plasmodium falciparum* infection in Owo, Ondo State, Nigeria reported a higher prevalence rate of 27.9 per cent for *P. falciparum* infection in pregnant women compared to 3 per cent in non-pregnant women population, but a much higher rate of 47.3 per cent among pregnant women with micronutrient deficiencies (Akinbo *et al.*, 2019).

Nutrition has also been recognized as a key factor in modulating malaria morbidity and mortality. The effects of protein energy malnutrition (PEM), widely prevalent in malarious areas worldwide, substantially increase the public health burden of malaria. Deficiencies in several specific micronutrients such as vitamin A and zinc also tend to aggravate malaria. Shankar (2000) suggests that improvements in dietary intake of both macronutrient and micronutrients are likely to have considerable impact on reducing the burden of malaria.

Malaria-malnutrition Interaction and its Impact on Pregnancy Outcomes: Overview of Possible Mechanisms

Very little is known about the exact mechanisms of nutrients affecting the pathophysiology of malaria infection, or malaria influencing malnutrition. However, there have been some reflections on possible underlying pathways explaining the malaria-malnutrition impact on pregnancy and some of these are discussed here. In a prospective study of pregnant Malawian women, McDonald *et al.* (2018) showed that MiP was associated with lower concentrations of L-arginine and higher concentrations of assymetric dimethyl arginine (ADMA) and symmetric dimethyl arginine (SDMA), which were further linked with adverse birth outcomes. In a model of experimental MiP, L-arginine supplementation led to decreased still-birth and increased birth weight as compared to controls, thereby improving birth outcomes. Building further from this observation, McDonald *et al.* (2018) and Beeson (2018) have shared new perspectives into the mechanisms of LBW caused by malaria and malnutrition. Amino acids constitute one of the important nutrients for fetal growth. Availability of amino acids to the foetus largely depends on maternal supplies and the capacity of the placenta to transport them to the foetus. L-arginine is an essential amino acid in pregnancy and an immediate precursor in the biosynthesis of nitric oxide (NO), which is crucial for endothelial tissue growth and function. Sufficient bioavailabilityof L-arginine and NO are, therefore, key for the proper development of the placental vascular space. Undernutrition in pregnancy can result in a decrease in bioavailable L-arginine, which dysregulates NO biosynthetic pathways, thereby leading to a reduced birth weight. NO generation and bioavailability can also be affected by ADMA and SDMA, which are metabolites found in the blood plasma and act as endogenous inhibitors of NO biosynthesis. An increased concentration of ADMA during malaria in pregnancy can, therefore, reduce NO bioavailability and lead to reduced placental vascular development and function.

Amino acid transport in the placenta, is also regulated by mTOR (mechanistic target of rapamycin) signalling. Placental mTOR signalling is in turn regulated by maternal nutrition and certain other amino acids such as leucine and arginine. With lower levels of bioavailable L-ariginie due to malnutrition, mTOR signalling is inhibited and placental nutrient transport is also reduced. All of this eventually leads to impaired fetal growth and low birth weight. Figure 8.2 gives a schematic representation of the possible mechanistic pathways discussed above.

Unger *et al.* (2016) has also discussed that undernutrition may have a possible role in reducing the immunity imparted by antimalarial antibodies, thereby increasing risk of malaria. Moreover, malaria and malnutrition may also affect the cellular immune responses. While placental malaria causes generation of local cytokine and chemokines for regulating immune responses to infection or inflammation, macronutrient undernutrition has also been associated with decreased T-cell numbers, reduced T-cell activation, implying a leser resistance to infection.

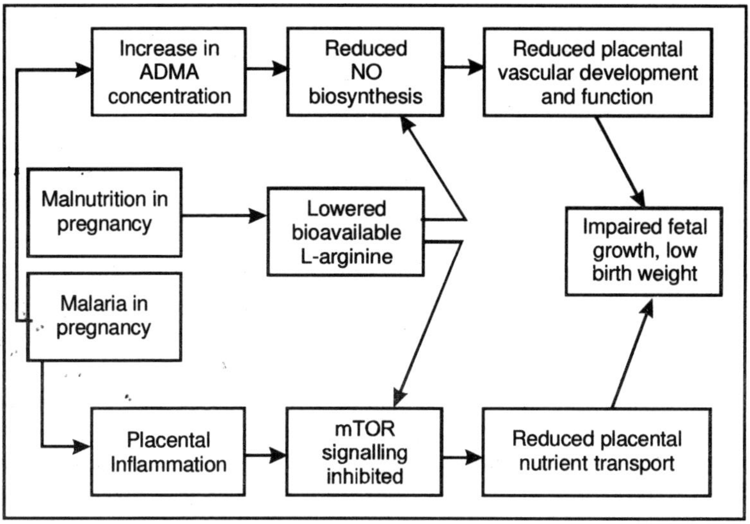

Fig. 8.2.: Mechanistic pathways of malaria and malnutrition during pregnancy leading to adverse birth outcomes [adapted from Beeson *et al.* (2018)]

The immunomodulatory properties of micronutrients such as vitamins A and B complex, zinc, and folate are also likely to play a role in affecting the immunity and pathophysiology of malaria infection (Shankar, 2000). Pathologic processes in malaria could also be influenced by other factors such as effect of the nutrient on the parasite biology or on gene regulation etc.

Addressing Malaria and Malnutrition in an Integrated Manner for Improved Pregnancy Outcomes

The relationship between malaria, malnutrition and maternal health are together complex. A better understanding of the interactions between malaria and malnutrition is essential for the design of optimal and targeted interventions. It is important that selective interventions for malaria and malnutrition are carefully integrated for their timely management and improved pregnancy outcomes.

Prevention of Malaria

Reducing the burden of MiP involves a three pronged approach, namely prevention, treatment and effective case management. The prevention strategies for malaria include vector control (prevention of exposure to mosquitoes) and chemoprevention (use of medication) approaches. Exposure to mosquitoes is largely prevented by the use of insecticide treated bed nets (ITNs) or Long Lasting Insecticidal Nets (LLINs). In 2017, half of people at risk of malaria in Africa were found to be sleeping under an ITN, and about 50 per cent of the African population was protected by this intervention (World Health Organization, 2018). However, the low utilization of ITNs against malaria among pregnant women, possibly be due to lack of awareness or inability to afford them is an issue of concern (Gunasekaran *et al.,* 2009; Odoko *et al.,* 2017; Taremwa *et al.,* 2017; Yitayew *et al.,* 2018). Appropriate awareness campaigns on use and benefits of ITNs need to be carried out while engaging different stakeholders such as the government, community, health-workers. Specific efforts should be directed towards pregnant women to help them understand the risk of MiP and the need to improve uptake of malaria prevention methods.

Another preventive strategy is the Indoor Residual Spraying (IRS), which involves spraying the walls of the households with insecticide to reduce human exposure to mosquitoes. This has also been shown to improve outcomes of MiP. Dichlorodiphenyl-trichloroethane (DDT) formulations have been one of the insecticides used for IRS (Sharma *et al.,* 2005; Hamusse *et al.,* 2012; Kasinathan *et al.,* 2019). However, according to the WHO, IRS protection declined from 5 per cent in 2010 to 3 per cent in 2017 globally, with decreases seen across all WHO regions (World Health Organization, 2018). Strategies for chemoprevention include intermittent preventive treatment in pregnancy (IPTp) which consists of providing anti-malarial medication to all pregnant women beginning in the 2nd trimester. Sulfadoxine-pyrimethamine (SP) has been the drug of choice for IPTp, and IPTp-SP has, therefore, been used by many countries in sub-Saharan Africa (Nwaefuna *et al.,* 2015, Orish *et al.,* 2015; Bouyou-Akotet *et al.,* 2016; Fokam *et al.,* 2016). In malaria endemic areas in Africa, WHO recommends provision of IPTp-SP to all women in their first or second pregnancy as part of antenatal care. Due to increasing resistance of *P. falciparum* to SP, alternative strategies for chemoprevention such as use of artemisinin-based combination therapy (ACT) are, therefore, being tested. Similar to ITNs and IRS, the uptake of IPTp has remained limited. In 2017, only 22 per cent of pregnant women from among 33 African countries received the recommended 3 or more doses of IPTp (World Health Organization, 2018). Barriers to access include the long distances required to travel to reach antenatal clinics, transportation costs, difficulty in accessing IPTp due to stock-outs, lack of awareness or insufficient information provided by health workers. In areas beyond Africa, where malaria transmission is comparatively lower, prophylaxis with mefloquine or chloroquine has been explored.

Treatment of Malaria

The WHO guidelines for the treatment of malaria provide a detailed description of trimester specific and species specific treatment strategies for malaria in pregnant women in first, second and third trimesters (World Health Organization, 2015). For the 1st trimester treatment of *P. falciparum* malaria, a 7-day treatment course of quinine with clindamycin is recommended. Treatment of uncomplicated malaria in the 2nd and 3rd trimester of pregnancy follows the same guidelines as treatment of malaria in non-pregnant adults. Pregnant women in 2nd and 3rd trimesters are also more likely to have severe malaria than other adults. Parenteral antimalarial drugs should be given to pregnant women with severe malaria in full doses without delay. Parenteral-artesunate is recommended for all trimesters, without delay. The WHO guidelines also recommend alternative treatment approaches in case the above recommended treatments are not available.

Addressing Inadequate Nutrition in Pregnant Women

Improved dietary patterns with better macronutrient and micronutrient intakes will be crucial for positively influencing maternal and fetal health during pregnancy. Hence, a healthy and balanced diet for the mother needs to be ensured for safe pregnancy, and for averting the risks of malnutrition. Generation of necessary awareness campaigns on the importance of maternal nutrition before and during pregnancy, education about effects of anaemia during pregnancy, especially among women of reproductive age is necessary for improving health of the pregnant mother. Other strategies such as referral to a better health care service or better management of delivery for pregnant women could be helpful.

Current Efforts in Tackling Malaria and Malnutrition in India

The Ministry of Health and Family Welfare (MoHFW), Government of India, through its National Vector Borne Disease Control Programme (NVBDCP) has been playing a key and continuous role in malaria management and eradication. The National Framework for Malaria Elimination in India (2016-2030) has set an aim to eliminate malaria from India by 2030 in a phased manner (MoHFW). Based on this, the National Strategic Plan for Malaria Elimination in India (2017-2022) provides a roadmap on progress towards malaria elimination (MoHFW). An Operational Manual for Malaria Elimination in India is also in place to assist states and Union territories in transitioning from malaria control to elimination over the next few years (MoHFW). In addition, the NVBDCP also provides several guidelines and training modules for effective management of malaria in the country.

There have been several government initiatives to tackle malnutrition in women. India's National Nutrition Strategy provides interventions for maternal care, health and nutrition (National Institution for Transforming India). These include improved supplementary nutritional support during pregnancy and lactation, improved health and nutrition counselling as part of antenatal care, promotion of iron and folic acid supplementation, consumption of adequately iodized salt and management of severe anaemia. Interestingly, this national strategy also talks about the need for prevention and treatment of malaria as part of community nutrition initiatives. In 2017-18, the Government of India commenced the National Nutrition Mission (also referred to as Rashtriya Poshan Abhiyaan), under the Ministry of Women and Child Development. The Mission will aim to reduce stunting, undernutrition, anaemia and low birth weight among women and children. Similarly, the National Health Mission (NHM) of the Ministry of Health and Family Welfare provides nutrition based interventions through the Reproductive, Maternal, New-born, Child and Adolescent Health (RMNCH+A). The programme seeks to ensure comprehensive and continuous care for women and children. Village Health Nutrition Day (VHND), another major initiative under the NHM, aims to mobilize villagers (especially women and children in rural parts of India) at a common Anganwadi Centre to enable them to interact freely with the local health personnel (Anganwadi workers, Accredited Social Health Activists etc.) and obtain basic services and information. VHNDs, therefore, provide a key platform to create necessary awareness on the importance of nutrition and the need for appropriate maternal nutrition throughout pregnancy.

Conclusion and Future Perspectives

The burden of malnutrition and malaria during pregnancy has been rightfully addressed as a "dangerous dyad" (Unger *et al.*, 2016). A greater understanding of the interaction between these two during pregnancy will add to the growing knowledge base. Further, it will also be helpful for informing policy decisions, and enabling design of targeted interventions in this regard. The present chapter outlines malnutrition-malaria linkages and discusses possible mechanism of action that could lead to adverse birth outcomes. Although strong evidences are yet to emerge, malnutrition and malaria do play a joint role in influencing pregnancy. The chapter also reflects that while new perspectives are emerging, there lies a huge scope for in-depth research to decipher such interactions and their implications in short as well as long term.

Globally, as well as nationally, there is a continued global momentum to addressing these two barriers in pregnancies. Guidelines are in place to tackle the malaria or malnutrition burden in women of reproductive age as well as pregnant women. These are also reflected in national level action plans, programmes or strategies, as evident in case of India. With rigorous efforts by national governments and international agencies, the burden of malnutrition and malaria has declined, but there is still a long way to go. It is important that interventions being implemented through such channels are integrated appropriately, particularly in low and middle income countries which are at a greater health risk. The

WHO's Sustainable Development Goals include ending hunger and malnutrition, as well as ending infections such as malaria. In order to achieve SDGs, nutritionists and malaria experts need to join hands together and come forward to tackle these twin challenges through right policies followed by their timely and effective implementation.

Acknowledgements

The authors are grateful to Dr. P.K Meherda, IAS, Commissioner-*cum*-Secretary, Department of Health and FW, Govt. of Odisha and Dr M.M Pradhan, Additional Director, Dept. of Health and FW, Govt. of Odisha for their valuable inputs.

REFERENCES

Akinbo, F.O., Alabi, L.O., Aiyeyemi, J.A. 2019. "Micronutrient deficiencies among pregnant women with Plasmodium falciparum infection in Owo, Ondo State, Nigeria." *African Journal of Clinical and Experimental Microbiology.* **20**: 127-36.

Bauserman, M., Conroy, A.L., North, K., Patterson, J., Bose, C., Meshnick, S. 2019. "An Overview of Malaria in Pregnancy." *Semin Perinatol.* **43**: 282-290

Beeson, J.G., Scoullar, M.J., Boeuf, P. 2018. "Combating low birth weight due to malaria infection in pregnancy." *Sci Transl Med.* **10**:eaat1506.

Boeuf, P., Aitken, E.H., Chandrasiri, U., Chua, C.L., McInerney, B., McQuade, L., Duffy, M., Molyneux, M., Brown, G., Glazier, J., Rogerson, S.J. 2013. "Plasmodium falciparum malaria elicits inflammatory responses that dysregulate placental amino acid transport." *PLoS Pathogens.* **9**:e1003153.

Bouyou-Akotet, M.K., Mawili-Mboumba, D.P., Kendjo, E., Moutandou Chiesa, S., Tshibola Mbuyi, M.L., Tsoumbou-Bakana, G., Zong, J., Ambounda, N., Kombila, M. 2016. "Decrease of microscopic Plasmodium falciparum infection prevalence during pregnancy following IPTp-SP implementation in urban cities of Gabon." *Trans R Soc Trop Med Hyg.* **110**: 333-342.

Cates, J.E., Unger, H.W., Briand, V., Fievet, N., Valea, I., Tinto, H., D'Alessandro, U., Landis, S.H., Adu-Afarwuah, S., Dewey, K.G., TerKuile, F.O. 2017. "Malaria, malnutrition, and birthweight: A meta-analysis using individual participant data." *PLoS Medicine.* **14**:e1002373.

Cetin, I., Laoreti, A. 2015. "The importance of maternal nutrition for health." *In Proceedings of the 11th International Workshop on Neonatology and Satellite Meetings: From the womb to the adult.* Hygeia Press. **4**: 1-11.

Das, D., Grais, R.F., Okiro, E.A., Stepniewska, K., Mansoor, R., Van Der Kam, S., Terlouw, D.J., Tarning, J., Barnes, K.I., Guerin, P.J. 2018. "Complex interactions between malaria and malnutrition: a systematic literature review." *BMC Medicine.* **16**: 186.

Development Initiatives. 2018. 2018 Global Nutrition Report. Available online at: https://globalnutritionreport.org/reports/global-nutrition-report-2018/, accessed 15 June, 2019.

Dobson, R. 2000. "Mosquitoes prefer pregnant women." *Br. Med. J.* **320**: 1558.

Farhadi, S., Ovchinnikov, R.S. 2018. "The relationship between nutrition and infectious diseases: A review." *Biomed Biotechnol Res. J.* **2**: 168.

Fokam, E.B., Ngimuh, L., Anchang-Kimbi, J.K., Wanji, S. 2016. "Assessment of the usage and effectiveness of intermittent preventive treatment and insecticide-treated nets on the indicators of malaria among pregnant women attending antenatal care in the Buea Health District, Cameroon." *Malar J.* **15**: 172.

Gunasekaran, K., Sahu, S.S., Vijayakumar, K.N., Jambulingam, P. 2009. "Acceptability, willing to purchase and use long lasting insecticide treated mosquito nets in Orissa State, India." *ActaTropica.* **112**: 149-155.

Hamusse, S., Balcha, T., Belachew, T. 2012. "The impact of indoor residual spraying on malaria incidence in East Shoa Zone, Ethiopia." *Glob. Health Action.* **5**: 11619.

Kasinathan, G., Sahu, S.S., Nallan, K., Tharmalingam, V., Swaminathan, S., Behera, K.P., Pradhan, M.M., Purusothaman, J. 2019. "Comparative efficacy of two rounds of indoor residual spraying of DDT 75%@ 1g/m^2 with that of DDT 50%@ 1g/m^2 against the malaria vectors in India." *Acta Trop.* **194**: 123-134.

Katona, P., Katona-Apte, J. 2008. "The interaction between nutrition and infection." *Clin Infect Dis.* **46**: 1582-1588.

Landis, S.H., Lokomba, V., Ananth, C.V., Atibu, J., Ryder, R.W., Hartmann, K.E., Thorp, J.M., Tshefu, A., Meshnick, S.R. 2009. "Impact of maternal malaria and under-nutrition on intrauterine growth restriction: a prospective ultrasound study in Democratic Republic of Congo." *Epidemiol Infect.* **137**: 294-304.

Macallan, D. 2009. "Infection and malnutrition." *Medicine.* **37**: 525-528.

McDonald, C.R., Cahill, L.S., Gamble, J.L., Elphinstone, R., Gazdzinski, L.M., Zhong, K.J., Philson, A.C., Madanitsa, M., Kalilani-Phiri, L., Mwapasa, V., terKuile, F.O. 2018. "Malaria in pregnancy alters L-arginine bioavailability and placental vascular development." *Sci Transl Med.* **10**:eaan6007.

Ministry of Health and Family Welfare. 2015-2016. National Family Health Survey-4. Available online at: http://www.indiaenvironmentportal.org.in/files/file/national%20family%20health%20survey%20-%20India%20fact%20sheet.pdf, accessed 15 June, 2019.

Ministry of Health and Family Welfare[a], Government of India. National Framework for Malaria Elimination in India (2016-2030). Available online at: https://www.nvbdcp.gov.in/WriteReadData/l892s/National-framework-for-malaria-elimination-in-India-2016%E2%80%932030.pdf, accessed 15 June, 2019.

Ministry of Health and Family Welfare[b], Government of India. National Strategic Plan for Malaria Elimination in India (2017-2022). Available online at: https://www.nvbdcp.gov.in/WriteReadData/l892s/nsp_2017-2022.pdf, accessed 15 June, 2019.

Ministry of Health and Family Welfare[c], Government of India. 2016. Operational Manual for Malaria Elimination in India. Available online at: https://www.nvbdcp.gov.in/WriteReadData/l892s/5232542721532941542.pdf, accessed 15 June, 2019.

National Institution for Transforming India, Government of India. Nourishing India: National Nutrition Strategy. Available online at: https://niti.gov.in/writereaddata/files/document_publication/Nutrition_Strategy_Booklet.pdf, accessed June 15, 2019.

Nwaefuna, E.K., Afoakwah, R., Orish, V.N., Egyir-Yawson, A., Boampong, J.N. 2015. "Effectiveness of intermittent preventive treatment in pregnancy with sulphadoxine-pyrimethamine against Submicroscopic falciparum malaria in Central Region, Ghana." *J Parasitol Res.* http://dx.doi.org/10.1155/2015/959427

Odoko, J.O., Nwose, E.U., Igumbor, E.O. 2017. "Utilization of insecticide treated nets against malaria among pregnant women in Southern Nigeria." *International Journal of Research in Medical Sciences.* **5**: 4661.

Orish, V.N., Onyeabor, O.S., Boampong, J.N., Afoakwah, R., Nwaefuna, E., Acquah, S., Sanyaolu, A.O., Iriemenam, N.C. 2015. "Prevalence of intermittent preventive treatment with sulphadoxine-pyrimethamine (IPTp-SP) use during pregnancy and other associated factors in Sekondi-Takoradi, Ghana." *Afr Health Sci.* **15**: 1087-1096.

Ramachandran, P. 2002. "Maternal nutrition—effect on fetal growth and outcome of pregnancy." *Nutr Rev.* **60**(suppl_5): S26-34.

Schaible, U.E., Kaufmann, S.H.E. 2007. "Malnutrition and infection: complex mechanisms and global impacts." *PLoS Medicine.* **4**:e115.

Scrimshaw, N.S., Taylor, C.E., Gordon, J.E. 1968. *Interactions of nutrition and infection.* World Health Organization.

Shankar, A.H. 2000. "Nutritional modulation of malaria morbidity and mortality." *J. Infect. Dis.* **182**(Supplement_1):S37-53.

Sharma, S.N., Shukla, R.P., Raghavendra, K., Subbarao, S.K. 2005. "Impact of DDT spraying on malaria transmission in Bareilly District, Uttar Pradesh, India." *J. Vector Borne Dis.* **42**(2): 54.

Taremwa, I.M., Ashaba, S., Adrama, H.O., Ayebazibwe, C., Omoding, D., Kemeza, I., Yatuha, J., Turuho, T., MacDonald, N.E., Hilliard, R. 2017. "Knowledge, attitude and behaviour towards the use of insecticide treated mosquito nets among pregnant women and children in rural South-western Uganda." *BMC Public Health.* **17**: 794.

Uneke, C.J. 2012. "Malaria during pregnancy: incidence, manifestations, therapy, and prevention." *Current Women's Health Reviews.* **8**: 326-36.

Unger, H.W., Ashorn, P., Cates, J.E., Dewey, K.G., Rogerson, S.J. 2016. "Undernutrition and malaria in pregnancy–a dangerous dyad?" *BMC Med.* **14**: 142.

Unger, H.W., Ome-Kaius, M., Karl, S., Singirok, D., Siba, P., Walker, J., Wangnapi, R.A., Mueller, I., Rogerson, S.J. 2015. "Factors associated with ultrasound-aided detection of suboptimal fetal growth in a malaria-endemic area in Papua New Guinea." *BMC Pregnancy Childbirth.* **15**: 83.

White, N.J. 2018. "Anaemia and malaria." *Malar. J.* **17**: 371.

World Health Organization. 2015. *Guidelines for Treatment of Malaria.* Third Edition. Available online at: https://www.who.int/malaria/publications/atoz/9789241549127/en/, accessed 15 June 2019.

World Health Organization. 2017. *Malaria in pregnant women.* Available online at: https://www.who.int/malaria/areas/high_risk_groups/pregnancy/en/, accessed 15 June 2019.

World Health Organization. 2018. *World Malaria Report 2018.* Available online at: https://www.who.int/malaria/publications/world-malaria-report-2018/en/, accessed 15 June 2019.

Yitayew, A.E., Enyew, H.D., Goshu, Y.A. 2018. "Utilization and Associated Factors of Insecticide Treated Bed Net among Pregnant Women Attending Antenatal Clinic of Addis Zemen Hospital, North-Western Ethiopia: An Institutional Based Study." *Malar. Res.Treat.* https://doi.org/10.1155/2018/3647184.

9

Maternal Mortality Ratio
What Can We Learn from Kerala?

Mitravinda Aneesh

Introduction

Maternal health is a reflection of a nation's overall growth and development. Maternal Mortality Ratio (MMR) of a country speaks volumes about its commitment towards human life. MMR is defined as the number of maternal deaths per 1,00,000 live births due to causes related to pregnancy or within 42 days of termination of pregnancy, regardless of the site or duration of pregnancy. Underdeveloped and developing countries are seen to have higher MMR levels. Worldwide, countries have been striving to reduce the maternal deaths through various means. Taking cognisance of the issue, United Nations introduced Millennium Development Goals followed by Sustainable Developments Goals in an effort to reduce MMR and improve maternal health.

Millennium Development Goals and their Impact

In September 2000, through the United Nations Millennium Declaration, the world leaders committed to eight main goals to be achieved by the year 2015. One of the main Millennium Development Goals (MDGs) was to improve maternal health and reduce child mortality. The MDG had set a target to reduce the maternal mortality ratio by 75 per cent by the year 2015. The global MMR had declined by nearly half from 1990 to 2015. In 1990, the MMR was 385 maternal deaths per 1,00,000 live births. In 2015, this figure had come down to 216 maternal deaths per 1,00,000 live births. The developing nations had achieved a 46 per cent reduction in MMR while the developing nations had brought about 37 per cent drop. Figure 9.1 illustrates the change in the MMR from 1990 to 2013 in the different regions of the world. Among all the nations, the greatest reduction in MMR was seen in Eastern Asia (65%) followed by Southern Asia (64%). Sub-Saharan Africa has been a region with the highest MMR in the world. However, it had made remarkable efforts to be able to bring down the MMR by 49 per cent.

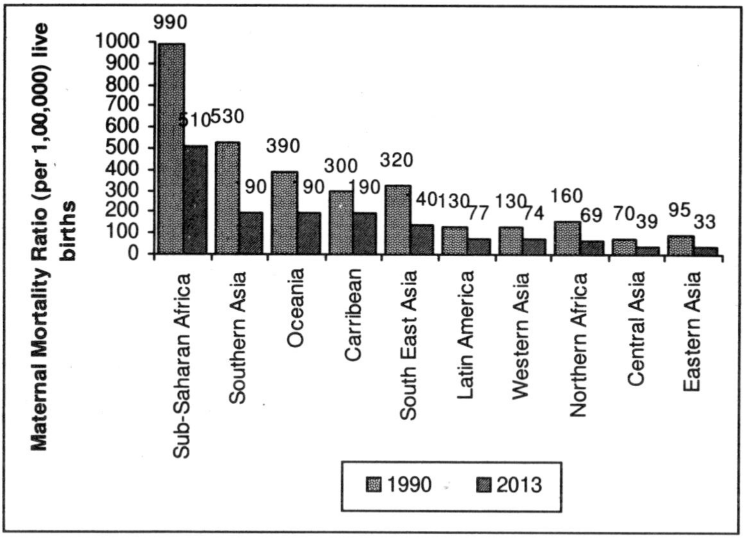

Fig. 9.1: Maternal Mortality Ratio of the different regions of the world in 1990 and 2013 (WHO, 2014).

Though the MDG helped the nations work towards and streamline the strategies to reduce maternal mortality, the high MMR particularly in the developing nations continued to pose a challenge. About 86 per cent of the maternal deaths were found to be concentrated in sub-Saharan Africa and Southern Asia. Therefore, in September 2015, the United Nations General Assembly adopted the 2030 Agenda for Sustainable Development Goals (SDGs). According to the third SDG, by 2030, the global mortality ratio should be less than 70 per 1,00,000 live births.

Global Strategies for reducing MMR

Worldwide, the prime cause for high maternal deaths in developing countries is haemorrhage. Other major complications include – infections, high blood pressure during pregnancy, complications during delivery and unsafe abortions (WHO, 2014). In view of these issues, a number of strategies have been employed to bring down the MMR such as (i) delivery with skilled health professionals, (ii) antenatal care, (iii) use of contraception, and (iv) reducing adolescent pregnancies. There have been steady improvements in the above measures. For instance, there has been a rise in proportion of deliveries attended by skilled health professionals between 1990 (59%) to 2014 (71%). WHO recommends a minimum of four antenatal visits during pregnancy. By 2014, in the developing countries, 52 per cent of pregnant women received the recommended number of antenatal care visit as compared to 36 per cent in 1990. The proportion of women using contraceptive measures to prevent unintended pregnancies rose from 55 per cent in 1990 to 64 per cent in 2014. With regards to birth rate among adolescents, the figure has dropped from 59 births per 1000 girls in 1990 to 51 births per 1000 girls in 2014. However, regional disparities persist in the coverage of these measures. In regions such as sub-Saharan Africa and Southern Asia, only half the numbers of deliveries were attended by skilled health professionals. A little over one-third pregnant women received the recommended antenatal care check-ups in Southern Asia while only 28 per cent of women reported use to contraceptive measures in sub-Saharan Africa. Likewise, large inequalities exist in availability, access and utilization of reproductive health services in urban and rural areas in these regions (WHO, 2014).

Maternal Mortality Ratio in India

High maternal mortality ratio has always been a concern in India. However, there is lack of sufficient reliable and valid estimates to substantiate this. Available reports suggest that India's MMR was 2000 maternal deaths per 1,00,000 live births (GoI, 1946). Since then, there has been a gradual decline in the number of maternal deaths. In the subsequent years, the MMR has came down to 1000, 800 and 500 in the 1950s, 1970s and 1980s respectively (GoI, 1961;

Bhat *et al.*, 1995; Bhat, 2002; Vora *et al.*, 2009). Given the concerns regarding reliability and validity, from the year 1997, the direct estimates of MMR have been obtained from Sample Registration Survey data.

Figure 9.2 shows the trends in the MMR from 1997 to 2016 in India (Rai and Tulchinsky, 2012, Niti Ayog, 2018). From 1997-98 to 2014-16, India witnessed 67 per cent decline in the MMR. India is a diverse country in many facets. This diversity is also reflected in the MMR of different states. In order to understand the regional variations, states with similar MMR were grouped together. Thus,

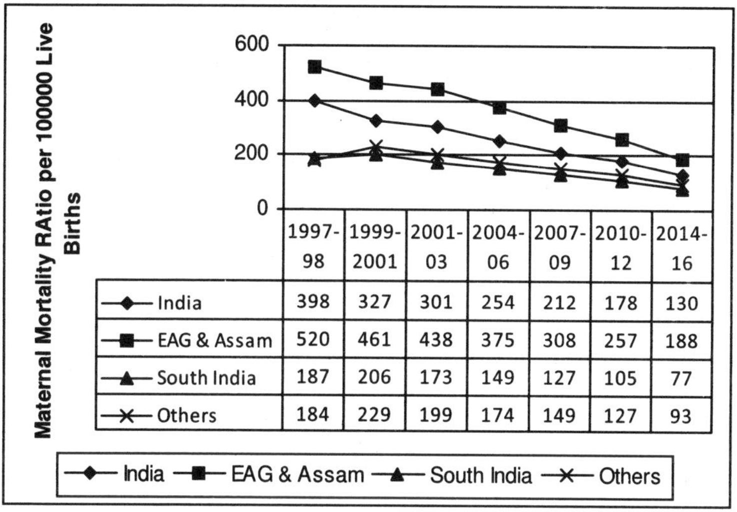

	1997-98	1999-2001	2001-03	2004-06	2007-09	2010-12	2014-16
India	398	327	301	254	212	178	130
EAG & Assam	520	461	438	375	308	257	188
South India	187	206	173	149	127	105	77
Others	184	229	199	174	149	127	93

Fig. 9.2: Maternal Mortality Ratio (per 1,00,000 live births) in India, EAG and Assam, South and Other States (1997–2016).

the states were grouped in to three categories—'Empowered Action Group (EAG)' comprising Bihar, Jharkhand, Madhya Pradesh, Chhattisgarh, Odisha, Rajasthan, Uttar Pradesh, Uttarakhand and Assam; 'Southern' states that includes Andhra Pradesh, Telangana, Karnataka, Tamil Nadu and Kerala and 'Others' comprising Gujarat, Maharashtra, Punjab, West Bengal, other North East states and Union territories.

Empowered Action Group comprises nine states which amount to 48 per cent of the Indian population. These nine states along with Assam receive high focus owing to their poor socio-economic indices coupled with high fertility and mortality rates.

From 1997-98 to 2014-16, EAG and Assam showed nearly 64 per cent reduction in the MMR. Among the states, highest decline during 2004-06 to 2014-16, was seen in the northern state of Uttar Pradesh and Uttarakhand (54.3%) followed by Assam (50.6%) and Rajasthan (48.7%). The Southern states have had a comparatively lower MMR than national average. From 1997-98 to 2014-16, the four southern states witnessed nearly 59 per cent drop in the MMR. In 2014, the state of Andhra Pradesh spilt to form Telangana. The MMR for Andhra Pradesh and Telangana have been presented separately for the years 2014-16. So, the per cent change cannot be computed for these states. Among the remaining, Kerala has always had the lowest MMR in the whole country. During 2004-06 to 2014-16, Kerala showed nearly 52 per cent drop in the MMR with the MMR in 2014-16 being 46 maternal deaths. Karnataka and Tamil Nadu saw a decline of 49 per cent and 40.5 per cent respectively in the years 2004-06 to 2014-16.

The MMR in the 'Other' states dropped by nearly half during 1997-98 to 2014-16. Among these states, during the years 2004-06 to 2014-16, highest reduction in MMR was seen in Maharashtra (53%) while the least was in West Bengal (28%) followed by Punjab (36.4%). The other North-eastern states and Union territories witnessed nearly 53 per cent fall in the MMR. In 2014-16, among all the Indian states, the highest MMR was recorded in Assam (237) followed by Uttar Pradesh/Uttarakhand (201) while the lowest was in Kerala (46) followed by Maharashtra. Three states in India—Kerala, Maharashtra and Tamil Nadu have already attained the SDG of achieving the MMR below 70 maternal deaths per 1,00,000 live births.

Kerala has for long had the MMR lower than the national average. A closer look at the health indicators of the state reveals its high development in comparison to the rest of the nation. What seems to have worked for Kerala is a host of factors including—smaller area (in comparison with the other Indian states), geographic location, excellent socio-demographic indicators, public reforms and most importantly, gender equality.

Kerala—An Example to Follow

Kerala is a unique state located in the southern part of the country. Kerala is surrounded by the Arabian Sea on the west and the

Western Ghats (Sahyadri ranges) on the east. The area of the state is 38,863 sq. km. About 48 per cent of the land is covered by the Western Ghats. This is the place where tea, coffee, spices (mainly cardamom) and rubber are largely cultivated. Besides, in the mainland, i.e. the land between the Ghats and the coast, cashew, arecanut, coconut, banana, tapioca and a wide variety of vegetables are grown. The coastal belt has the most fertile land where rice and coconuts are abundantly grown.

Kerala has a high Human Development Index (HDI) of 0.770 which is close to that of countries like Mexico and Cuba. It is in fact the only state in India with a high HDI. India, on the other hand, has a rank of 130 with HDI of 0.640. This striking difference in the HDI is owing to the socio-demographic, health and economic profile of the state. The high HDI of Kerala reflects high literacy, life expectancy and economic growth. There are several factors which make Kerala stand out. Some of them are given below:

(i) *Poverty*—As per the available data, the per cent individuals below poverty line in Kerala is around 17.4 as compared to the national average of 21.8 (MSME 2015, Ministry of Statistics and Programme Implementation, 2017). Interestingly, the extent of individuals below poverty line in rural Kerala is nearly half of that in urban Kerala (Rural—9.6% *vs* Urban—16.4%) (MSME 2015). This is a strange contrast to the national scenario.

(ii) *Basic Amenities*—Nearly 96 per cent of households receive electricity as compared to 80 per cent households all over India. The electrification of households is even throughout the state irrespective of rural and urban areas. On the other hand, the national figures for electrification of households is much lesser in rural India (73%) *versus* urban India (96%) (Ministry of Statistics and Programme Implementation, 2017). Likewise, 76 per cent of the households in Kerala receive drinking water as compared 56 per cent of the households' country wide. Kerala is better connected by roads than the rest of the country. The road density (km/million individuals) is nearly double in Kerala than the national average (MSME, 2015).

(iii) *Literacy*—Kerala has the distinction of being the state with highest levels of literacy in India. The literacy rate does support this claim. Among males, 94 per cent are literate in Kerala while it is 75 per cent in the whole country. Even among females, 87 per cent women in Kerala are literate while the overall national literacy rate is 53 per cent (MSME 2015, Ministry of Statistics and Programme Implementation 2017)(Fig. 9.3).

(iv) *Gender Equity*—Kerala has a much better sex ratio as compared to Assam, Uttar Pradesh and overall India. As also the per cent share of females in the total population in Kerala is 52 while the India stands at 48 per cent (Ministry of Statistics and Programme Implementation, 2017). The gender inequality in Kerala is dismally low. This is evident in the male and female literacy rates as well. Further, women do hold key decision-making positions. For instance, Kerala is one of the states where women have one-third participation in the local self-government bodies including village-level meetings. Moreover, 10 per cent of the development funds received by local government is supposed to be utilized for development of women is to be managed by female representatives of village council (Kabeer, 2005).

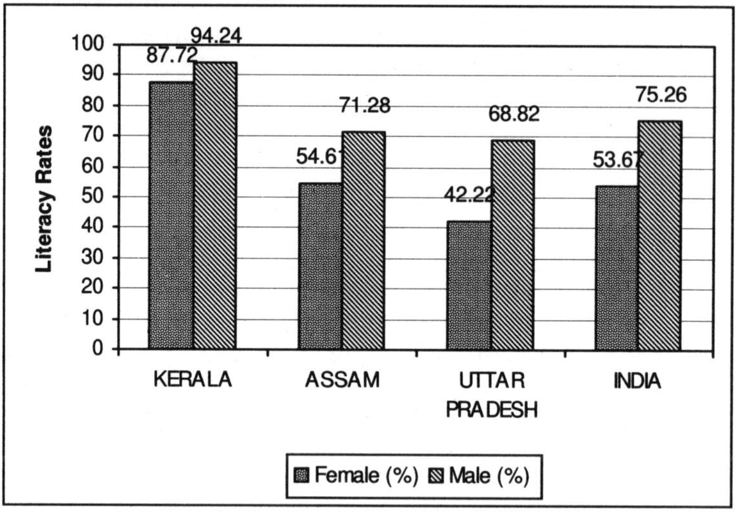

Fig. 9.3: Female and Male Literacy Rates in Kerala, Assam, Uttar Pradesh and India.

Kerala's Health Profile

Owing to the factors discussed in the previous section, Kerala has way better health indicators than the national average and other Indian states (Figure 9.4). The life expectancy of men and women in Kerala surpasses that of India (ICMR, 2017). The infant mortality rate (IMR) of India is thrice that of Kerala (SRS, 2017). The prevalence of stunting (low height-for-age) of India is twice that noted in Kerala (Raykar *et al.*, 2015). The under-five mortality per 1000 live births of India is thrice that of Kerala. In fact, the under-five mortality of certain states such as Assam and Uttar Pradesh are nearly four times that of Kerala (ICMR, 2017). Likewise, maternal mortality ratio in Kerala has met the SDG while most of the other states of India are still long way away.

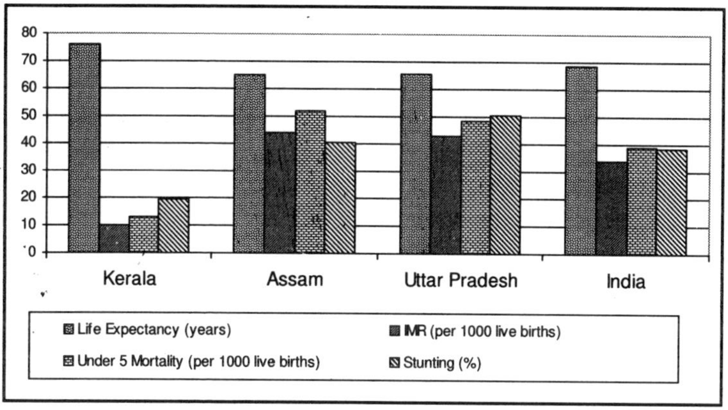

Fig. 9.4: Health Statistics of Kerala, Assam, Uttar Pradesh and India.

The social fabric of the state has contributed immensely to Kerala's progress. This exemplary development of the state in spite of having low per capita income has caught the attention of not only India but also, world over. Kerala's progress and development is unique and has been a subject for study for eminent economists, public health specialists, policy makers and several others.

Kerala Model of Development

Kerala's high HDI is a lesson for the rest of the country. Kerala's experience was noted and documented as early as in 1975 by researchers from Centre of Developmental Studies, Thiruvananthapuram. This example set by Kerala is popularly known as Kerala Model of Development. The model is defined as "Kerala's high standard of living (comparable to US or Europe) at very low per capita income which is only 1/80th of US citizens' per capita income" (Nithya, 2013).

Many factors seem to have contributed to Kerala's development. These include—

(i) Socio-political and socio-religious movements in the pre- and post-colonial era.
(ii) Peasants and workers's movement.
(iii) Role of Christian missionaries.
(iv) Public participation and action (rather than the mere policies) have been pivotal in transforming the state.
(v) Programmes such as Kudumbashree for poverty eradication and women empowerment at village-level.
(vi) Emigration from Kerala to other countries has boosted the per capita income and the overall state economy (Kumar, 2013; Nithya, 2013).

Kerala Model of Development improved the health indicators through its large network of public health care system encompassing Primary Health Centres, Community Health Centres, Taluk/District Hospitals and Medical College Hospitals at the primary, secondary and tertiary levels. This resulted in universal health coverage across the sections of the society. In addition to Modern Medicine, Ayurveda, Homoeopathy, and other alternative systems are also very popular in Kerala.

This model has also drawn some criticism with regards to land-agricultural policies, industrial stagnation which have led to a drop in the per capita income and rise in the educated unemployed. However, these critical views are beyond the purview of this Chapter.

Kerala's Sustained Efforts in reducing the MMR

In 1997, the MMR in Kerala was 54 deaths per 1,00,000 live births. As compared to the national average MMR, Kerala has always fared better. However, from 1997 to 2012, there was no marked improvement in the MMR. This was despite higher rates of institutional deliveries (98%), female literacy (94%) and low fertility levels (1.6%). This prompted the state to look deeper into the issue of maternal deaths. In view of this mounting concern, the Kerala Federation of Obstetrics and Gynaecologists (KFOG) decided to conduct Confidential Review of Maternal Deaths (CRMD). CRMD was modelled on the protocol followed by United Kingdom Confidential Enquiries into Maternal Deaths (CEMD). CEMD is possibly the best example of self-audit and serves as a reference standard for such reviews.

Confidential Review of Maternal Deaths (CRMD)

The Department of Health, Government of Kerala is being supported by KFOG in the maternal death review process. All government and private hospitals in the state were expected to report every maternal death and provide complete case details in a pre-structured format. The format helped in identifying medical issues as also non-medical factors such as education and social characteristics that may be potentially related to maternal deaths. Every death was allotted a code number to maintain the anonymity. Every case report was critically assessed by a team of experts that included practicing obstetricians, physicians, cardiologists, anaesthesiologist and neurologists. The analyses of all the case reports were collated to arrive at the total number of maternal deaths, their causes and measures for prevention of future deaths.

Paily and colleagues (2014) published the findings of the CRMDs between the years 2004 and 2009 indicated as:

(i) Most common causes of maternal deaths were haemorrhage (22.5%) as well as pre-eclampsia and eclampsia (15.6%).
(ii) Guidelines for the management of third stage of labour and hypertensive disorders were not routinely followed.
(iii) Lack of protocols for managing hypertensive disorders in many hospitals.
(iv) Problems in providing round-the-clock medical care at peripheral centres and smaller district hospitals.
(v) Lack of ambulance referral for emergency cases.

(vi) Higher incidence of amniotic fluid embolism (AFE) than other countries. Committee members were suspicious if the doctors were using AFE as a diagnosis to escape the blame of negligence. The diagnostic criteria of AFE were, therefore, well-defined.

(vii) Maternal deaths were also caused by postpartum sepsis. This was possibly due to lack of aseptic practice and adequate policy on the use of antibiotics.

(viii) Among the non-obstetric causes, cardiac disease emerged as one of the leading reasons for maternal death.

Following the CRMD, the below given programmes were implemented on priority basis—

(i) Training of the health care staff for carrying out labour aseptically as per KFOG standard protocols and management of postpartum haemorrhage. KFOG along with NRHM started a certified course of Emergency Obstetric Care and Life Support (EMOCALS) for obstetricians and nurse/midwives.

(ii) Simplified standard protocol for management of postpartum haemorrhage, pregnancy-induced hypertension, eclampsia were disseminated.

(iii) A new technique to manage placenta previa accrete was developed.

(iv) Referral transport services for emergency care.

(v) Availability of life-saving drugs in all the peripheral maternity units.

The entire experience of CRMD received willing participation of the health care staff. One of the main reasons for this was the assurance of confidentiality of the case reports. However, there was little support from the hospital administrative staff owing to the lack of knowledge.

Development and Implementation of Quality Standards

National Institute of Health Care Excellence (NICE), United Kingdom along with Government of Kerala and KFOG were involved in the process of development and implementation of Quality Standards (QS) based on clinical guidelines to reduce maternal mortality. Quality standards were concise sets of prioritised statements in order to facilitate measurable quality improvements (Vlad *et al.*, 2016). They provide "health policymakers, health insurers, service providers, health care professionals and patients with definitions of what high quality health care looks like in practice; and related performance measures that are reliable and meaningful to the local setting in which they are used" (NICE International, 2014). The QS consisted of ten evidence-based guidelines to reduce post-partum haemorrhage (PPH) and pregnancy-induced hypertension (PiH), the two most prominent causes of maternal mortality in the state (Maloney, 2019).

A pilot study was undertaken at eight hospitals in the state. One-day training programme was conducted for the health care providers which addressed issues such as PPH and PIH with emphasis on preventive care outcomes—active management of third stage of labour (AMTSL), measurement of blood loss and fourth stage monitoring. During the pilot study, the value of precise, detailed and explicit QS was appreciated by the participants. However, a few challenges were encountered—insufficient staff, variability in practice (Vlad *et al.*, 2016).

Following this, QS programme was rolled out to 22 hospitals that provided antenatal and delivery services. In the hospitals that were a part of the pilot, improvements were seen in quantitative measurement of blood loss and recording of BP and pulse rate during fourth stage of labour. However, no improvements were seen in the rates of PPH, PiH, pre-eclampsia and eclampsia. Several barriers in the QS implementation were identified such as—lack of infrastructure, storage of qualified staff, adherence to old methods, poor confidence among the staff and lack of equipment needed for the implementation of QS (Maloney, 2019). The report of the roll-out phase puts forth a set of recommendations to counter the barriers noted. In spite of having achieved the SDG, Kerala's sustained efforts in micro-analyses of the problem, identification of barriers, implementation of recommended measures following by monitoring and evaluation should be appreciated.

Strategies by India to reduce MMR

No doubt India has achieved a marked reduction in the MMR. However, it failed to meet the MDG of reducing the MMR by 75 per cent by 2015. Nevertheless, several factors contributed in achieving the reduction in MMR. Government of India schemes such as National Rural Health Mission (NRHM) and Janani Suraksha Yojana (JSY) have contributed immensely in reducing the MMR. JSY's cash transfer policy was successful in increasing the institutional delivery to 78.9 per cent in 2015-16 from 38.7 per cent in 2005-06. Further to this NRHM, increased the number of deliveries by Skilled Birth Attendants, referral services including linkages with the Comprehensive Emergency Obstetric and Newborn Care Centres (CEmONC) centres were also noted to be primary drivers behind the decline in MMR. In spite of this, regional inequalities and inadequate quality health care remain the main barriers (Kansal, 2018). India is now working towards achieving SDG. In its effort towards this goal, Government of India has launched new initiatives Ayushman Bharat, health and wellness centres, Anaemia Mukt Bharat, Poshan Abhiyaan, Labour Room Quality Improvement Initiative (LAQshya), Prime Minister Safe Motherhood Abhiyaan (PMSMA).

Maternal Death Surveillance and Response (MDSR)

Maternal Death Review (MDR) was mentioned in Reproductive and Child Health (RCH) Phase-I (1997–2004), and was subsequently included in RCH Phase-II (2005–2012). However, great disparity has been noted among the states that implemented MDR. A report in this regard by GoI (2018) has identified three gaps—under-reporting of maternal deaths, lack of quality MDR, and absence of response or action taken. In view of this and the WHO guidelines, GoI has revised the guidelines and introduced Maternal Death Surveillance and Response (MDSR) to include surveillance (to improve reporting), response (to improve analysis and action planning) and incorporation of confidential death review. GoI has reiterated that MDSR should not be fault-finding exercise and no disciplinary action would be taken against the service providers (Kansal *et al.*, 2018).

What should India Learn from Kerala?

The Government of India has launched several programmes all throughout the country in an effort to reduce the high MMR. It has even succeeded to a great extent. Nevertheless, there are several factors that have held it back from emulating Kerala. Kerala had achieved what India is now striving to achieve a long way back. Kerala Model of Development is the outcome of superior quality health care with low per capita income. This was feasible mainly due to greater public expenditure/investment in health, public involvement and most importantly gender equality.

Social Determinants of Health care—Gender Equality, Literacy and Women's Empowerment

Gender equality that is displayed by Kerala is unique. It exists across the urban-rural areas and socioe-conomic strata. This equality is reflected in terms of high literacy rates among females and males. Higher education empowers the women to make informed decisions for their own welfare and that of their family. The picture in the rest of the nation is of a complete contrast. In India, the status of women in urban areas seems to be improving lately. Nevertheless, there exists great disparity across the socio-economic sections in the urban areas. The status in rural areas is far grimmer. Women are seldom decision-makers even if it is regarding their own marriage, health or education. Lack of education increases their ignorance regarding matters of finance, health and self-care. Most of them are unaware about the importance of antenatal care, iron-folic acid supplements, tetanus toxoid injections, institutional delivery and pregnancy-related complications. What makes things worse is the ignorance on the part of the husband and/or other head of the family (usually a male). Lack of education also leads to poor self-esteem which makes women believe that they are inferior and do not deserve respect. There are two studies from Uttar Pradesh and North-east states that highlight the presence of obstetric violence (Chattopadhyay *et al.*, 2017, Joshi, 2019). Instances like these, act as a huge deterrent to public utilization of maternal health services.

One of the main challenges faced by EAG states is universal coverage, i.e. to make sure that every pregnant woman receives the antenatal, perinatal and post-natal services. NRHM and JSY with the help of accredited social health activists (ASHA) have been able to increase the number of institutional deliveries. However, many pregnant women directly come to the hospital for delivery without sufficient antenatal check-ups. Antenatal services are crucial in timely identification of women at-risk or with pregnancy-related complications. Timely identification and adequate treatment helps in preventing undue risk to the mother's health and life. Lack of antenatal services or its utilization is one of the major 'delays' that needs to be addressed at the earliest.

Role of Government, International Agencies and Medicos

A strong public health care system is the backbone of Kerala's remarkable success. A well-spread network of primary, secondary and tertiary health centres is pivotal in disseminating timely medical services. High literacy rate and public awareness have contributed to the effective utilization of services to keep up the demand. Both, Central as well as Government of Kerala has introduced a number of programmes in an effort to reduce the MMR. Kerala's strength lies in effective implementation followed by monitoring and evaluation which is crucial to measure the efficacy of the programmes. Timely data collection, analysing, identifying the pitfalls, use of corrective measures and publishing reports in this regard is a proof of their sustained efforts in monitoring and evaluation.

International collaborations with WHO, NICE (UK), CEMD (UK) have provided the required guidance and assistance in planning, development and implementation of Confidential Maternal Death Review and Quality Standards. India is now working towards the implementation of MDSR. India is yet to work to strengthen its public health care network. Uniform distribution of primary, secondary and tertiary health centres in urban and rural areas is imperative. Infrastructure, equipments, trained medical and paramedical staffs are essential for smooth functioning of these centres. Further, timely referral and transport services in rural areas will improve the utilization of services. Empathetic staff and easily accessible services will encourage public to avail the services. All this requires increase in government investment in the health care sector. Along with investment, periodic monitoring and evaluation of the services/programmes will help improve the quality of the overall system. Another crucial factor that has worked in Kerala's favour is the relatively small geographic area which helps in uniform implementation, monitoring and evaluation. Nevertheless, as mentioned earlier, Kerala's untiring sustained efforts have made it possible to attain a low MMR. India has a long way to go. Focus on education, gender quality, universal health coverage with sufficient committed skilled manpower along with adequate infrastructure is the need of the hour. This is not merely the Government's responsibility. Unequivocal support and participation from every section of the society will indeed make a huge difference.

REFERENCES

Bhat, P.N.M., Navaneetham, K., Rajan, S.I. 1995. "Maternal mortality in India: Estimates from a regression model." *Studies in Family Planning.* **26**(4): 217–32.

Bhat, P.N.M. 2002. "Maternal mortality in India: An update." *Studies in Family Planning,* **33**(3): 227–36.

Chattopadhyay, S., Mishra, A., Jacob, S. 2017. "Safe, yet violent? Women's experiences with obstetric violence during hospital births in rural Northeast India: Culture, Health and Sexuality." *Culture, Health and Sexuality.* doi: 10.1080/13691058.2017.1384572.

Government of India. 1946. *Report of the Health Survey and Development Committee.* New Delhi: Manager of Publications.

Government of India. 1961. *Report of the Health Survey and Planning Committee.* New Delhi: Manager of Publications.

Government of India. 2018. *Guidelines for Maternal Death Surveillance and Response.* http://www.nhm.gov.in/images/pdf/programmes/maternal health/guidelines/Guideline_for_MDSR.pdf. Accessed on September 8, 2019.

Indian Council of Medical Research, Public Health Foundation of India, Institute for Health Metrics and Evaluation Disease. 2017. *India: Health of the Nation's States—The India State-Level Disease Burden Initiative.* New Delhi: ICMR, PHFI and IHME.

Joshi, D. 2019. *Women's Experiences of Childbirth: A Study in Rural Uttar Pradesh.* Unpublished Doctoral dissertation. Tata Institute of Social Sciences.

Kabeer, N. 2005. "Gender equality and women's empowerment: A critical analysis of the third millennium development goal 1." *Gender and Development.* **13**:1: 13-24, DOI:10.1080/13552070512331332273

Kansal, A., Garg, S., Sharma, M. 2018. "Moving from Maternal Death Review to Surveillance and Response: A Paradigm Shift." *Indian Journal of Public Health.* **62**: 299–301. doi: 10.4103/ijph.IJPH.

Kansal, A., Kandpal, S.D. 2018. "India's Story of Reducing Maternal Mortality—Achievement so far and Commitments Ahead." *Indian Journal of Community Health.* **30**(02): 107-10.

Kumar S.K. 2013. Kerala Model of Development – Critical Analysis and a Design for the Future. Unpublished Doctoral dissertation. BITS, Pilani.

Maloney, S., Ghosh, R., Jose, J. and Kurian, V. 2018. *Impacts of an intervention to reduce maternal mortality in Kerala, India, 3ie Grantee Final Report.* New Delhi: International Initiative for Impact Evaluation (3ie).

Ministry of Statistics and Programme Implementation. 2017. *Selected Socio-economic Statistics India 2017.* New Delhi: Ministry of Statistics and Programme Implementation.

MSME Development Institute. 2015. *State Profile of Kerala.* Thrissur: MSME.

NICE International. 2014. *Principles for developing clinical Quality Standards in low- and middle-income countries.* London: NICE International.

Nithya, N.R. 2013. "Kerala Model of Health: Crisis in the Neo-liberal Era." *International Journal of Science and Research.* **2**(8):201–203.

Niti Ayog. 2018. *Maternal Mortality Ratio (Per 100000 Live Births).* Available at https://niti.gov.in/content/maternal-mortality-ratio-mmr-100000-live-births. Accessed on August 16, 2018.

Paily, V.P., Ambujam, K., Nair, V.R., Thomas, B. 2014. "Confidential review of maternal deaths in Kerala: a country case study." *BJOG,* **121** (suppl 4): 61–66. doi: 10.1111/1471-0528.13000.

Rai, R.K., Tulchinsky, T.H. 2012. "Addressing the Sluggish Progress in Reducing Maternal Mortality in India." *Asia-Pacific Journal of Public Health,* DOI: 10.1177/1010539512436883

Raykar, N., Majumdar, M., Laxminarayan, R., Menon, P. 2015. *India Health Report: Nutrition 2015.* New Delhi: Public Health Foundation of India.

Sample Registration System. 2017. *SRS Bulletin.* Vol. 51 (1). New Delhi: Registrar General of India.

Vlad, I., Paily, V., Sadanandan, R., *et al.* 2016. "Improving quality for maternal care—a case study from Kerala, India." *F1000 Research.* **5**: 166. doi: 10.12688/f1000research.7893.1.

World Bank. 2017. *Kerala—Indicators at a Glance.* Available at http://documents.worldbank.org/curated/en/339981504162153632/Kerala-Indicators-at-a-glance. Accessed on September 17, 2018.

World Health Organization. 2014. *Trends in maternal mortality: 1990 to 2013. Estimates by WHO, UNICEF, UNFPA, The World Bank and the United Nations Population Division.* Geneva: WHO.

10

Impact of Household Income on Child Mortality among the Pnars and Sakacheps

Junali Kropi

Introduction

Child mortality is a leading indicator of child health and overall development of a nation, as it reflects the social, economic, and environmental conditions in which children (and others in society) live, including their health care (McGuire, 2006). Child mortality may be defined as "mortality or death during the age of one to four years" (Kabir et al., 1995). It has been steadily increased with decreasing socio-economic position but then tended to jump notably amongst the lowest socio-economic strata. Societies with greater differences in income distribution have multiple worse health outcomes that include different causes of death, for example, diseases which are sensitive may be more influenced by income (Birchenall, 2007; Subramanian et al., 2007). The study of child mortality recognition has inspired international organizations as well as national governments to intensify their efforts to lower the level of mortality and raise the level of child survival (Jain and Visaria, 1988). Analysis of various national-level surveys revealed the lower economic condition of the family, was likely to be disadvantaged in terms of child survival (Baruah and Borah, 2017). Several studies confirm the importance of income for child health (O'Hare *et al.*, 2013; Yu *et al.*, 2018, Nguyen *et al.*, 2019). Women of reproductive age in low and middle-income countries are more vulnerable to both communicable and non-communicable diseases than those in high-income countries (Gebretsadiki and Gabreyohannes, 2016). Similarly, there has been the risk of under-five mortality for a child whose mother earns less than her husband is higher as compared with those who earn more. This could be due to the fact that mothers who earn more have the chance to spend money any time they wish without waiting for their husbands to provide care for their child found income of mother to be a determinant factor (Abir *et al.*, 2015). The effect of the age of the mother on child health outcomes has been explored in several studies in low- to middle-income countries (Wang *et al.*, 2009; Raj *et al.*, 2010, Finley *et al.*, 2011, Kirigia *et al.*, 2015, Bazile *et al.*, 2015). In low- to middle-income countries, 26.5 per cent of women have their first birth before the age of 18, and 83.1 per cent before age 24 (DHS, 2011).

In worldwide, 5.9 million children below five years of age died in 2015. The risk of a child dying before completing five years of age is still the highest in the World Health Organization (WHO) Low-income countries reported 76 deaths per 1000 live births, about 11 times the average rate in high-income countries (7 deaths per 1000 live births) (WHO, 2015). A recent systematic review and meta-analysis reported that the risk of child mortality associated with maternal death was 4·1 (95%CI: 2·4–7.0) (Chikhungu *et al.*, 2017). Although the number of under-five deaths worldwide has declined from 12.7 million in 1990 to 5.9 million in 2015–16,000 everyday compared with 35,000 in 1990 (UNICEF, 2015). In spite of this progress, India continues to be the region with the high under-five mortality rates. In the present study, an attempt has been made to understand the effect of the interaction of household income with mother's age on child mortality among the Pnar and Sakachep of Jaintia Hills, Meghalaya.

Material and Method

The present study is preliminary. It was carried out among Pnar and Sakachep tribal communities of Saitsama village in Jaintia Hills district of Meghalaya, North-east India. Meghalaya is a hilly state in North-east India (25°02′ to 26°06′ North latitude and 89°48′ to 92°50′ East longitude). A cross-sectional sample of 197 mothers (112 Pnar; 87 Sakachep) aged 18 to 70 years were included in the present study. The Pnar is one of the Khasi sub-groups, who follow the matrilineal system of society and speak the Mon-Khmer language of Austro-Asiatic language family. Although they still maintain their unique religion called *Niam-Tre*, a majority of the Pnar of Saitsama village have embraced Christianity. On the other hand, Sakachep is one of the Kuki tribes who had lived in Vairengte (Mizoram) and migrated to Tripura around 300 years ago. It is narrated that the Sakachep migrated from Tripura to Meghalaya in the early 19th century. All the Sakachep tribes embraced the Christian religion. The Saitsama village in Jaintia Hills is a village where both the Pnar and Sakachep live together. The Sakachep followed patrilineal whereas the Pnar followed the matrilineal system. The Pnar dialect is the main language spoken by the people in the village. However, the Sakachep have their own dialect without any script, which is akin to Hmar and other Lushai group of languages. Agriculture is the main occupation of both communities. Rice is their staple food and they consume different varieties of vegetables, fish, and meat.

Mortality Data

The nature of data collected was based on parameters suggested by the World Health Organization (1964 and 1968) and Mahadevan (1986). These are as follows: *Individual records, Fertility, Mortality,* and *Socio-economic correlates*. A cross-sectional sample of 197 mothers (112 Pnar; 87 Sakachep) aged 18 to 70 years were included in the present study. The individuals of both the communities found within the age range of 18 to 70 years were grouped under three categories based on their ages for easy assessment classified as people belonging < 35 years, people between the age of 35-45 and the people who are > 45 years. Data on household monthly income were collected directly from the heads of households, using a structured schedule for household economic conditions. The per capita monthly income of the households for classifying the three economic groups (Khongsdier, 1997) as follows:

Above ('X + 4SD/N) = High income group (HIG)
('X – 4SD/N) to (Mean + 4SD/N) = Middle income group (MIG)
Below ('X + 4SD/N) = Low Income group (LIG)

Results and Discussion

Table 10.1 shows the baseline characteristic of the participant in the present study. Out of 197 mothers, there were 112 Pnar and 85 Sakachep tribes which composed of 56.85 per cent and 43.15 per cent of the total participant respectively. The Table shows that about 55.84 per cent, 17.77 per cent and 26.40 per cent of the mothers belong to the age group >35 years, 35 – 45 years and < 45 years respectively.

Table 10.1: Baseline characteristics of participants

Characteristic	*Number/Percentage*
Community	
Pnar	112 (56.85)
Sakachep	85 (43.15)
Age Group	
<35	110 (55.84)
35-45	35 (17.77)
>45	52 (26.40)
Income Group	
Lower Income Group	87 (44.16)
Middle Income Group	52 (26.40)
High Income Group	58 (29.44)
Reproductive history of mother	
Number of Live Birth	961
Number of Child Mortality	38

With regard to income group, about 44.16 per cent, 26.40 per cent and 29.44 per cent of the mothers belong to LIG, MIG, and HIG respectively. The Table also shows the reproductive history of the mothers where live birth and child mortality accounted as 961 and 38 in number respectively.

Table 10.2 shows the percentage frequency of child mortality among the Pnar and Sakachep mother. The overall child mortality percentage of both the population is 3.95 per cent. It is observed from the Table that the child mortality percentage is higher among the Pnar (5.02%) than the Sakachep (2.59%). However, the Chi-square test indicates no statistical significance between the Pnar and Sakachep (χ^2=2.66, df=1, p>0.05).

Table 10.2: Child Mortality among the Pnar and Sakachep

Tribe	*No. of mother*	*No. of Live birth*	*Child Mortality*	*Child Mortality (%)*
Pnar	112	537	27	5.02
Sakachep	85	424	11	2.59
Total	197	961	38	3.95

χ^2=2.66, df= 1, p>0.05

Table 10.3 shows the percentage frequency of child mortality among the Pnar and Sakachep by the mother's age group which is divided into three age group, i.e. <35 years, 35-45 years and >45 years respectively. Among the Pnar, the percentage of child mortality whose age is >35, 35-45 and >45 years were 5.31 per cent, 5.10 per cent, and 4.74 per cent respectively. About 3.09 per cent, 3.64 per cent and 1.32 per cent of child mortality occurred among the Sakachep mother whose age group belongs to >35, 35-45 and above 45 years respectively. The child mortality percentage is observed higher in the age group below 35 years among the Pnar mother, however, in the case of Sakachep, it is higher in 35-45 years of age group. The χ^2 test indicates that mother's age group is insignificant in both Pnar (χ^2= 2.93, df=2, p>0.5) and Sakachep (χ^2= 0.89, df=2, p>0.5) mothers respectively.

Table 10.3: Child Mortality by mother's age group

Age group	*No. of mother*	*No. of Live birth*	*Child Mortality*	*Child Mortality (%)*
Pnar				
<35 years	66	207	11	5.31
35–45 years	15	98	5	5.10
>45 years	31	232	11	4/74
χ^2= 2.93, df= 2, p>0.05				
Sakachep				
<35 years	44	162	5	3.09
35–45 years	20	110	4	3.64
>45 years	21	152	2	1.32
χ^2 =0.89, df = 2 , p>0.05				

Table 10.4 shows the percentage frequency of child mortality by household income group. Among the Pnar, there were 35

mothers, 34 mothers and 43 mothers belonging to the category of LIG, MIG, and HIG respectively. The child mortality percentage is higher among mothers belonging to LIG (6.70%), followed by MIG (5.46%) and HIG (2.06%). The chi-square χ^2 test shows its statistical significant (χ^2=7.82, df =2, p<0.5).

Table 10.4: Child Mortality by mother's income group

Income group	*No. of mother*	*No. of Live birth*	*Child Mortality*	*Child Mortality (%)*
Pnar				
LIG	35	209	14	6.70
MIG	34	182	10	5.46
HIG	43	146	3	2.06
χ^2= 7.82, df = 2 , p<0.05				
Sakachep				
LIG	52	291	8	2.75
MIG	18	86	2	2.33
HIG	15	47	1	2.13
χ^2= 0.68, df = 2 , p>0.05				

It is also revealed from the Table that about 52, 18 and 15 Sakachep mothers belong to LIG, MIG, and HIG respectively. Similarly, like the Pnar, the child mortality percentage is found to be higher among the women belonging to the category of LIG (2.75%), followed by MIG (2.33%) then HIG (2.13%) respectively. However, the χ^2 test indicates it is not statistically significant among the Sakachep (χ^2= 1.65, df=2, p>0.5).

Table 10.5 shows the results of the analysis of variance on the effect of age and household income on child mortality. Although, in Table 10.4 the chi-square shows statistically significant in income among the Pnar mothers, however, the effect of income is insignificant after controlling the effect of age in Table 10.5 (F=2.10, p>0.05). The eta^2 shows that about 0.039 or 3.9 per cent of the variance accounted for by household income whereas age accounted for only 0.010 or 1 per cent of the variance in child mortality respectively. Further, the Table also shows the interaction between age and income (age+ income) accounted for about 4.8 per cent (F=1.29, p>0.05) on child mortality respectively.

In the case of Sakachep, there is no statistical significance with age (F = 1.29, p>0.05) and income (F=0.55, p.0.05). The eta^2

Table 10.5: Results of the analysis of variance on the effect of age and household income on child mortality

Source of variance	*Sum of squares*		*df*		*Mean sum of squares*		*F- value*		*p-value*		*Eta²*	
	Pnar	*Sakachep (Skp)*	*Pnar*	*Skp*	*Pnar*	*Skp*	*Pnar*	*Skp*	*Pnar*	*Skp*	*Pnar*	*Skp*
Age	0.42	0.08	2	2	0.21	0.04	0.55	0.89	0.58	0.75	0.010	0.007
Income	1.62	0.16	2	2	0.81	0.08	2.10	0.55	0.13	0.58	0.039	0.014
Age+Income	2.10	0.36	4	4	0.50	0.09	1.29	0.62	0.28	0.62	0.048	0.031
Error	39.78	10.99	103	76	0.39	0.45						
Total	44.99	11.58	111	84								

shows that about 0.014 or 1.4 per cent of the variance accounted for by household income and age accounted for 0.7 per cent of the variance respectively. The interaction between household income and age (Income+age) accounted for by 3.1 per cent respectively. It is observed that after controlling the effect of age and income, the variation shows higher among the Sakachep. However, compared to their counterpart, the effect of age and income on child mortality is lower among the Sakachep than the Pnar.

Discussion

The absolute risk of poor child health outcomes is lower when mothers are in a high SES household, there remains a high RR of poor child health outcomes for young mothers even in high SES households. The persistence of the age gradient across the SES groups highlights that child and maternal health issues associated with the age of the mother cut across socio-economic lines and the children of young rich women are not shielded from the RR of a poor health outcome. This indicates that the biological immaturity of young mothers also affects child health outcomes in addition to the social disadvantage young mothers often face (Finlay *et al.*, 2011). In the present study, mother's age has statistically insignificant in both the study population with regard to child mortality which may be attributed due to the rural setting of the environment. Better income promotes access to better health care which in turn lowers child mortality. Studies have shown that low economic status is associated with increased rates of child mortality (Gwatkin *et al.*, 2007; Wagstaff, 2000).

The trend of child mortality percentage decreases with increasing income among the Pnar and Sakachep. The present population is consistent with the studies reported among the rural Kabui Naga of Manipur (Kamei, 2017), Idu Mishmi of Arunachal Pradesh (Das and Das, 2017), Jaintias of the Meghalaya (Limbu *et al.*, 2017). Among the Pnar mothers although age had no significant effect on child mortality it appears that the interaction effect with household income on child mortality cannot be totally ignored as the present study shows that about 3.9 per cent of the variance accounted for by household income whereas age accounted only 1 per cent of the variance in child mortality respectively. Further, the interaction between age and income (age+income) accounted for about 4.8 per cent ($F=1.29$, $p>0.05$) on child mortality respectively. The Sakachep mothers, on the other hand, had no significant effect on age and income but the effect of variance is observed more when both age and income are taken into account. There is about 1.4 per cent of the variance accounted for by household income and age accounted for 0.7 per cent of the variance respectively. The interaction between household income and age (Income+age) accounted for by 3.1 per cent respectively. The nature of variation on child mortality in LIG was higher than the middle and high-income groups in both the study population. It is observed that after controlling the effect of age and income, the variation shows higher among the Sakachep but when both the population is taken into consideration, the effect of age and income on child mortality is lower among the Sakachep than the Pnar.

Conclusion

The present study suggests that the effect of the interaction between household income and age on child mortality is more clearly perceptible more among the Pnar than the Sakachep mothers. In other words, children born to mothers who were in better economic conditions had higher survival rates when compared between the two study populations. It also provides us with a comprehensive database of two heterogeneous ethnic groups living in the same geographical conditions that have very close relations with each other. However, it was not clear from the data to what extent the beneficial effect resulted from maternal socio-economic status. As the study could not adjust the analysis for disease-specific risk factors of the children and the health status of mothers, the association remains subject to further exploration. Nonetheless, the findings provide important insight into health policymakers in the country. Future studies should focus on assessing the relationship by including a more diverse range of maternal and child health-related variables among the women of North-east India. Therefore, governments, the private sector and development partners should in solidarity sustainably and equitably provide the resources necessary to build resilient national health systems and structures affecting the determinants of health to facilitate the provision of basic needs to end preventable child morbidity and mortality.

REFERENCES

Abir, T., Agho, K.E., Page, A.N., Milton, A.H., Dibley, M.J. 2015. "Risk factors for under-5 mortality: evidence from Bangladesh Demographic and Health Survey, 2004-2011." *BMJ Open.* **5**(8):e006722.

Baruah, R., Borah, M. 2017. "Social determinants of morbidity during infancy: Results from a cross-sectional study in rural areas of Assam, India." *Indian J Child Health.* **4**(1): 79-84.

Bazile, J., Rigodon, J., Berman, L., Boulanger, V.M., Maistrellis, E., Kausiwa, P., Yamin, A. 2015. "Intergenerational impacts of maternal mortality: Qualitative findings from rural Malawi." *Reprod Health.* 12 Suppl **1**:S1.

Birchenall, J.A. 2007. "Economic development and the escape from high mortality." *World Development.* **35** (5): 43–68

Chikhungu, L.C., Newell, M.L., Rollins, N. 2017. "Under-five mortality according to maternal survival: a systematic review and meta-analysis." *Bull World Health Organ.* **95**(4): 281–287.

Das, N.K., Das, R. 2017. "Assessment of Demographic and Socio-economic Factors on Child Mortality by Using Verbal Autopsy." *In Child Health in India.* New Delhi, Omsons Publications. pp. 42-52.

Finlay, J.E., Özaltin, E., Canning, D. 2011. "The association of maternal age with infant mortality, child anthropometric failure, diarrhea and anaemia for first births: evidence from 55 low- and middle-income countries." *BMJ Open.* **1**(2):e000226.

Gebretsadik, S., Gabreyohannes, E. 2016. "Determinants of Under-Five Mortality in High Mortality Regions of Ethiopia: An Analysis of the 2011 Ethiopia Demographic and Health Survey Data." Hindawi Publishing Corporation. *Intern. J. Pop. Res.* 1602761.

Gwatkin, D.R., Johnson, S.R., Suliman, K.E., Wagstaff, A., Amouzou, A. 2007. *Socio-economic Differences in Health, Nutrition and Population within Developing Countries: an Overview,* The World Bank, Washington DC.

ICF Macro. "DHS final reports." In: *DHS M,* ed. Calverton 2011.

Jain, K.A., Visaria, P. 1988. *Infant Mortality in India: Differentials and Determinants.* New Delhi: Sage Publications.

Kabir, M., Chowdhury, R.I., Amin, R. 1995. "Infant and child mortality levels and trends in Bangladesh." *Journal of Bio-social Science.* **27**(2): 179-192.

Kamei, C. 2017. "Influence of Demographic and Socio-economic Factors on Infant and Child Mortality among the Rural Kabui Nagas of Manipur." In *Child health in India.* New Delhi, Omsons Publications: 112-119.

Khongsdier, R. 1997. "The War Khasi of Meghalaya: Implication of variation in adult body dimensions." *Journal of Human Ecology,* Vol.**6**: 299-305.

Kirigia, J.M., Muthuri, R.D., Nabyonga-Orem, J., Kirigia, D.G. 2015. "Counting the cost of child mortality in the World Health Organization African region." *BMC Public Health.* **15**:1103.

Limbu, D.K., Khual, G.K., Syngkon, H. 2017. "Influence of Biosocial Factors on Child Mortality among the Jaintias of the Jaintia Hills District, Meghalaya." In *Child health in India.* New Delhi, Omsons Publications. pp. 87-96.

Mahadevan, K. 1986. *Mortality, Biology and Society: Analytical, Framework and Conceptual Model.* New Delhi; Tejeswar Singh for Sage Publication Pvt. Ltd. pp. 239-287.

McGuire, J.W. 2006. "Basic health care provision and under-5 mortality: a cross-national study of developing countries." *World Development.* **34**(3): 405–425.

Nguyen, D.T.N., Hughes, S., Egger, S., Scott LaMontagne, D., Simms, K., Castle, P.E., Canfell, K. 2019. "Risk of childhood mortality associated with death of a mother in low and middle-income countries: a systematic review and meta-analysis." *BMC Public Health.* **19:** 1281

O'Hare, B. Makuta, I., Chiwaula, L, Bar-Zeev, N. 2013. "Income and child mortality in developing countries: a systematic review and meta-analysis." *J R Soc Med.* **106**(10): 408-414.

Raj, A., Saggurti, N., Winter, M., Labonte, A., Decker, M.R., Balaiah, D., Silverman, J.G. 2010. "The effect of maternal child marriage on morbidity and mortality of children under 5 in India: cross-sectional study of a nationally representative sample." *BMJ.* **340**: b4258.

Subramanian, S., Kawachi, I., Smith, G.D. 2007. "Income inequality and the double burden of under-and overnutrition in India." *J Epidemiol Community Health.* **61**(9): 802-809.

Wagstaff, A. 2000. "Socio-economic inequalities in Child Mortality: Comparisons across Nine Developing Countries." *Bull World Health Organ.* **78**(1): 19-29.

Wang, S.C., Lee, S.H., Lee, M.C., Wang, L. 2009. "The effects of age and aboriginality on the incidence of low birth weight in mountain townships of Taiwan." *J. Public Health (Oxf).***31**:406-412.

WHO, 1968. Research in human population genetics. WHO technical report series No. 387. Geneva: WHO.

WHO, 1964. Research in population genetics of primitive groups. WHO Technical Report Series No. 279. Geneva: WHO.

World Health Organization, Report, Global health observatory (GHO) data. 2015.

Yu, F., Yan, Z., Pu, R., Tang, S., Ghose, B., Huang, R. 2018. "Do Mothers with Lower Socio-economic Status Contribute to the Rate of All-Cause Child Mortality in Kazakhstan?" *BioMed Research International.* 3629109.

SECTION-III

Reproductive Health, Indigenous Healthcare Practices and Health Services

11

Reproductive Health of Angami Naga Challenges and Issues

Viserano Peseyie and *Sudipta Ghosh*

Introduction

Reproductive health represents a state of complete physical, mental and social well-being, and not merely the absence of reproductive diseases or alterations. It involves all of the reproductive processes, functions and systems at all stages of human life. Both men and women have the right to be informed and to have access to safe, effective, affordable and acceptable methods of family planning of their choice that are not against the law (UN, 1995; WHO, 2009). Women's right to the enjoyment of the highest standard of health must be secured throughout the life cycle in equality with men. Women are affected by many of the same health conditions as men, but women experience them differently (UN, 1995). Furthermore, men and women should have access to appropriate health care services that will enable women to go safely through pregnancy and childbirth, as well as to provide couples with the best chance of having a healthy infant (UN, 1995). Reproductive health is a universal concern, but is of special importance for women particularly during the reproductive years. Women's health during the reproductive or fertile years (between the ages of 15 and 49 years) is relevant not only to women themselves, but also has an impact on the health and development of the next generation. Many of the health challenges during this period are ones that only young girls and women face (WHO, 2009). Women's health involves their emotional, social and physical well-being and is determined by the social, political and economic context of their lives, as well as by biology. However, health and well-being elude the majority of women. A major barrier for women in achieving the highest attainable standard of health is inequality, both between men and women and among women in different geographical regions, social classes and indigenous and ethnic groups. Reproductive health is a fundamental component of an individual's overall health status and a central determinant of quality of life (UN, 1995; WHO, 2009). It is intricately linked to issues of women's and children's health, the spread of sexually transmitted diseases, poverty, education, gender equality and human rights (UN, 1995). Reproductive health is thus, a condition in which the reproductive process is accomplished in a state of complete physical, mental and social well-being and is not merely the absence of disease or disorders of the reproductive process (UN, 1995; Fathalla, 1997). With these important issues about reproductive health in mind, the present chapter aims to understand the reproductive health and related issues in Angami Naga women.

Materials and Methods

The Angami Naga are an indigenous population from Kohima and Dimapur districts of Nagaland, North-East India. The morphological traits of Angami reflect Mongoloid characteristics in general. Linguistically, they come under the group of Tibeto-Burman family. The Angami society is patriarchal and patrilineal society. Data was collected from 42 ever married Angami women of Jotsoma Village, Kohima district, Nagaland, using simple random sampling method. The participants those were interviewed were in their reproductive age ranging from 21-48 years. These women were informed about voluntary participation and their right to withdraw at any time during the study without giving any reason to do so. Written and oral information regarding the study was given and also written informed consent was obtained from all the women who volunteered for this study. They were assured of anonymity and confidentiality about their identity throughout the study. Information was collected using both closed and open ended questionnaires. Basic socio-demographic data was collected from all the participants. Reproductive health related questions like age at menarche, menstrual cycle details, age at marriage, age at first childbirth, maternity history, use of contraceptive methods for prevention of pregnancy were asked to each participant. The questions pertaining to women's perceptions, opinions and attitudes towards family planning were open-ended.

Results and Discussion

The reproductive characteristics of Angami Naga women reveal that mean age of attaining menarche is 15.00±2.16 years and the range is generally between 12-18 years of age (Table 11.1). More than half of the participants (61.90%) had attained menarche at the age of 14 years (Figure 11.1). It is evident from the results that Angami Naga is similar with Anal (14.94 years, Khiloni, 2009); Mao Naga (14.59 years, Maheo, 2004); Ao Naga (15 years, Purnungla and Sengupta, 2002) and Kabui Naga (15.40 years, Singh, 2006) in attaining menarche. However, the mean ages at menarche among Indian women in general (13.76 years, Pathak *et al.*, 2014) and the Meitei women (13.60 years, Singh, 2006) are earlier than Angami Naga. The mean age at marriage of these women are found to be 26.50±5.34 years ranging from 18-35 years of age (Table 11.1); which is later than the Anal (22.4 years, Khiloni, 2009), Kabui Naga (20.0 years) and Meitei of Manipur (19.98 years) (Singh, 2006). Correspondingly, the mean age at first child birth among Angami women is found to be 27.00±5.63 with range from 18-36 years of age (Table 11.1). However, many of the participants (16.67%) had their age at marriage at the age of 23 years (Figure 11.2). Similarly, majority of the participants (21.43%) had their first child birth at the age of 24 years (Figure 11.3). The mean for total number of pregnancies from all the participants is 3.50±1.87 with a range from 1-6 pregnancies (Table 11.1). For women with more than one child, the mean of duration between pregnancies is 5.50±3.03 and the range is generally found to be between 1-10 years between two pregnancies (Table 11.1).

Table 11.1: Reproductive characteristic of Angami Naga women

Variables	*Mean*	*Standard deviation*	*Minimum*	*Maximum*
Age at menarche (years)	15	2.16	12	18
Age at marriage (years)	26.5	5.34	18	35
Age at first child birth (years)	27	5.63	18	36
Total number of pregnancies (no.)	3.5	1.87	1	6
Duration between pregnancies (years)	5.5	3.03	1	10

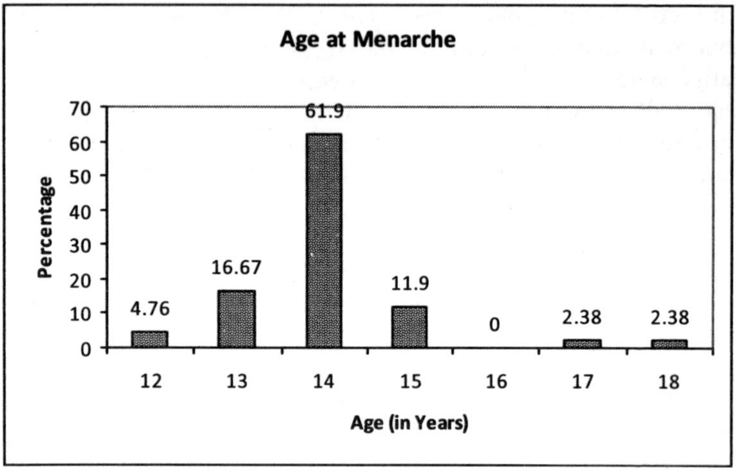

Fig. 11.1: Frequency distribution of age at menarche of Angami Naga

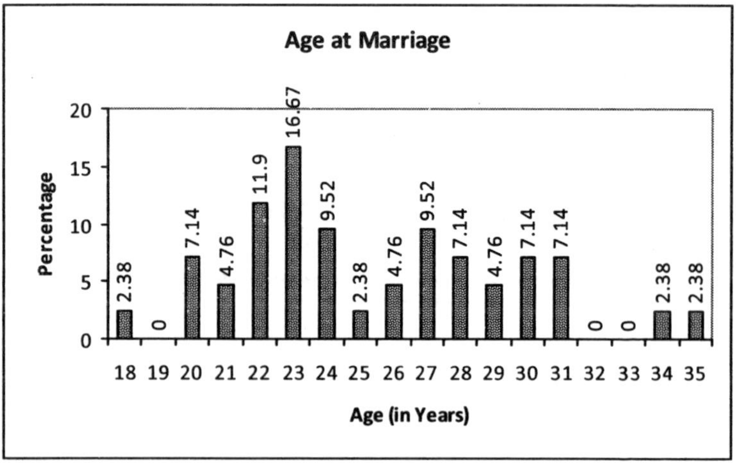

Fig. 11.2: Frequency distribution of age at marriage of Angami Naga

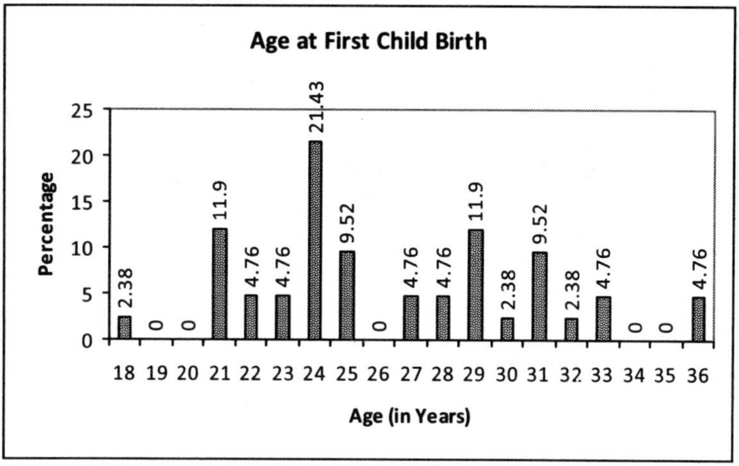

Fig. 11.3: Frequency distribution of age at first childbirth among Angami Naga.

The women in general, reported that their menstrual bleeding days lasts for 4 (38.10%) or 5 (33.33%) days (Table 11.2). During menstruation (Table 11.3), the common illness reported by the women includes backache (14.29%), headache (4.76%), abdominal cramping (42.86%) and fatigue (4.76%). Some reported abdominal cramping and backache (16.67%), backache and headache (2.38%), fatigue with headache (2.38%) and also abdominal cramping and backache with poor appetite (2.38%). Only few women (9.52%) reported of not suffering such menstrual illness (Table 11.3). Almost all the participants (92.86%) reported negative intake of any painkillers during menstruation. However, very few women (7.14%) reported the use of painkillers during menstrual period.

Table 11.2: Menstruation cycle of Angami women

Number of bleeding days	*Frequency*	*Percentage*
3	9	21.43
4	16	38.10
5	14	33.33
6	2	4.76
7	1	2.38

Table 11.3: Menstrual illnesses and related issues among Angami Naga women

Menstrual Illnesses and Related Issues	*Frequency*	
	*Yes**	*No**
Menstrual period without any illness	4 (9.52)	38 (90.47)
Usage of painkillers during period	3 (7.14)	39 (92.86)
Backache	6 (14.29)	36 (85.71)
Headache	2 (4.76)	40 (95.24)
Abdominal cramping	18 (42.86)	24 (57.14)
Fatigue	2 (4.76)	40 (95.24)
Abdominal cramping, backache	7 (16.67)	35 (83.33)
Backache, headache	1 (2.38)	41 (97.62)
Fatigue, backache	1 (2.38)	41 (97.62)
Weak appetite, abdominal cramping, backache	1 (2.38)	41 (97.62)

* Percentages are given in the parentheses.

Regarding the use of contraceptives, Chandhik *et al.* (2003) in a survey conducted by Indian Council of Medical Research (ICMR) reported that many potential informational barriers exist to contraceptive use. It is important that women must be aware of the methods available, know where supplies of these methods can be obtained and they must know how to use the method they choose because lack of such knowledge is strongly associated with unmet need for contraception. With regard to family planning and use of contraceptive method in the present study, only one woman (2.38%) reported use of contraceptive method for prevention of pregnancy (Table 11.4). All the participants (100%) have mentioned

Table 11.4: Use of contraceptive methods among Angami Naga women

Variables	*Frequency*	
	*Yes**	*No**
Have you ever used any contraceptive method?	1 (2.38)	41 (97.62)
Do you think you can afford use of contraceptive method?	42 (100.00)	0 (0.00)
Support of husband for its use	41(97.62)	1 (2.38)
Do not use for religious reasons	1 (2.38)	41 (97.62)
Do not use for fear of side effects	11 (26.19)	31 (73.81)
Do not use for health problems	1 (2.38)	41 (97.62)
Inconvenient to use	19 (45.24)	23 (54.76)
Any other personal reasons	7(16.67)	35 (83.33)

* Percentages are given in the parentheses.

that they could afford the use of contraceptive method. However, on the basis of the use of contraceptive method with the knowledge of their husband and his opinion or support for its use; majority (97.62%) reported their husband's approval for its use if need be. Whereas, one participant (2.38%) said that her husband disapproves of the use of such methods for prevention of pregnancy. Nearly half of the participants (45.24%) found it inconvenient to use contraceptives while, some do not use such methods for fear of side effects (26.17%). Further, few do not practice these methods for religious reasons (2.38%) and for certain health conditions (2.38%) which was not disclosed. Also, few women (16.67%) did not disclose the reason for not adopting any contraceptive method. Thus, agreeing that knowledge and awareness does not always lead to the use of contraceptives (Prachi *et al.*, 2008). Also, majority (97.62%) of women wanted to adopt a contraceptive method only after achieving desired family size (Table 11.5) as several studies indicate that in rural areas the desired family size of most couples is still three or more children (Chandhik *et al.*, 2003). Perhaps, this may also be applicable to some women who had their reasons for not using contraceptive method until they reach a desired family size.

Table 11.5: Factors influencing decision making in family planning among Angami women

Variables	*Frequency*	
	*Yes**	*No**
Decision on family planning is taken solely by husband	2 (4.76)	40 (95.24)
Family planning decisions made jointly with husband	40 (95.24)	2 (4.76)
Is there any financial situation?	19 (45.24)	23 (54.76)
Inadequate housing?	0 (0.00)	42 (100.00)
Want as many children as possible	1 (2.38)	41 (97.62)
Desire for a son in the family	1 (2.38)	41 (97.62)
Desire for a daughter in the family	1 (2.38)	41 (97.62)
Family pressure on having lesser children	11 (26.19)	31 (73.81)
Availability or accessibility of family planning services	13 (30.95)	29 (69.05)
Social norms to have less children	25 (59.52)	17 (40.48)
Other personal reasons	7 (16.67)	35 (83.33)

* Percentages are given in the parentheses.

Family size seems to have changed with time; as earlier, the Angamis had larger family size as compared with the present day family size. The social norm relating to the change in adopting family planning of having lesser number of children at present may be because of economic reasons. It is evident from the results that Angami women play important roles in decision-making on family size with almost all (95.24%) of them making decision on their family size jointly with their husband (Table 11.5). While, only few (4.76%) reported that the decision was made solely by the husband. For many of the participants, financial situation (45.24%), availability and accessibility of family planning services (30.95%) and family pressure (26.19%) affects their decision on family size and spacing between children. Some (16.67%) had other reasons that affect their decision-making on family size. The increase in number of children in a certain family may be because of desire for a particular sex, for example, a son (2.38%) or a daughter (2.38%) in the family, as stated by few of the participants. Although, both the birth of a son or a daughter is not an unwelcome event since both sexes are always wanted in general in Angami community.

According to UN report of the Fourth World Conference on Women (1995), "Reproductive rights, rest on the recognition of the basic right of all couples and individuals to decide freely and responsibly the number, spacing and timing of their children and to have the information and means to do so, and the right to attain the highest standard of sexual and reproductive health and also, to make decisions concerning reproduction free of discrimination, coercion and violence." (p. 36). A woman's right to reproductive autonomy is often impaired because of her status in society. Enjoyment of this right depends on her right to act as an independent adult of full legal capacity to participate in civil society and to be free from discrimination in its various forms (Shalev, 2000). On the basis of the interview taken on each participant in the present study, it has been observed that—"Reproduction rights rest on the recognition of basic right of the couple", as shared by a forty year old mother. With regard to the right of a woman to make autonomous choices about her reproduction freely and without coercion, another forty year old participant replied, "It involves her body and mind and she only knows her health condition." Another agreed saying, "Yes, as a woman, we have our rights to make our choices. We should also live a healthy life." "Woman knows the problem of her health in regard to reproduction, therefore, she has the right to make her own choice", agreed one of the participants, who is a mother of three children. Another woman agreed saying, "Yes, by doing so, they seize better economic opportunities and fulfil their capabilities." Most of the participants are of the opinion that decision should be made by both husband and wife together to raise the less or more children they have, healthy and well with the capabilities they have and can provide their children with.

Nearly half of the participants (47.62%) reported on availing information on family planning services and consultations from their family itself (Table 11.6). While the others sought help and acquire information from Family Planning cabinet (21.43%), Maternal Hospital (19.05%) or Women's Consultation (11.90%). On the basis of the interview of the Health Centre Doctors, it has been observed that the Primary Health Centre of Jotsoma Village conducts Village Health Sanitation and Nutrition Day which is held every second Friday of the month every year. The programme gives health talks on women health, hygiene and Antenatal Check-up (ANC). It was reported that all ANC tests are done free of cost for pregnant women. Besides Antenatal Check-up, Health Centre provides information and requirements for family planning and use of contraceptive methods for prevention of pregnancies. It was reported from the Primary Health Centre that at present, there are two women who use Copper-T method for prevention of pregnancy and eight women registered on taking Oral contraceptive pills.

Table 11.6: Frequency table on Family Planning

Where do you avail information on family planning services or consultations?	*Frequency*	*Percentage*
Family planning cabinet	9	21.43
Maternal Hospital	8	19.05
Women's consultation	5	11.90
Family	20	47.62

Conclusion

In conclusion, the study highlights that on an average, the Angami Naga women even after being in a patriarchal society, play a crucial role in making decisions about family planning and maintaining and taking care of their reproductive health. They are aware of the importance of the positive health outcomes with contraceptive use and spacing of children which benefit not only men and women but also the future generation. The limitations for this study are fewer variables, time constraint and less sample size. It will be beneficial to other populations too if only further study is carried out in a larger area with more and deeper focus on the reproductive health of women.

REFERENCES

Census of India. 2011. Nagaland, District Census Handbook, Kohima, Series14, Part XII-B. Directorate of Census Operations, Nagaland. Available online at censusindia.gov.in. > 2011census > dchb, accessed 20 September, 2016.

Chandhick, N., Dhillon, B.S., Kambo, I., Saxena, N.C. 2003. "Contraceptive knowledge, practices and utilization of services in the rural areas of India" (An ICMR Task Force Study). *Indian J Med Sci.* **57**(7): 303-310.

Fathalla M.F. 1997. *Issues in Reproductive Health: Health and being a woman.* Available online at: http://www.un.org/womenwatch/daw/csw/issues.htm, accessed 8 January, 2017.

Khiloni, L. 2009. "Fertility Performance of the Anal Women of Lambung Village, Chandel District, Manipur." *Anthropologist.* **11**(4): 277-280.

Maheo, L.M. 2004. *The Mao Naga tribe of Manipur: A demographic Anthropological Study.* New Delhi: Mittal Publications.

Pathak, P.K., Tripathi, N., Subramanian, S.V. 2014. "Secular Trends in Menarcheal age in India—Evidence from the Indian Human Development Survey." *Plos one.* 9(11).

Prachi, R., Gupta, S.D., Barua, A., Jaju, S., Khati, B. 2008. "A study of knowledge, attitude and practice of family planning among the women of reproductive age group in Sikkim." *J Obstet Gynaecol India.* **58**(1): 63-67.

Purnungla, Sengupta, S. 2002. "Menarche and menopause among the Ao Naga women of Nagaland, India." *Journal of Human Ecology.* **13**(14): 323-234.

Shalev, C. 2000. "Rights to Sexual and Reproductive Health—the ICPD and the Convention on the Elimination of All Forms of Discrimination Against Women." *Health and Human Rights.* 4(2): 39-66.

Singh, J. 2006. "Ethnic variation in fertility patterns among four communities of Manipur." *Journal of Human Ecology.* 2(1), 1-9.

United Nations. Report of the Fourth World Conference on Women. 1995. Beijing, China. Available online at A/CONF.177/20/Rev.1, accessed 15 December, 2018.

World Health Organisation (WHO). 2009. Department of Reproductive Health and Research, Partner Brief. Geneva, Switzerland. Available online at WHO/RHR/09.02, accessed 10 May, 2019.

12

Reproductive Health Seeking Behaviour among the Khamtis of Assam

Juri Borah and *Sarthak Sengupta*

Introduction

Reproductive health is one of the important components of the overall health status of an individual. Hence, it is a crucial part of life too. Reproductive health is defined by the International Conference on Population and Development (ICPD) as "a state of complete physical, mental and social well-being and not merely the absence of disease or infirmity, in all matters relating to the reproductive system and to its functions and processes" (United Nations, 1994). Health depends upon our ability to understand and manage the biological requirements to effectively counteract with the prevailing situations. Individuals, families, communities, and societies are considered as the determinants of health, which in turn are influenced by various factors. Therefore, health is multifactorial which is affected by socio-cultural factors apart from depends on physical, clinical and biological factors.

Understanding human behaviour is considered a prerequisite to improving health practices. WHO (1998) defined health behaviour as "any activity undertaken by an individual, regardless of actual or perceived health status, for the purpose of promoting, protecting or maintaining health, whether or not such behaviour is objectively effective towards that end." The most illustrative definition was given by Gochman (1982), who defined it as "those personal attributes such as beliefs, expectations, motives, values, perceptions, and other cognitive elements; personality characteristics, including effective and emotional states and traits;

and overt behaviour patterns, actions and habits that relate to health maintenance, to health restoration and to health improvement." Thus, health behaviour is an individual's perceptions of health status or of improvement, recovery, or other changes in health status, which develop through traditions and specific to different cultural setup. Cultural belief and attitude greatly influence the health-seeking behaviour of the community (Thomlinson *et al.*, 2004). However, the medical practices have been reflected according to the medical belief and prevailing attitude to restore the healthy state of the community (Roy and Ali, 2001; Russel, 2005; Jain *et al.*, 2006; Mazumdar and Gupta, 2007; Shaikh *et al.*, 2008). Measures of socio-economic status like poverty, income, material deprivation, education, occupation etc. may be positively and negatively associated with health status (Marmot and Wilkinson, 1999; Lynch and Kaplan, 2000).

The present chapter is an attempt to understand the reproductive health-seeking behaviour among the Khamtis of Assam. In the present study reproductive health seeking behaviour is considered in terms of their perception and belief regarding health, health maintenance behaviour and also compares a few aspects with some proximate factors.

Materials and Methods

The findings of the present study are based on the data collected from 62 ever married Khamti mothers having at least one surviving child from four Khamti villages, namely Sri Bhuyan Khamti *Gaon*, Gosaibari Khamti *Gaon*, Borpathar Khamti *Gaon*, and Bor Khamti *Gaon* located in Lakhimpur district of Assam. Observation, interview, and case study are the methods applied to collect the information. The Khamti is one of the important branches of Tai speaking group of people. They are Mongoloid and are Buddhist by religion. Historians say that the Khamti people migrated to India from Myanmar and thereby settled on the bank of the river Tengapani. Later on, between 1780-1790 AD, they became the authority of Sadiya. However, in 1839 they were defeated by British and their authority went to British people. In 1843, a group of 500 individuals expatriate to Narayanpur area of Lakhimpur district, Assam and the rest were resettled in Sadiya which is now known as Namsai sub-division located in the lower regions of Lohit district, Arunachal Pradesh (Gait, 1905; Gogoi, 1971). In Assam, the Khamti people are numerically very meagre. At present, they are found mainly in Narayanpur area of Lakhimpur district, Assam. In Lakhimpur, they are sparsely scattered in four small villages, namely Bor Khamti *Gaon*, Gosaibari Khamti *Gaon*, Sri Bhuyan Khamti *Gaon*, and Borpathar Khamti *Gaon*.

Results and Discussion

The present age of the respondents ranges from 16 years to 67 years. A maximum number of mothers are found in the age group of 25-29 years (22.58%). The proportion of illiterate mothers is considerably high (24.19%). Most of the mothers have attained education up to high school standard (27.42%) and only a limited fraction of mothers have completed graduate level of education (3.23%). The Khamti mothers who engages in the job is also very nominal (3.23%). Most of the mothers remain busy with household activities only. In regard to the educational level of their male counterparts, it is found that the proportion of literate is appreciably high (98.39%), although the person with higher education is less in number. 24.19 per cent of the male individuals are engaged as a serviceholder in different government offices and private sectors. Moreover, 12.90 per cent of the individuals are earning by running a petty business. Among them, 53.23 per cent and 8.06 per cent of the individuals are found as cultivators and wage earners respectively.

Pregnancy, the most crucial period in the lifetime of a woman, in which proper care is required to ensure the well-being of both the expected woman and the foetus, to enhance safe birth and to identify and manage complications. Distribution of the Khamti mothers who sought prenatal care from a medical institution as per their background characteristics is shown in Table 12.1. In this regard, it is found that 72.58 per cent of the mothers have availed the facilities in the form of vaccination or folic acid, calcium tablet or combination of all. The residues although didn't seek medical assistance; almost all of them have followed some restrictions in terms of food habit and way of living as maintained by their oral traditional knowledge. Sarmah (2014) also reported the consciousness of Bodo Kachari women living in Guwahati, Assam during their conceiving stages. In Manipur also, Chanu (2007) from her study acknowledged the Loi women for their awareness and participation up to a great extent during their pregnancy period. Among the Khasi of Meghalaya, Purkayastha and Singh (2017) found that 48.0 per cent of women received antenatal check-ups during the three years preceding their survey.

Table 12.1: Background characteristics and prenatal care among the Khamti mothers

Background characters	*No. of mothers*	*Yes*	*%*	*No*	*%*
Present age (in years)					
≤20-29	19	18	94.74	1	5.26
30-39	8	8	100.00	0	0
40-49	15	11	73.33	4	26.67
≥ 50	20	8	40.00	12	60.00
Maternal education					
Illiterate	15	7	46.67	8	53.33
Primary	10	5	50.00	5	50.00
Secondary and above	37	33	89.19	4	10.81
Paternal occupation					
Cultivator	33	21	63.64	12	36.36
Service	15	12	80.00	3	20.00
Petty business	8	7	87.50	1	12.50
Wage earner	6	5	83.33	1	16.67

The proportions of the mothers who have taken medical assistance during pregnancy are found to be more among the young category (94.74%). Manna *et al.* (2011) and Purkayastha and Singh (2017) also observed less antenatal care among the mothers with higher age groups living in the tea garden areas in Jalpaiguri and Darjeeling districts of West Bengal and the Khasi of Ri Bhoi district of Meghalaya respectively. The frequencies of the mothers sought medical care during pregnancy are considerably higher among those who have attained education up to secondary level and above (89.19%). It gradually comes down from primary level educated mothers (50.00%) to illiterate section (46.67%). Earlier studies carried out by various scholars among different population groups such as Nanda and Niranjan (1999) among the Scheduled Tribes in India; Sunil *et al.* (2006) from different rural areas of India; Ram and Singh (2006) in rural Uttar Pradesh; Saikia and Singh

(2009) in different parts of India as a whole; Manna *et al.* (2011) in tea garden areas in Jalpaiguri and Darjeeling districts of West Bengal; Singh *et al.* (2012) among the married adolescent in rural India and the work of Purkayastha and Singh (2017) among the Khasi of Ri Bhoi district of Meghalaya also mentioned the improved status of antenatal care in accordance with advanced maternal educational status. The frequency of the mothers adopted prenatal care from a medical institution is more among those whose husbands are maintaining their livelihood by running a petty business (87.50%), followed by those who are engaged as serviceholders (80.00%). Taking the antenatal care up to a great extent among the families with the better economic condition was also reported by Manna *et al.* (2011) in tea garden areas in Jalpaiguri and Darjeeling districts of West Bengal and Purkayastha and Singh (2017) among the Khasi of Ri Bhoi district of Meghalaya.

During pregnancy, the Khamti mothers consider some food items as proscribed type such as chilly, sour food, taro, new rolled leaf blade of taro plant (local name: *fouk*, scientific name: *Colocasia esculenta*), white gourd (local name: *mapakmoun*, scientific name: *Benincasa hispida*), uncooked rice flour, too hot rice and tea, East Indian glory bower (local name: *Patak Khai*, scientific name: *Clerodendrum olebrookiannum*) and any food item appears as twin. They also believe that if a pregnant mother eats new rolled leaf blade of taro plant the child's behaviour will be of the aggressive type. Again, if the pregnant mother eats uncooked rice flour, the newborn comes out with cradle cap, they believe. During pregnancy, the mother is given curry made of the stalk of a particular kind of taro plant (*kola kochur thari*) for more secretion of breast milk. If a pregnant mother has a burning sensation during urination, she is given a mixture of juice made up of milk and grass known as *yaa paak khai* in Khamti language.

The restriction is observed with regard to their daily activities also. A pregnant mother is not allowed to cross a rope which is tied to a cow or any other animals. She is not allowed to go to that house if anyone dies. Although the husband is allowable to go, he can not touch the corpse. The spoon is not permitted to keep within the cooking utensils like *kerahi,* pot etc. They uphold these kinds of belief systems not to experience the delivery complicacy. After the preparation of the foodstuff like rice or any curry, the spoon is moved over the foodstuff at least once in order to avoid a baby with a mental disability. The ashes formed after preparing the foodstuff are not kept inside the cooking place (*chouka*) having the fear of a child with a big palate. The husband is not permitted to kill any life during the conceiving stage of his wife because a new life is coming to their family. When the husband goes outside and returns back, he is not permitted to come inside directly. He has to wait for a while in the outside and passes spittle at least once. Otherwise unnatural forces may affect his wife and the unborn baby too.

Place of delivery is also an important aspect since it determines whether the delivery is safe or not. Institutional delivery or delivery at home assisted by trained personnel is considered as safe delivery. Usually, Khamti mothers prefer to deliver their babies at home. The parturient mother tries herself to deliver a baby by force with the help of a rope. However, the elderly village women also provide helping hand as per the need. There is no traditional *dhai* as such among them. Among the respondents, out of the total delivery, the proportion of home delivery (71.28%) is the maximum. 25.53 per cent of the delivery is recorded at a government hospital and the remaining 3.19 per cent are in private nursing home. Among the Bharia women in Madhya Pradesh, a rare approach to doctors or ANM for help in delivery time was documented in the study conducted by Pandey and Tiwary (2001). Lack of finance and sometimes lack of faith were recorded as the main causes for underutilization of the help of ANM in delivery. Chanu (2007) also recorded higher incidences of home delivery among the Loi women living in rural areas of Manipur (72.84%). Studies conducted by Sharma (2007) recorded the proportions of deliveries at home as nearly 91.00 per cent among the Scheduled Tribes of Madhya Pradesh. Manna *et al.* (2011) also reported the unwillingness to visit the hospital for delivery among the mother inhabiting the tea garden areas in North Bengal. Grover and Chhabra (2012) highlighted the proportions of home delivery as two-thirds of total deliveries in the urban villages of Delhi. The study of Sarmah (2014) documented the highest number of home delivery among the Bodo Kachari women for which she considered poverty, lack of education, lack of transportation and interruption of husband or family members in institutional delivery as the basic causes. Contrary to it, Dutta and Das (2017-18) observed a lesser proportion of home delivery (3.9%) among the Sonowal Kachari women of Lakhimpur district, Assam. They reported the incidence of delivery by the expectant women as 1.9 per cent and also delivery at government and private hospital as 93.7 per cent and 0.5 per cent respectively.

Table 12.2 shows the background characteristics and place of delivery among the Khamti mothers. The proportion of home delivery is found to decrease substantially from the higher age groups to the lower one. Mothers belong to 30-39 years of age group (15.79%) are found to prefer the child deliveries at a private nursing home in comparison to the other age cohorts. The prevalence of delivery of a baby at a private nursing home is not recorded among the mothers who belong to 50 years or more. Not a clear picture of the place of delivery according to maternal education can be drawn. Among the Sonowal Kachari women of Lakhimpur district, Assam Dutta and Das (2017-18) could not find any significant relationship between maternal education and place of delivery. However, the incidence of home delivery was found to be more among the Sonowal Kachari mother with lower attainment of education. The proportion of home delivery is found as considerably higher among those whose husbands are

Table 12.2: Background characteristics and place of delivery among the Khamti mothers

Background characters	*No. of mothers*	*Home*		*Government hospital*		*Private nursing home*		*Total*
		No.	*%*	*No.*	*%*	*No.*	*%*	
Respondents Present age (in years)								
≥20-29	19	2	7.69	23	88.46	1	3.85	26
30-39	8	10	52.63	6	31.58	3	15.79	19
40-49	15	33	66.00	15	30.00	2	4.00	50
≥50	20	89	95.70	4	4.30	0	0	93
Maternal education								
Illiterate	15	67	91.78	6	8.22	0	0	73
Primary	10	29	39.19	39	52.70	6	8.11	74
Secondary and above	37	38	92.68	3	7.32	0	0	41
Paternal occupation								
Cultivator	33	88	77.88	23	20.35	2	1.77	113
Service	15	23	62.16	11	29.73	3	8.11	37
Petty business	8	15	62.5	8	33.33	1	4.17	24
Wage earner	6	8	57.14	6	42.86	0	0	14

cultivators (77.88%). On the other hand, the frequency of delivering a baby at a private nursing home is relatively higher among the mothers whose husbands are engaged as a service holder (8.11%), followed by the persons earn by running a petty business (4.17%). Interestingly, quite a good number of mothers among whom the husbands are wage earner (42.86%) have preferred to deliver their babies at a government hospital.

The instances of a normal delivery are the maximum (98.94%). Only a limited proportion of cases of cesarean are observed (1.06%). During the time of delivery, the mother is not permitted to tie her hairs. However, she is not permitted to use any garland also. Otherwise, delivery complications may occur, they believe. For incising the umbilical cord sharp bamboo strips are used in case of home delivery. Mustard oil is applied in the navel portion to make it dry. They preserved the navel cord of the newborn by wrapping with a cloth for future purpose. Dutta and Das (2017-18) also reported the higher incidence of normal delivery (67.5%) among the Sonowal Kachari women of Lakhimpur district, Assam.

The gap between two subsequent childbirths is known as birth spacing. It is required for the better health of the mother and the child too. Maximum numbers of the Khamti mothers are found to deliver their babies with a gap of 1-2 years (38.83%), followed by 1 year (28.19%) of the gap (Table 12.3). They disposed of the afterbirth materials by digging the area where the stair of the residential house is constructed. They have a belief that deeper the pit delays of the next pregnancy. The same custom to bring the larger gap between two issues is also reported among the Tai Khamyangs of Assam (Barua, 1998) and Bharias of Madhya Pradesh (Pandey and Tiwari, 2001).

Table 12.3: Duration of birth spacing among the Khamti mothers

Birth Spacing (in years)	*No.*	*%*
1	53	28.19
1-2	73	38.83
2-3	36	19.15
3-4	8	4.26
4	18	9.57
Total	188	100.00

Post-natal care of the mother and the child is of equal importance for the betterment of the mother as well as the newborn child. Table 12.4 shows the background characteristics and post-natal immunization of the children among the Khamti mothers. The mothers are categorized into three groups. Some mothers (75.81%) got immunized all of their children and some of them (14.52%) did not immunize all of their children. However, there are Khamti mothers (9.68%) who did not prefer to give immunization to their children. All the younger mothers (100.00%) are found to immunize all of their newborn children. Conversely,

Table 12.4: Background characteristics and post-natal immunization among the Khamti mothers

Background characters	*No. of mothers*	*Yes*		*Incomplete*		*No*	
		No.	*%*	*No.*	*%*	*No.*	*%*
Present age (in years)							
≥20-29	19	19	100.00	0	0	0	0
30-39	8	8	100.00	0	0	0	0
40-49	15	13	86.67	1	6.67	1	6.67
≥50	20	7	35.00	5	25.00	8	40.00
Maternal education							
Illiterate	15	5	33.33	5	33.33	5	33.33
Primary	10	7	70.00	0	0	3	30.00
Secondary and above	37	35	94.59	1	2.70	1	2.70
Paternal occupation							
Cultivator	33	21	63.64	5	15.15	7	21.21
Service	15	15	100.00	0	0	0	0
Petty business	8	6	75.00	1	12.50	1	12.50
Wage earner	6	5	83.33	0	0	1	16.67

the proportion of mothers who either did not immunize their children (40.00%) or did not give immunization to all of their children (25.00%) is quite high among those in which the present age is 50 years or more. 94.59 per cent of the women having education up to secondary level and beyond that have immunized all of their children. In this regard, the frequency of the mothers is found to decrease as their level of education decreases from primary level education (70.00%) to illiterate section (33.33%). However, the proportion of the mothers who has not vaccinated to all of their children (33.33%) or did not immunize a single child

(33.33%) is observed as more among the illiterate categories. Dyavarishetty and Kowli (2012) also mentioned the influence of the educational status of the mother on the timely vaccination of the child. Their study observed the higher proportions of the illiterate mothers who delayed vaccination of the child than those who had been to school. Similarly, the work of Patra (2013) also noted the influence of the educational status of Indian women on the uptake of vaccination. All the mothers whose husbands are service holder are found to immunize all of their children. The proportions of the mothers who did not immunize their children are found as considerably higher among those whose husbands are cultivators (21.21%), followed by the wage earners (16.67%).

Food items from climbing plants such as white gourd (Local Name: *mapakmoun*, scientific Name: *benincasa hispida*), ridged gourd (local name: *ma hoy*, scientific name: *lagernaria siceraria*), bitter gourd (local name: *makkhai khum*, scientific name: *momordica charantia*), yard-long bean (local name: *thosai*, scientific name: *Vigna unguiculata sesquipedalis*) etc. are forbidden to have right after delivery up to 3rd month if a mother delivers a boy child. They believe that the newborn baby will experience a gynaecological problem (*ekoniya*) if the mother consumes such food items. In the case of a girl child, no such restriction is followed. After delivery, till 2-3 months the mother is not permitted to eat black gram, ground dry fish etc. because it may affect the navel cord of the mother. During breastfeeding mother is not permitted to eat East Indian glory bower (local name: *patak khai*, scientific name: *Clerodendrum olebrookiannum*) because they believe it soaks the mother's breast milk. On the contrary, if a woman has an excessive amount of breast milk it is prescribed as medicine. Fried, spicy and oily foods right after delivery are also prohibited among the Bodo Kachari women of Assam (Sarmah, 2014).

A newborn is not allowed to bring outside right after birth. In case of a boy child, it is permitted after 5 days and 3 days while a girl child is born. It is tried to follow if the delivery occurs in the medical institution also. The newborn is not permitted to touch by other family members up to 1 week. Even the husband is also not allowed to touch the baby. One can touch the newborn after removing his/her hair. The incised hairs are put within a ball made of cow dung and either kept on the wall of their house or throw in the root of the tree *musa balbisiana colla* (*aathiya kol*). It is not allowed to throw in another place. When a mother goes outside the residence with the newborn, a white coloured thread (*kecha suta*) is tied to the newborn baby's hand for that it would protect them against unwanted forces. That thread is sanctified with holy water already brought from their Buddhist temple and preserved since long.

If a newborn cries a lot, it is believed that the baby has a stomach problem (*aalukhuni*). The preserved navel cord is kept in a glass of water for a while and is given to drink to the suffered child. However, occasionally some other dose is also prescribed. The bark of a tree named *kadamba* (local name: *kadam*, scientific name: *Neolamarckia cadamba*) is removed carefully from the tree with a machete from lower to higher height and the bark is cut into seven pieces from one end to the other. It is kept in a glass of water for a few minutes and is given to drink.

Adoption of family planning measures has utmost importance to limit the family size. The proportion of Khamti mothers using family planning measures are found as low. Only 25.81 per cent of mothers are found to use contraceptive measures. Among the respondents, 17.74 per cent are using various hormonal medicines to reduce their birth and 8.06 per cent of the mothers have adopted the process of sterilization. Among the Jaintias of Meghalaya, Chakrabarty (1995) reported the frequency of users of family planning devices as only 22.46 per cent. Das (2002) in her study found the acceptors of family planning measures as 49.32 per cent among the Karbis of Assam. Chanu (2007) mentioned the frequency of family planning adopters as about 41.76 per cent among the Loi women in Manipur. She recorded the use of condom and loop as the most common methods among the Loi women living in both rural and urban areas of Manipur. In Assam, Gogoi (2013) reported the adopters of family planning measures as 93.0 per cent, 92.0 per cent, and 79.0 per cent among the Assamese Caste Hindus, Boro Kachari and the Muslim respectively. Sarmah (2014) in her study among the *Bodo Kachari Women in Assam* recorded the female sterilization (45.90%) as a well-accepted family planning measure, which is followed by the use of the oral pill (18.85%). The adopters of family planning devices are found as lesser (41.95%) than the non-adopters (58.05%) among the Sonowal Kachari women of Assam studied by Saikia (2015). Among the married women in rural Haryana, Ahamed *et al.* (2015) found the frequency of women using any contraceptive method as 55.2 per cent, where tubectomy (22.1%) and copper-T (14.8%) record the common beings. Among the Dibongiya Deori women of Assam, Borah (2017) recorded the users of family planning measures as 55.06 per cent in the rural and 63.64 per cent in urban areas respectively.

Table 12.5 shows the level of maternal education all level and adoption of family planning measures among the Khamti mothers. The frequency of the contraceptive users is found to be more among those who have attained education up to secondary and above level (35.14%). In this regard, only a minor difference between the illiterates and the mothers having a primary level of education is observed. Among the illiterate mothers (13.33%), the proportion of users is slightly higher than the mothers having a primary level of education (10.00%). In a study carried out by Deka (2012) among the adolescent girls of Meghalaya shows the significant relationship between educational status and users of family planning. The study reports the mother's educational status as an influential factor behind the knowledge of family planning among adolescent girls. The statistical positive association between knowledge of family planning and educational status among the women of the Assamese Caste Hindus and the Boro Kacharis in Assam was also reported by Gogoi (2013). The proportion of family planning users was recorded as 98.00 per cent among the literate Sonowal Kachari women (Saikia, 2015).

Table 12.5: Maternal education all level and adoption of family planning measures among the Khamti mothers

Maternal education	*No. of mothers*	*Yes*	*%*	*No*	*%*
Illiterate	15	2	13.33	13	86.67
Primary	10	1	10.00	9	90.00
Secondary and above	37	13	35.14	24	64.86

Conclusion

The reproductive health-seeking behaviour of the Khamti population is intimately related to their cultural tradition. They are bound up with a number of belief systems related to reproduction. The information detailed so far also supports the influence of various factors on their reproductive health-seeking behaviour. The present study emphasizes on improved health services in the form of health education by developing effective communication strategies on health education and health care. Although the study is based on the micro-level investigation, nevertheless, it is hoped to be helpful in undertaking positive strategies by the government in the near future.

REFERENCES

Ahamed, F., Lohiya, A., Kankaria, A., Silan, V., Kharya, P., Rizwan, S.A. 2015. "Menstrual disorders and its determinants among married women of Rural Haryana." *Journal of Clinical and Diagnostic Research,* **9**(9): 06-09.

Barua, I. 1998, "Socio-cultural and environmental factors of health and economy: a case study of Tai Khamyangs of Assam" in *Contemporary Studies in Human Ecology,* eds. M.K. Bhasin and S.L. Malik, Indian Society for Human Ecology, Delhi.

Borah, J. 2017, A study on the reproductive health of the Dibongiya Deori women of Assam. Ph.D. thesis, Department of Anthropology, Dibrugarh University.

Chakrabarty, M. 1995, Differential fertility and infant mortality among the Jaintias of Meghalaya: a study on bio-social correlates. Ph.D. thesis, Department of Anthropology, Gauhati University.

Chanu, T.J. 2007. A study of reproductive and child health among the Lois of Imphal Valley. Ph.D. thesis, Department of Anthropology, North Eastern Hill University.

Das, R. 2002. "A study of family planning practices among the Karbis of Kamrup, Assam." *South Asian Anthropologists,* **2**(1): 9-15.

Deka, K. 2012. Awareness and attitudes towards family planning among the adolescent girls of Meghalaya. Ph.D. thesis, Department of Anthropology, North Eastern Hill University.

Dyavarishetty, P.V., Kowli, S.S. 2012. "A facility based study on timely immunization of the infants, in a health center in Mumbai." *Indian Journal of Maternal and Child Health,* **15**(1):1-8.

Gait, E.A. 1905. *History of Assam,* Messers Thacker Spink, and Co., Kolkata, and Shimla.

Gochman, D.S. 1982. "Labels, systems, and motives: some perspectives on future research." *Health Education Quarterly,* **9**:167-174.

Gogoi, L. 1971. *The Tai Khamtis,* Chowkhamoon Gohain, Chowkham, Arunachal Pradesh.

Gogoi, M. 2013. A study on family planning practices in a multi-ethnic setting in Goalpara district, Assam. Ph.D. thesis, Department of Anthropology, Gauhati University.

Grover, P., Chhabra, P. 2012, "Neonatal care practices in urban villages." *Indian Medical Gazette,* January, pp. 32-38.

Jain, M., Nandan, D., Misra, S.K. 2006. "Qualitative assessment of health-seeking behaviour and perceptions regarding the quality of health care services among the rural community of district Agra." *Indian Journal of Community Medicine,* 31:140-144.

Lynch, J., Kaplan, G. 2000. *Socio-economic Position in Social Epidemiology,* eds L.F. Berkman and I. Kawachi, Oxford University Press, New York, pp. 13-35.

Manna, P.K., De, D., Ghosh, D. 2011. "Knowledge attitude and practices for antenatal care and delivery of the mothers of a tea garden in Jalpaiguri and Darjeeling districts, West Bengal." *National Journal of Community Medicine,* **2**(1): 4-8.

Marmot, M. and Wilkinson, R.G. 1999. *Social Determinants of Health,* Oxford University Press, New York.

Mozumder, P.G., Gupta, K. 2007. "Indian system of medicine and women's health: a clients perspective." *Journal of Biosocial Science,* **39**: 819-841.

Nanda, S., Niranjan, S. 1999. "Utilization of antenatal care (ANC) service by the Scheduled Tribes in India." *Journal of Human Ecology,* **10**(2): 99-104.

Pandey, G.D., Tiwary, R.S. 2001. "Socio-cultural reproductive health practices of primitive tribes of Madhya Pradesh: some observations." *The Journal of Family Welfare,* 47(2): 27-33.

Patra, N. 2013. "Universal immunization programme in India: the determinants of childhood immunization." Available from: SSRN: https://ssrn.com/abstract=881224 or http://dx.doi.org/10.2139/ssrn.881224.

Purkayastha, P., Singh, K.N. 2017. "Fertility preferences and antenatal check-ups among the rural Khasi women of Ri Bhoi district, Meghalaya (India)." *International Journal of Recent Scientific Research,* **8**(8): 19423-19427.

Ram, F., Singh, A. 2006. "Is antenatal care effective in improving maternal health in rural Uttar Pradesh? evidence from a district level household survey." *Journal of Biosocial Science,* **38**(4): 433-448.

Roy, B., Irshad Ali, A.N.M. 2001. "Medical pluralism and pattern of acceptance of the different medical options among the Dimasa Kacharis of North Cachar Hills in Assam." *Journal of Human Ecology,* **12**: 25-32.

Russell, S. 2005. "Treatment seeking behaviour in urban Sri Lanka: trusting the state, trusting the private providers." *Social Science and Medicine* **61**: 1396-1407.

Saikia, N., Singh, A. 2009. "Does the type of household affect maternal health?: evidence from India." *Journal of Biosocial Science,* **41**(3): 329-353.

Saikia, N. 2015. Fertility performance and blood group incompatibility among the Sonowal Kacharis of Dibrugarh district, Assam. Ph.D. thesis, Department of Anthropology, Dibrugarh University.

Sarmah, L. 2014. Reproductive health-seeking behavior among the Bodo-Kachari women in North Guwahati Area, Assam. Ph.D. thesis, Department of Anthropology, Gauhati University.

Shaikh, B.T., Haran, D., Hatcher, J., Azam, S.I. 2008. "Studying health-seeking behaviours: collecting reliable data, conducting comprehensive analysis." *Journal of Biosocial Science*, **40**: 53-68.

Sharma, R.K. 2007. "Newborn health among tribes of Madhya Pradesh—an overview." *Biannual Newsletter of Regional Medical Research Centre for Tribals Jabalpur*, **4**(1): 1-12.

Singh, P.K., Rai, R.K., Alagarajan, M., Singh, L. 2012. "Determinants of maternity care services utilization among married adolescents in Rural India." *PLoS ONE*, **7**(2):e31666, doi:10.1371/journal.pone.00316662.

Sunil, T.S., Rajaram, S., Zottarelli, L.K. 2006. "Do individual and program factors matter in the utilization of maternal care services in rural India?: a theoretical approach." *Social Science and Medicine*, **62**(8): 1943-1957.

Thomlinson, E., McDonagh, M.K., Crooks, K.B., Lees, M. 2004. "Health belief of rural Canadians: implications for practice." *Australian Journal of Rural Health*, **12**(6): 258-263.

United Nation. 1994. *Report of the International Conference on Population and Development*, Cairo.

World Health Organization (WHO) 1998, *Health Promotion Glossary*, WHO, Geneva. Accessed from:http://www.who.int/healthpromotion/about/HPR%20Glossary%201998.pdf.

13

Maternal and Child Health Care Services in Assam
An appraisal

Himangi Kalita, Nitish Mondal and *Kh. Narendra Singh*

Introduction

The improving well-being of mothers, infants and children is an important public health goal for the world and well-being determines the health of the next generation and can help predict future public health challenges for the families, communities and health care system. India, with a population of more than 1.21 billion, has the highest maternal mortality in the world (45,000 in 2015) (WHO, 2015) and child death is 1.2 million in 2015 (United Nations Children's Fund, 2015). India has made an appreciable progress in improving the overall health status of its population but in the field of maternal and child health it is far from satisfaction. Quality aspects in maternal health care have long been ignored in the Indian public health system. Though with the launch of the National Rural Health Mission (NRHM) has made efforts to address lacunae associated with quality of maternal care in the public health system, there is scope for improvement. Therefore, maternal and child health continues to be a matter of concern in the country. Assam occupies a distinctive place due to its geographical, historical, social, cultural and political feature which is situated in the North-east region of the country. Assam is the largest among the states of North-East India. The population of Assam is about 31 million making the 14th most populated state in India with a growth rate of about 17 per cent which is very close to the national growth rate of 17 per cent (Census, 2011).

The literacy rate in the state is improved tremendously to 73 per cent from the last decade which was 63.25 per cent. The sex ratio in the state is 954 females to 1000 males and the child sex ratio is 962. The state is infamous for its high maternal mortality ratio which stands as high as 328 maternal deaths per hundred thousand mothers per year during 2010-12 is the highest in the country (all-India average: 178, with Kerala having the lowest MMR), the corresponding national attainment level is 178 (SRS, 2011- 13). As per National Family Health Survey (NFHS-4), a total of 30.8 per cent women are married before 18 years of age in Assam. This in turn, leads to early pregnancy and contributes to high maternal mortality rate. The Sample Registration System (SRS) survey also revealed that infant mortality rate in the state went down from 47 deaths in 2015 to 44 in 2016. However, it is still much higher than the national average of 34. All these factors indicate the poor maternal and child health care services in the state.

Poor access to quality health care facilities is one of the most important reasons of high maternal and neonatal mortality in India. Some of the factors for underutilization of maternal care services include: young maternal age; religion; poor education; unskilled occupation; poverty; low caste; parity (higher birth order were less likely to access antenatal services); lack of autonomy; poor familial support; lack of access to transport; and the high cost of care and when it is accessed, its poor quality (such as shortages of supplies and staff, mistreatment by staff, or poor training or limited experience of staff as availability of skilled human resources is an important aspect to provide quality maternal and newborn care) (Kumar *et al.*, 2013; Kassebaum *et al.*, 2014; Goudar *et al.*, 2015; Kaur *et al.*, 2019). Moreover lack of skilled staff, inadequate infrastructure and lack of accountability have been recognized as some other key reasons for the failure of referral systems in India (Gupta *et al.*, 2017).

Maternal and Child Care Situation in Assam

The condition of North-eastern states in terms of various health care facilities and well trained man power resources are very grim and unsatisfactory. The lack of human resources is as responsible for inadequate provision for health care services as lack of physical infrastructure, especially in rural areas. The state Assam is infamous due to its high maternal mortality ratio which stands as high as 390 maternal deaths per hundred thousand mothers per year during 2007-09 (ORGI, 2011). High fertility, abortion, transport, and emergency care are among the key determinants of maternal mortality. Far distance to health facility discouraged people towards institutional births. Instead adequacy of essential equipment/laboratory services required for maternal care significantly encouraged deliveries at public health facility (Patel and Ladusingh, 2015). At the same time, poor infrastructure and ineffective public health services is also responsible for low inadequate obstetric care indicating an urgent public health concern (Singh and Badaya, 2014). Vidler *et al.* (2016) in their study in rural Karnataka reported that health facility infrastructure should also be enhanced to ensure a consistent power supply and improved cleanliness on the wards. Essential maternal health care during pregnancy, delivery and post-natal periods could reduce the chance of maternal death and improve overall health not only of mother but also of new-born (Koblinsky *et al.*, 1999, Graham *et al.* 2000; Sinha *et al.*, 2014; Lassi *et al.*, 2016). The objectives of the present chapter are to evaluate and assess the situation of maternal and child health status and related health care services in rural areas of Assam. Several research investigations have shown that maternal health is essential component to ensure the desired reproductive performance and health of children in population. Researchers have reported that several mothers suffer from lack of access to health, poor conditions, rural residence and poor quality of life—especially in developing countries like India. The regular utilization of maternal health care services are necessary which may take good care of mother and their children and can reduce maternal morbidity and mortality (Kifle *et al.*, 2017). The present chapter will evaluate the current situations and aware the people about importance of maternal and child health status and cater attention of the government, policy maker and bureaucrats about present scenario of maternal and child health care services in real existence.

Methodology

The present chapter is based on secondary sources which are collected from Statistical Hand Book, Assam. 2014, NFHS-3,

NFHS-4, SRS 2011, SRS 2013, Census 2011 and related literature from various research journals, articles, internet etc. Online data bases were also searched to collect the necessary information of the demography and data related to maternal and child health. National census data and several published reports were used to analyze and discuss the objectives of the present study. The analysis carried out in this chapter is qualitative and descriptive. The data has been analyzed with the help of frequencies, percentages, rates and ratios and are presented in table and figure.

Results and Discussion

World Health Organization (WHO) estimates that more than half a million women lose their lives in the process of reproduction worldwide every year; of these deaths, about 99 per cent are from developing countries including India. World Bank clarifies that maternal mortality can be avoided in India by giving proper obstetric care and most of these mortalities are avoidable if mothers have access to maternal health care services properly. However, a large proportion of women and child still do not receive antenatal check-ups inability to meet the cost related to visiting a health facility, their thinking that it is not necessary, lack of knowledge and inadequate health services (IIPS, 2002). In Assam, mothers who had antenatal check-up in the first trimester is 68.5 per cent in urban area whereas in rural areas of Assam it is only 53.5 per cent (NFHS-4). Mothers who had full antenatal care are 6.7 per cent in NFHS-3 and it is 18.1 per cent in NFHS-4. Institutional births have increased from 22.4 per cent in NFHS-3 to 70.6 per cent in NFHS-4. Births assisted by doctor/nurse/LHV/ANM/other health personnel are 31.0 per cent (NFHS-3) and increased to 74.3 per cent in NFHS-4. Though data shows the improvement in health seeking behaviour of mother still it failed to overcome the problem of maternal and child mortality (Table 13.1). Assam is one of the states having high infant and child mortality, maternal mortality and has regional disparities of maternal and child health care. The IMR and MMR is much higher especially in the rural areas and mainly attributed to lack of adequate health care facilities, lack of knowledge about health, hygiene, awareness of health care services and less institutional delivery and acute shortage of doctors and medical staff in the hospitals. Moreover, health care centres are

Table 13.1: Health status and health care of mother and their children

Sl. No.	Indicators	NFHS-4 (2015-16) Urban	NFHS-4 (2015-16) Rural	NFHS-4 (2015-16) Total	NFHS-3 (2005-06) Total
1.	Women age 20-24 years married before age 18 years (%)	23.9	33.9	32.6	38.0
2.	Total fertility rate (children per woman)	1.5	2.3	2.2	2.4
3.	Infant mortality rate (IMR)	28	50	48	66
4.	Under-five mortality rate (U5MR)	40	58	56	84
5.	Mothers who had antenatal check-up in the first trimester (%)	68.5	53.5	55.1	40.0
6.	Mothers who had at least 4 antenatal care visits (%)	60.4	44.8	46.5	23.5
7.	Mothers who consumed iron folic acid for 100 days or more when they were pregnant (%)	44.0	30.5	32.0	10.3
8.	Mothers who had full antenatal care(%)	30.4	16.6	18.1	6.7
9.	Registered pregnancies for which the mother received Mother and Child Protection (MCP) card (%)	95.6	96.4	96.3	na
10.	Mothers who received post-natal care from a doctor/nurse/LHV/ANM/midwife/ other health personnel within 2 days of delivery (%)	71.5	51.9	54.0	13.2
11.	Mothers who received financial assistance under Janani Suraksha Yojana (JSY) for births delivered in an institution (%)	42.4	69.9	66.1	na
12.	Average out of pocket expenditure per delivery in public health facility (Rs.)	4,501	3,054	3,210	na
13.	Children born at home who were taken to a health facility for check-up within 24 hours of birth (%)	1.8	1.9	1.9	0.0
14.	Children who received a health check after birth from a doctor/nurse/LHV/ ANM/midwife/other health personnel within 2 days of birth (%)	24.8	22.7	22.9	na
15.	Institutional births (%)	92.9	68.2	70.6	22.4
16.	Institutional births in public facility (%)	61.7	59.8	60.0	13.0
17.	Births assisted by doctor/nurse/LHV/ ANM/other health personnel (%)	94.1	72.1	74.3	31.0

Source: National Family Health Survery-4.

also less in Assam in comparison to the number of population in the state. Total number of subcenters in the state is 4621, PHCs is 1014, CHCs is 151, Sub-District hospital is 14 and District hospital is 25 according to the Health and Family Welfare Department, Government of Assam. District-wise detailed numbers of health centres in the state are mentioned in Table 13.2.

Table 13.2: District-wise number of government hospitals in Assam

Sl. No.	*District*	*No. of SCs*	*No. of PHCs*	*No. of CHCs*	*No. of Sub-District hospitals*	*No. of District hospitals*
1.	Barpeta	264	51	6	1	1
2.	Baksa	157	41	5	0	1
3.	Bongaigaon	84	30	3	0	1
4.	Cachar	270	33	5	0	1
5.	Chirang	86	25	3	0	1
6.	Darrang	163	30	6	0	1
7.	Dhemaji	98	22	4	0	1
8.	Dhubri	246	44	8	2	1
9.	Dibrugarh	231	30	7	0	0
10.	Goalpara	151	41	5	0	1
11.	Golaghat	144	40	4	1	1
12.	Hailakandi	105	13	3	0	1
13.	Jorhat	144	44	5	2	0
14.	Kamrup(M)	51	25	3	0	1
15.	Kamrup®	280	71	11	1	1
16.	Karbi Anglong	145	46	5	1	1
17.	Karimganj	218	29	5	0	1
18.	Kokrajhar	161	45	4	1	1
19.	Lakhimpur	156	30	8	1	1
20.	Morigaon	123	36	5	0	1
21.	Nagaon	354	80	15	0	1
22.	Nalbari	121	47	9	0	1
23.	Dima Hasao	65	11	2	0	1
24.	Sivsagar	219	45	4	2	1
25.	Sonitpur	275	58	7	2	1
26.	Tinsukia	164	23	6	0	1
27.	Udalgubri	146	24	3	0	1
	Assam	4621	1014	151	14	25

Source: Government of Assam, Health and Family Welfare.

The supply constraints of healthcare services, demand-side factors (social, economic and cultural) create limitation in health care utilization among mothers. It is found from the several studies that rural health care services are poorer than urban health care services and it can also be seen in Assam also which is shown in Table 13.1. According to experts, the state of Assam still lags behind in terms of quality health care provided by the government, especially in rural areas. Communication facilities, availability of medical staff and drugs, laboratory equipments and services, infrastructural facilities, drinking water facilities—all these facilities are very poor in rural health care systems. A study shows high doctor-patient ratio in Assam which is much higher than the national average. Currently, there is one doctor per more than two thousand patients in Assam whereas, according to the World Health Organization (WHO) norms, there should be one doctor per one thousand patients. In view of the above, therefore an attempt has been made to study the differentials, accessibility, utilization pattern and factors affecting on utilization of maternal and child health care services in rural areas of Assam.

However, utilization of these services in most developing countries is constrained due to various cultural, socio-economic, and demographic factors (Addai, 2000). Explanatory factors for underutilization of maternal care services are numerous, and include: young maternal age; superstitious beliefs; poor education; unskilled occupation; poverty; low caste; parity (higher birth order were less likely to access antenatal services); lack of autonomy; poor familial support; lack of access to transport; and the high cost of care and when it is accessed, its poor quality (such as shortages of supplies and staff, mistreatment by staff, or poor training or limited experience of staff) (Kumar *et al.*, 2013; Kassebaum *et al.*, 2014; Goudar *et al.*, 2015). While recognizing the importance of health infrastructure in improving health, the Government of India launched the National Health Policy in 2002 and the National Rural Health Mission (NRHM) in 2005 to strengthen the rural health care infrastructure in the country along with the state of Assam but the improvement in health infrastructure has been quite uneven across regions with large-scale inter-state variations (Baru *et al.*, 2010; Kumar, 2013; Hazarika, 2013; Raj *et al.*, 2015).

Causes of Poor Maternal Health Care in Assam

Within India, there is marked variation in MMR and health care access between regions and in socio-economic factors (IIPS, 2010; Barros *et al.*, 2012). Several research studies have reported that mothers are too young and they are receiving minimal antenatal care (Sugathan *et al.*, 2001; Fikree *et al.*, 2002; Singh, 2012; Ponna *et al.*, 2017) and a large proportion of the women are found to be undernourished (Fikree *et al.*, 2002; Ackerson and Subramanian, 2008; Bisai, 2010; Sen *et al.*, 2010) and results in malnutrition and ill health (Talukdar and Das, 2016) and suffering from different grades of anaemic during pregnancy (Ahmed 2000; Bentley and Griffiths, 2003; Girija, 2008; Ackerson and Subramanian, 2008; Nisar *et al.*, 2015; Rakesh, 2017). There is the issue of scarcity of medicines in government hospitals. Instead of getting free medicines, patients have to purchase everything. Moreover, district hospitals still lack special care units, medicines and laboratories to deal with any epidemic. The IMR and MMR is much higher especially in the rural areas and mainly attributed to lack of adequate health care facilities, lack of knowledge about health, hygiene, awareness of health care services and less institutional delivery and acute shortage of doctors and medical staff in the hospitals. Along with the supply constraints of health care services, demand-side factors (social, economic and cultural) create limitation in health care utilization among mothers. It is found from the several studies that rural health care services are poorer than urban health care services. According to experts, India still lags behind in terms of quality health care provided by the government, especially in rural areas. Communication facilities, availability of medical staffs and drugs, laboratory equipments and services, infrastructural facilities, drinking water facilities—all these facilities are very poor in rural health care systems.

Determinants of Maternal Health Care Utilization in Assam

Several factors tending to increase maternal death (i.e., MMR) include obstructed labour, malnutrition, poverty, overwork, lack of primary health care, parasitic disease. Moreover, many cultural and social factors also promote maternal death (Stokoe, 1991). Thus, the socio-economic determinants of maternal health care utilization are educational attainment, parity level, health insurance coverage, ethnicity, household wealth and geographic region are statistically significant factors that affect the use of health care services (Celik *et al.*, 2000). Similarly, it is seen that most maternal deaths were among those with low levels of literacy and poor socio-economic strata. In addition, ignorance, hesitation, long queues at formal facility, non-availability of persons at home to taking care of pregnant women as well as heavy workloads are barriers to avail maternal and child health care services. Husband restriction is not independent to unresponsive doctors and non-availability of female health provider (Dutta and Sengupta, 2018). Good quality ANC should be able to avoid many maternal deaths. But it is seen that antenatal care visit is poor, customarily they think that it is not necessary or may be due to illiteracy and ignorance. In a study among the Karbis of Guwahati city revealed that mother's education is positively related to awareness of antenatal care and place of delivery (Mazumder, 2016). Rane *et al.* (2019) found in their study that Pregnancy Induced Hypertension (PIH) found as important cause of high MMR needs to be addressed properly as only 56 per cent studied population had their blood pressure checked during antenatal period, which indicates need to improve quality ANC. Therefore, suggested intervention is quality ANC with risk referral services. Besides this, delivery care services by health institutions are criticized by non-availability of female health providers and ambulance reduces the probability of maternal health seeking care (Rane *et al.*, 2019). Along with this, poor infrastructural facilities, long waiting period, unavailability of drugs and laboratory facilities, rude behaviour of health personnel etc. demotivated and distracts the patients towards health care services. Post-natal care (PNC) is another determinant of maternal health care utilization and post-natal deaths were more indicating need to improve quality of PNC and provision of quality antenatal and post-natal services with fully functional primary care facility are necessary in order to improve the health status (Dutta and Sengupta, 2018; Rane *et al.* 2019). ANC visits, place of delivery and PNC, the covariates considered were age of the women, type of family, working status of the women, mass-media exposure, number of contacts with the health worker during ANC period, SHG membership and marginalization etc. are the determinants of maternal health care utilization.

Recommendation to Improve the Current Health Care Situations

In the interest of public health, basic public care determiners like safe drinking water, environmental sanitation and adequate nutrition should have to be given priority. Some approaches to reverse the tragedy of maternal death and to improve health care situation include antenatal care with risk referral, training and supervision of traditional birth attendants, maternity waiting homes, decentralized maternal-child health care, provision of legal medical abortion, preferably contragestational agents and prostaglandins, blood banks at delivery units and standardized obstetric care. A report on assessment of *Janani Suraksha Yojana* in Assam during 2007 suggested for quality improvement of the primary health care services to normal deliveries, sufficient payment to cover all the expenses to *Janani Suraksha Yojana* beneficiaries, proper arrangement for transport facilities. The knowledge on new born health care providers at Sub-Health Centres should be enhanced. Besides it can also be seen the inequality in infrastructural facilities in different health centres. So the infrastructure gap in all the health care facilities should be met. Thus, the provision of quality antenatal and post-natal services with fully functional primary health care facility and easy access to emergency obstetric care along with assured referral system needs to be in place.

Conclusion

It is seen that rural health care services are poorer which leads to poor maternal and child health. In general, poorer health is highly associated with the availability and use of health care services in numerous populations. Therefore, safe motherhood practices and child survival programmes are important in a region like Assam having high infant and child mortality. Use of intensive health care services reduces health complications. Therefore, it is necessary to improve community awareness on maternal health to motivate women to use more antenatal care services to reduce health complications during the reproductive time span. Moreover, health and development are intimately connected. While insufficient development leads to poverty, inappropriate development results in prevalence of environmental health problems. Health in general and maternal and child health in particular is an aspect which is highly associated with the growth and development of a country. A broad and balanced growth of the society is dependent on the desirable level of health status of the mother and their child. Thus, to promote the health status of the mother and their child, the health care services should be proper and easily accessible to all parts of a region. India's health and welfare ministry has come out with different schemes in this regard, but the message has not reached the illiterate people. People should aware about proper health care for the pregnant woman, new mothers and children.

REFERENCES

Addai, I. 2000. "Determinants of use of maternal-child health services in rural Ghana." *Journal of Biosocial Science,* vol. 32, no. 1, pp. 1-15.

Ann, L., Montgomery, Usha Ram, Rajesh Kumar, Prabhat Jha and for the Million Death Study Collaborators, 2014. "Maternal mortality in India: Causes and health care service use based on a Nationally Representative Survey." *PLoS ONE.* **9**(1): e83331

Baru, R., Acharya, A., Acharya, S., Shiva Kumar, A.K. and Nagaraj, K. 2010. "Inequities in Access to Health Services in India: Caste, Class and Region." *Economic and Political Weekly.* **45**(38): 49-58.

Barros, A.J.D., Ronsmans, C., Axelson, H., Loaiza, E., Bertoldi, A.D., *et al.* 2012. "Equity in maternal, newborn and child health interventions in countdown to 2015: a retrospective review of survey data from 54 countries." *Lancet.* **379**: 1225-1233.

Celik, Y. and Hotchkiss, D.R. 2000. "The socio-economic determinants of maternal health care utilization in Turkey." *Soc Sci Med.* **50**(12): 1797- 806.

Centre for Operations Research and Training (CORT) (2007). *Assessment of Janani Suraksha Yojana in Assam.* Vadodara: Race Course Circle.

Dutta, P. and Sengupta, B. 2018. "Barriers of Maternal Health Seeking Behavior: A Bayesian Analysis." *Journal of Women's Health Care.* DOI: 10.4172/2167-0420.1000439.

Gogoi, M., Unisa, S. and Prusty, R.K. 2014. "Utilization of maternal health care services and reproductive health complications in Assam." *India. J Public Health.* DOI 10.1007/s10389-014-0614-y. ISSN 2198-1833.

Goudar, S.S., Goco, N., Somannavar, M.S., Vernekar, S.S., Mallapur, A.A., Moore, J.L., Wallace, D.D., Sloan, N.L., Patel, A., Hibberd, P.L., Koso-Thomas, M. 2015. "Institutional deliveries and perinatal and neonatal mortality in Southern and Central India." *Reproductive Health.* **12** (Suppl 2):S13.

Graham, W.J., Bell, J.S., Bullough, C.H.W. 2000. "Can skilled attendance at delivery reduce maternal mortality in developing countries?" *Studies in Health Services Organization and Policy.* **17**: 97-130.

Gupta, A.K., Talati, S., Sudip Bhattacharya, A,S. 2017. "Health system Strengthening-focusing on referrals: an analysis from India." *JOJ Nurs Heal Care* 2.

Hazarika, I. 2013. "Health workforce in India: assessment of availability, production and distribution." *South-East Asia Journal of Public Health.* **2**(2): 106-112.

IIPS. 2002. Reproductive and Child Health Project: District Level Household Survey. (Nasik District), Mumbai.

IIPS. 2010. District level household and facility survey (DLHS-3) 2007-2008: India. Mumbai: International Institute for Population Sciences.

Kassebaum, N., Bertozzi-Villa, A., Coggeshall, M., Shackelford, K., Steiner, C., Heuton, K., *et al.* Akademin Hälsa och samhälle, Medicinsk vetenskap and Högskolan Dalarna. 2014. "Global, regional, and national levels and causes of maternal mortality during, 1990-2013: A systematic analysis for the global burden of disease study 2013." *Lancet.* **384**(9947): 980-1004. doi:10.1016/ S0140-6736(14)60696-6.

Kaur, J., Franzen, S.R.P., Lewis, T.N., Murphy, G. 2019. "Readiness of public health facilities to provide quality maternal and newborn care across the state of Bihar, India: a cross-sectional study of district hospitals and primary health centres."

Kifle, D., Azale, T., Gelaw, Y.A., Melsew, Y.A. 2017. "Maternal health care service seeking behaviors and associated factors among women in rural Haramaya District, Eastern Ethiopia: a triangulated community-based cross-sectional study." *Reproductive Health,* Vol. 14, Article number: 6.

Koblinsky, M., Campbell, O., Heichelheim, J. (1999) "Organizing delivery care-what works for safe-motherhood?" *Bulletin of World Health Organization.* **77**(5): 399-406.

Kumar, J.R. 2013. "Role of Public Health Systems in the Present Health Scenario: Key Challenges." *Indian Journal of Public Health.* **57**(3): 133- 137.

Kumar, C., Singh, P.K., Rai, R.K. 2013. "Coverage gap in maternal and child health services in India: assessing trends and regional deprivation during 1992- 2006." *J Public Health.* **35**(4): 598.

Lassi, Z.S., Kumar, R., Bhutta, Z.A. 2016. "Community-Based Care to Improve Maternal, Newborn, and Child Health." *International Bank for Reconstruction and Development / The World Bank.* PMID:27227219

Mazumder, M.N. 2016. "Utilization of maternal health care services among the Larbis of Guwahati City." *Indian Journal of Research.* **5**: 404-406.

ORGI, 2011. *Special Bulletin on Maternal Mortality in India 2007-09.* Sample Registration System, Office of Registrar General, India (ORGI), New Delhi.

Patel, R. and Ladusingh, L. 2015. "Do Physical Proximity and Availability of Adequate Infrastructure at Public Health Facility Increase Institutional Delivery? A Three Level Hierarchical Model Approach." *PLoS One.* **10**(12):e0144352. doi: 10.1371/journal.pone.0144352. eCollection 2015.

Rabha, A.P. 2017. "Quality assessment of maternal and child health care services at Primary health care level in Kamrup District of Assam." *International Journal of Biomedical Research.* **8**(08): 479-483. ISSN: 0976-9633 (Online); 2455-0566 (Print).

Raj, S.S., Manthri, S., Sahoo, P.K.. 2015. "Emergency referral transport for maternal complication: lessons from the community based maternal death audits in Unnao district, Uttar Pradesh, India." *Int J Health Policy Manag.* **4**(2): 99-106. doi: 10.15171/ijhpm.2015.14. eCollection 2015 Feb.

Rane, T.M., Mahanta, T.G., Baruah, M., Baruah, S.D. 2019. "Epidemiological study of maternal death in Assam." *Clinical Epidemiology and Global Health.* 2213-3984/©2019 INDIACLEN. Published by Elsevier, a division of RELX India, Pvt. Ltd. All rights reserved.

Singh, S. and Badaya, S. 2014."Health care in rural India: A lack between need and feed." *South Asian J Cancer.* **3**(2): 143-144.

Sinha, L.N., Kaur, P., Gupta, R., Dalpath, S., Goyal, V., Murhekar, M. 2014. Newborn care practices and home-based post-natal newborn care programme—Mewat, Haryana, India, 2013." *Western Pac Surveill Response J.* **5**(3):22-9. doi: 10.5365/WPSAR.2014.5.1.006. eCollection 2014.

Stokoe, U. 1991. "Determinants of maternal mortality in the developing world." *Aust N Z J Obstet Gynaecol.* **31**(1): 8-16.

United Nations Children's Fund. 2015. Level and trends in child mortality: estimates developed by the UN Inter-agency group for child mortality estimation, New York.

Vidler, M., Ramadurg, U., Charantimath, U., Katageri, G., Karadiguddi, C., Sawchuck, D., Qureshi, R., Dharamsi, S., Joshi, A., von Dadelszen, P., Derman, R., Bellad, M., Goudar, S., Mallapur, A. 2016. "Utilization of maternal health care services and their determinants in Karnataka State, India." *Reprod Health.* 13 Suppl **1**:37. doi: 10.1186/s12978-016-0138-8

World Health Organization (WHO). 2015. Trends in maternal mortality: 1990 to 2015: estimates by WHO, UNICEF, UNFPA, World Bank group and the United Nations Population Division, Geneva.

14

Birth Spacing
A Study Among the Shia Muslims Women of Lucknow

Madhushree Dey, Sarvendra Yadav and *Rajesh K. Gautam*

Introduction

Clinically, birth spacing or interpregnancy interval is an optimal gap between two successive births. It is one of the essential methods to change the size and structure of a population. Additionally, it creates a link with various dimensions, viz. maternal and child health as well as development, nutritional status, morbidity and mortality rate. Concurrently, birth spacing also aids in regaining the healthiest living condition from a previous birth, labour and lactation, and also maintains/facilitates a better family condition.

Problems can be easily identified/noticed if a woman gets pregnant frequently following a previous birth even at a young age or undergo for abortion either spontaneous or induced, faces the risk of anaemia (Shakya, *et al.* 2011). Some shreds of evidence are also there which showed that shorter birth intervals increase the risk of preterm birth, low birth weight, small gestational age of a child, and shorter birth spacing would lead to premature rupture of membranes, third-trimester bleeding and puerperal endometritis which put the woman into a great risk of haemorrhage, and these are the evident problems which increase the maternal death (Hailu and Gulte, 2016; Yadav and Pandey, 2017). So, adequate birth spacing is a fruitful decision as it acts as an indicator of determining the future physical and mental capacities of the child as well as look into the health of the mothers.

Besides the biological problem related to women and their child's health, inadequate birth spacing tends to accelerate the population growth. As a result, the socio-economic development of an area slows down. A shorter birth interval will possibly be imprinted a destructive footprint not only on the individual but a nation will also get trapped into this worst set of circumstances. On the other side, unplanned birth spacing may impair the fertility levels and become a barrier to show their contribution to economic development (Yadav and Pandey, 2017). Not only the birth interval with a minimal gap has a negative impact but also a maximal space shows certain impairment in foetal condition. Even families with multiple children also come across to the shorter or longer birth interval.

Therefore, to have proper birth spacing, various determinants play important role behind it such as educational status, early marriage, contraceptive usage and economic condition (Shakya, *et al.* 2011). Understanding the nature of the reproductive pattern, fertility behaviour and knowledge on birth spacing can only be gained through effective family planning strategies. So, for the better health status of mother and child, and to control/check the population growth, the Indian Family Welfare Programme had initiated several new initiatives such as adoption of various contraceptive methods among the couples which not only help in achieving the desired family size, but also reduce the chances of the occurrence of maternal and infant mortality rate. Through research, it has been found out that spacing between births of at least 3 to 5 years could increase the survival chances of infants and mothers by 2.5 times. Even the Millennium Development Goals (MDGs) of United Nations aims to promote the Healthy Timing and Spacing of Pregnancy (HTSP), and it is considered as an important family planning intervention. It has also been found out that the decision making, abortion, age at marriage, and women empowerment also play a significant role in lengthening the birth interval which directly influences the health of both mothers and neonates, and also helps in shaping the economy, environment and political map of any nation (Starbird *et al.* 2016).

In the above background, the present study is carried out in Lucknow city of Uttar Pradesh (UP) state of the Indian Union which is situated along the banks of river Gomti, lies in between

26° 30′ to 27° 10′ North latitude and 80° 30′ to 81° 13′ East longitude. It is accessible from every part of India through air, rail and road. It is the capital city of Uttar Pradesh and also popularly known as the City of *Nawabs*, Golden City of the East and the City of *Tahzeeb* (https://lucknow.nic.in/about-district/). The City of *Nawabs* with the majority population of *Shia* Muslims where this study was accomplished. The *Shias* are one of the two sects of Islam. They are the followers of the Islamic Prophet Muhammad's family. They are largely distributed in the state of UP and Bihar. In this background, there is an attempt to gain insights of the pattern and determinants of birth spacing among *Shia* women and it aids in bringing more awareness about the physiological and socio-economic benefits of optimal birth spacing among the couples, individuals and community at large.

Materials and Methods

A cross-sectional study was conducted in the areas of Victoria Street, *Mehtab Bagh* and City Station of Lucknow in the month of May in 2019. The study population was composed of 150 married women with age-range of 15 to 59 years. To meet the objectives, a semi-structured interview schedule was designed and it had been administered to obtain information on socio-economic status, reproductive and other demographic profile through personal interviews, survey method and most of the interviews were conducted during day time between 11.00 am—5.00 pm according to their convenience.

Ethical guidelines were followed as per the Helsinki Declaration (2008). The survey was carried out with the consent of the Principal of Shia Women College, head of the family and the respondents. Besides, the study protocol included the cover letter with the details of the potential risks of participating in the study and explained that all the data collected were confidential and that participation was voluntary. Subjects were selected based on purposive and snowball sampling method which worked significantly among them.

After data collection, it was entered into Excel and SPSS for further calculation and analysis. The outcomes were reported as mean±Standard Deviation (SD) for continuous variables and percentages for categorical variables. One-sample t-test, linear regression and Chi-square tests were used to interpret the findings. P-value of less than 0.05 was considered to be statistically significant.

Results

It is evident from Table 14.1 that the mean of the current age of the married women was 38.92±10.63 years, mean age at marriage was 21.28± 4.55 years, mean age at first birth was 19.76±7.92 years, the total number of pregnancies, total number of live births and the total number of living children were 3.06±2.13 years, 2.31±1.74 years and 2.25±1.66 years respectively. The mean age of spacing between first and second child was 2.18±2.20 years with a maximum age of 12 years.

Table 14.1: Central Tendency of some selected demographic variables

Variables	*Mean*	*Standard Deviation*	*Minimum*	*Maximum*
Current Age (in years)	38.92	10.63	20	59
Age at Marriage (in years)	21.28	4.55	13	42
Age at her first Birth (in years)	19.76	7.92	13	35
Total Number of Pregnancies	3.06	2.13	0	9
Total Number of Live Births	2.31	1.74	0	8
Total Number of Living Children	2.25	1.66	0	8
Spacing Between First and Second Child	2.18	2.20	0	12

A total of 22.7 per cent of women in the age group 20-30 years had birth spacing less than 2 years, while 16.7 per cent of women in 31-40 years of age group had 6-12 years of birth spacing. In the 41-50 years and 31-40 years of age group, 70.8 per cent of women had 2-3 years and 33.3 per cent of women had 4-5 years of birth spacing respectively (Figure 14.1).

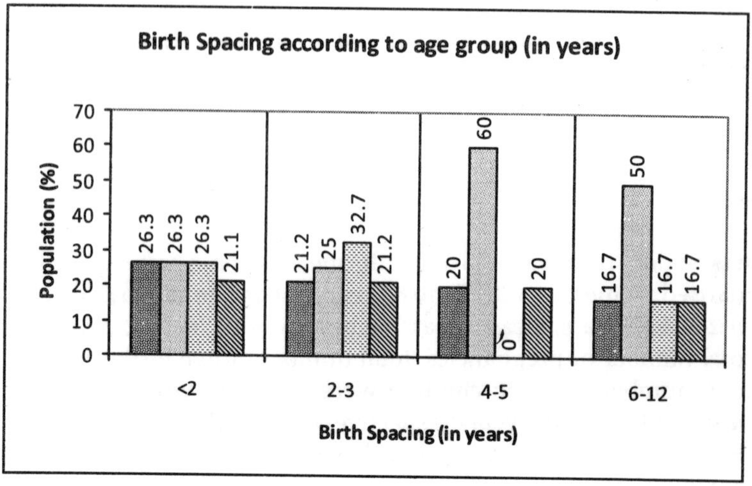

Fig. 14.1: Birth spacing according to age group of mothers.

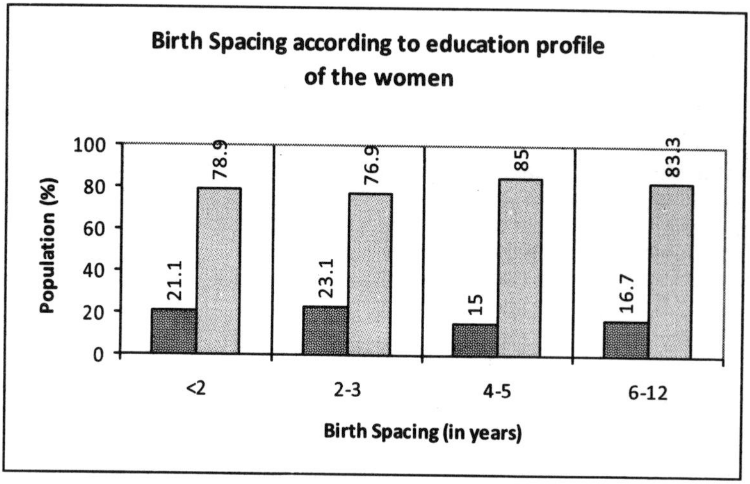

Fig. 14.2: Birth Spacing according to education profile of mothers.

The further analysis (Table 14.2) indicates that the lengthening of the birth interval had happened due to abortion (38%). And the prevalence of abortion was found higher among the educated women (84.2%); while only 15.8 per cent uneducated women opted for abortion. Again, within the educated population of women, the prevalence of non-abortion is high. Out of 150

Table 14.2: Educational Profile and Prevalence of Abortion

Abortion	*Education Profile of the Women*			
	Uneducated		*Educated*	
	N	*%*	*N*	*%*
Not experienced	16	17.2	77	82.8
Experienced	9	15.8	48	84.2

women, 77 educated women did not abort their fetus, but 48 educated women aborted their foetus. Poor physiological and economic conditions were the reasons of abortion.

Comparison of birth spacing between educated and uneducated women is presented in Figure 14.2. It is evident that higher proportion of uneducated women have 2-3 years of birth spacing (57%) as compared to 48.8% of educated women. <2 years of birth spacing was almost similar in both the cohort. Among educated women 4-5 years and 5-12 years of spacing is higher (20.7% and 12.2%) as compared to uneducated women (14.3% and 9.5%).

Further to elucidate the relationship between birth spacing (target) and other variables (predictors) like age at first birth, the total number of pregnancies, total number of living children, total number of children and the total number of abortion, linear regression analysis was computed for the target population. The analysis was done keeping the birth spacing as dependent and the rest 4 predictors as an independent variables. Birth spacing was dependent on age at first birth (R^2= 0.086; $P< 0.001$), the total number of pregnancies (R^2=0.202; $P< 0.001$), the total number of living children (R^2= 0.110; $P< 0.001$) and the total number of abortion (R^2=0.106, $P<0.001$) as displayed in (Table 14.3).

Chi-square test was performed to understand the relationship between the prevalence of previous and present use of contraceptive along with educational and occupational status of the couples with birth spacing. After the statistical analysis, depicted in Tables 14.4 and 14.5, insignificant relation between these categorical variables were found with $p >0.05$.

Table 14.3: Regression analysis between birth spacing and other studied variables

Independent Variable	*Dependent Variable*	*Bivariate Linear Regression Analysis*		*df*	*F-Value*	*t-Value*	*P-Value*
		R^2	*B±SE*				
Total number of pregnancies	Birth Spacing	0.202*	0.464±0.076	149	37.364	6.113	0.001
Age at first birth		0.086*	0.082±0.022	149	13.972	3.738	0.001
Total number of living children		0.110*	0.439±0.102	149	18.383	4.228	0.001
Total number of abortion		0.106*	0.645±0.154	149	17.512	4.185	0.001

* Linear Regression analysis is significant at P< 0.001 level.

Table 14.4: Mean birth spacing and family planning method

Categories Contraceptive use		*Birth spacing in years*								*χ^2*
		<2		*2-3*		*4 -5*		*6-12*		
		N	*%*	*N*	*%*	*N*	*%*	*N*	*%*	
Previous use	Yes	7	14.9	23	48.9	10	21.3	7	14.9	1.233*
	No	11	20.4	28	51.9	10	18.5	5	9.3	
Current use	Yes	6	13.0	23	50.0	11	23.9	6	13.0	2.323*
	No	13	22.8	29	50.9	9	15.8	6	10.5	

* Chi-square test is insignificant (P>0.05).

Hence, it can be inferred from the above data that the existence of birth spacing was mainly influenced by the predictors like age at first birth, the total number of living children, total number of pregnancies and total number of abortions. The role of contraceptive usage, educational and occupational status of the couples were seemed to be less dominant in maintaining an adequate birth spacing and could be better understood from the given Tables 14.4 and 14.5.

One sample t-test was performed to determine the statistical indifference of the mean birth spacing (2.1867) years with the mean birth spacing of India (1.10 years= 22 months) and mean age at first birth of the women of Uttar Pradesh (18.4) years (NFHS-4,

Table 14.5: Mean birth spacing and general profile of the target population

General profile of the women	Categories	Birth spacing in years								χ^2
		<2		2-3		4 -5		6-12		
		N	%	N	%	N	%	N	%	
Educational Status of the informant	Uneducated	4	19	12	57.1	3	14.3	2	9.5	0.023*
	Educated	15	18.3	40	48.8	17	20.7	10	12.2	
Occupational status of the informant	Not Working	15	18.3	42	51.2	16	19.5	9	11	0.607*
	Working	2	13.3	7	46.7	4	26.7	2	13.3	
Educational Status of the spouse	Uneducated	2	22.2	4	44.4	2	22.2	1	11.1	0.296*
	Educated	15	18.3	42	51.2	14	17.1	11	13.4	
Occupational Status of the spouse	Not Working	0	0.0	1	100	0	0.0	0	0.0	0.784
	Working	8	19.0	20	47.6	7	16.7	7	16.7	

* Chi-square test is insignificant (P>0.05).

2015-16). After analysing the available data, it was found that the mean birth spacing and mean age at first birth of the target population is significantly different from mean birth spacing of India, and mean age at first birth at P< 0.05 level. The proper illustration has been given in Table 14.6.

Table 14.6: Analysis of age at the first birth and spacing between first and second child through one-sample test among 150 women of Shia Muslims of Lucknow, 2019

Variables	*N*	*df*	*Test Value*	*Mean*	*t*	*P-Value*
Spacing between first and second child (in years)	150	149	1.10	2.1867	6.043	0.000
Age at her first birth (in years)	150	149	18.4	19.7600	2.102	0.037

Discussion

This study had focused on birth spacing and tried to determine all the possible factors responsible for birth intervals among the *Shia* women of Lucknow. From this study, sufficient information was collected through using various tools and techniques. Mean current age of the target population was found 38.92 years, mean age at marriage was 21.28 years, mean age at first birth was 19.76 years, mean of the total number of pregnancy was found 3.06, mean of a total number of live births was 2.31, mean of the total number of living children 2.25 and spacing between first and second child was found 2.18 years. The mean value of both the variables, i.e. age at first birth and spacing between first and second child was higher than the national average, i.e. 19.76 years and 2.1867 years respectively. A study of Shakya, Pokharel and Yadav (2011) showed that the educational status of the couples was associated with the birth spacing. But the findings of this study uttered a different story. The educational and occupational status were insignificant with the average birth spacing as p>0.05. Even the family planning methods did not show much positive result as P>0.05 through chi-square test.

In several studies, it has been estimated that birth interval shows a difference according to the age of the mother. This study also had similar findings. Prevalence of the lowest birth interval was found in the younger mother, while highest in the older. A total of 22.7 per cent of women of the age group 20-30 had <2 years of birth spacing; while 33.3 per cent of women in the age group 31-40 years had 4-5 years of birth spacing. Comparison of educated and uneducated women demonstrates that higher proportion of educated women (84.2%) opt for abortion, whereas only 15.8 per cent uneducated women opted abortion. Prevalence of abortion was mainly due to physiological and economic problems. On the other hand, it was found that most of them consider a child as a gift from Allah so opting for an abortion equals to committing some sort of sin. So, few uneducated women went for sterilization which prevented them from foeticide and this observation was in consonance with the study of Kanojia *et al.* (1996).

Bivariate linear regression analysis indicates that the birth spacing among *Shia* muslim women of Lucknow is determined by the total number of pregnancies (20.2%), age at first birth (8.6%), the number of living children (11%) and the total number of abortion (10.6%).

Conclusion

It has been found that the average birth spacing is relatively higher than the national average of birth spacing among the *Shia* Muslims of Lucknow. Majority of the women were found to have 2-3 years of birth spacing. But around 30 per cent of married women practised short term birth interval <2 years, which was below the recommended optimal birth spacing, i.e. 3-5 years. So, they needed to maintain the healthiest birth interval for attaining safe motherhood. It was also found that the occurrence of foetal loss was the reason behind the birth spacing, rather than due to the use of spacing methods or adoption of the family planning method. Moreover, age at marriage, age at first birth, total number of pregnancies, children ever born and number of abortions were found as predictors for birth spacing.

REFERENCES

Hailu, D. & Gulte, T. (2016). "Determinants of Short Interbirth Interval among Reproductive." *International Journal of Reproductive Medicine, 2016*, 1-19. Retrieved from http://dx.doi.org/10.1155/2016/6072437

International Institute for Population Sciences (IIPS) and ICF. 2017. *National Family Health Survey (NFHS-4), India, 2015-16: Uttar Pradesh*. Mumbai: IIPS.

Kanojia, J.K., Nirbhavane, N.C., Toddywala, V.S., *et al.* (May-June, 1996) "Dynamics of contraceptive practice amongst urban Indian women." *The National Medical Journal of India*. **9**(3): 109-112.

Shakya, S., Pokharel, PK., and Yadav, BK. (2011). "Study on birth spacing and its determinants among women of Kirtipur Municipality of Kathmandu District." *International Journal of Nursing Education*, **3**(1): 56-60. Retrieved from https://www.researchgate.net/publication/301220757

Starbird, E., Norton, M., and Marcus, R. (2016). "Investing in Family Planning: Key to Achieving the Sustainable Development Goals." *Global Health: Science and Practice*, **4**(2).

WHO, 2005. *Report of a WHO Technical Consultation on Birth Spacing*. Department of Making Pregnancy Safer, Department of Reproductive Health and Research. Geneva, Switzerland: WHO.

Yadav, B., and Pandey, S. (2017). "Study of knowledge, attitude, and practice regarding birth spacing and methods available for spacing in rural Haryana, India." *International Journal of Reproduction, Contraception, Obstetrics and Gynecology*, **7**(4): 1390. https://lucknow.nic.in/about-district/ Retrieved at 8:30 pm dated 9th June, 2020.

15

Ethnomedicinal Practices for Management of Post-natal Health in Golaghat District

Hriday Ranjan Gogoi and *Ajit K. Tamuli*

Introduction

Dependence of the village people on wild and domesticated plants as medicine for health care, diseases curing, healing practices and seeking processes is an established phenomenon. Ethnomedicine refers to the traditional medical practices concerned with the cultural interpretation of health, diseases and illness and also health care seeking process and healing practices (Krippner, 2003). The ethnomedicinal knowledge always comes continuously from forefathers to upcoming generations in oral form and hence, scientific valediction may not have been undertaken in this field. But in modern drug discovery ethnomedicinal knowledge plays an important role. The Ayurveda which means "Science of life", a oldest medicinal system in Indian subcontinent and has been practised since 12th century. It aims to accomplish physical, mental, social and spiritual well-being as holistic medicine (Anvar *et al.*, 2015). Around the world more than 35,000 plants species are being used for different cultural practices. According to WHO, about 80 per cent of the world population are still dependent on traditional system for primary health care (Karemore *et al.*, 2017; Anvar *et al.*, 2015). The term post-natal health is the stage of the mother and the child occurring after delivery of a child. Post-natal period can be defined as the first 6 (6-8) weeks after child birth which is critical to the lives of mother and her neonate (WHO, 2013; Chaturvedi *et al.*, 2017; Aishwarya *et al.*, 2018). In many villages and backward areas, there were no hospitals thus, the people are depended on the local herbal practitioners and on the plants in vicinity to take care of post-natal health. Therefore, a good number of plants were used as to ease delivery, to clean womb to induce labour and to protect child and mother from the evils (Peltzer, 2009).

Materials and Methods

Geography and Climate

Golaghat district mainly comprises sub-tropical climate. The total area of the district is approximately 3502 km^2 and it lies 100m above the mean sea level. Golaghat district is surrounded in the north by Brahmaputra river, in south by Nagaland, in the east by Jorhat, and the west by KarbiAnglong and Nagaon district. It is strategically positioned between 26°0´-27°.1´ N latitude and 93°0´-94°18´ E longitude (Barukial *et al.*, 2010). In Golaghat district there are a number of rivers flowing through the region. Dhansiri is the chief river of the district. Doyang, Nambor, Doigrung, and Kaliony are the main four streams of Dhansiri river. The river Kakodunga marks the border of Golaghat and Jorhat distict. Kaziranga, Nambor, Garampani, upper Doigrung, Bijuli etc. are the main forests in the district. Murphulani is the village present in East part of the district. The latitude 26.5222799 and longitude 93.9774371 are the geo-coordinate of the village. No.1 Murphulani is situated in East by Doigrung river and Nambor reserve forest, West by Bijuli reserve forest, North by No. 2 Murphulani and Doigrung river and South by Bogijan and Karbi Anglong hills. The climate of Golaghat is characterized by sufficiently high precipitation, moderate and high humidity. The climate may be termed as a humid mesothermal one. Climate, edaphic and biotic factors together determine the vegetation of an area. The climate is tropical with hot humid summer during April to September and dry winter during November to February. The area experience heavy rain of monsoon during May to August. The total rainfall is 100-120 cm. The area experience maximum temperature of 38°C and minimum temperature of 10°C. The area falls under evergreen and semi-evergreen forest zone but thick forest is absent due to habitation, urbanization, and agriculture.

The people and their habitat

The residents of No.1 Murphulani comprises Ahom, Chutia, Adivashi communities and few Sonowal Kachari and Kacharis. Though, the people of Sonowal Kachari are functionally slightly different, they use Assamese language and culture, they do not have their own dialect. It is said that during the reign of Ahom some of the Kacharis were engaged in washing gold particles from the sands of river, hence the prefix "Sonowal" was added to specify them (Konch Ritamoni *et al.* 2014). The study was undertaken in different habitats of No.1 Murphulani are Kalbarichuk, Saporichuk, Dohchuk, Chotionapathar, Dokhorapathar, Liksoniachuk and Borgaon. Most of the Ahom people are habitating in Kalbarichuk, Saporichuk, Dohchuk, Chotionapathar and Liksoniachuk and Adivashis are living in Borgaon and Dokhorapathar mostly. Sonowal Kachari and Kachari people are distributed in all the corner of the village. The village is located near the upper Doigrung Nambor reserve forest and Bijuli forest situated on the bank of river Doigrung. Therefore, availability of wild plants and vegetables are much more in this place, hence the people's dependency on it as their feeding habit.

Data Collection

The study was carried out during the period from February 2018 to September 2018 in 7 (seven) chuks of the village of Golaghat District. Data were collected from the informants and personal observations and some are from publications. 10 informants were randomly selected between ages of 50-70 years from each chuk. Out of 70 informants there were only 7 males and 63 females. Semi-structured interviews and personal observations were employed to collect data. Information was provided by sharing herbal prescriptions for management of post-natal health. Medicinal plants were collected from their natural habitats with the help of informants. The following tools were used for data collection:

Semi-structured interview: It included identification of medicinal plants, ethnomedicines, method of use, mode of preparation, dosages for management of post-natal health and recording.

Personal observation: It included attending the local medicine man during healing practices.

Statistical analysis: Data of medicinal plants used in post-natal health was analyzed using Informants consensus factor 9(Fic) and Fidelity level (FL).

Informants consensus factor (Fic): It is used to analyse the general use of plants. It was used to highlight the plants of a particular cultural relevance and agreement in the use of plants. Fic can calculate the level of homogeneity among informants (Trotter and Logan, 1986). The ranges of Fic values from 0 -1. Fic = (Nur-Nt)/(Nur-1) [Where, Nur= No. of use reports from informants for a particular plant use category. Nt = Number of species used for that plant use category for all informants].

Fidelity level (FL): It calculates the percentage of informants claiming the use of a certain plant into a particular disease (Alexiades, 1996). Higher the FL, higher preferences of that plant to treatment of the disease.

FL (%) = Np/N*100

Where, Np = number of informants that claim the use of a plant species to treat particular disease.

N = number of informants that claim the use of a plant species as a medicine to treat any disease.

Results and Discussions

Traditional medicines are the chief sources of primary health care in this village. There are various approaches that used to improve the maternal health. Traditionally Drinking herb for post-natal care is of two phases, first phase is post-natal maternal phase, applied in morning after second or third day of giving birth. It carried out recovery process. Second phase is Recovery treatment for vital organs, treatment was used as liquid and pill forms (Zumaidar *et al.*, 2019). After 3 days of child birth, there is a ritual of healings in order to manage the post-natal health is called the "*Kochujaal*" (Assamese). The term *Kochujaal* is because on that day *Colocasia esculenta* plant (*Kochu*) with fruits of *Piper nigrum* are cooked together and give it to the mother to eat.After fallen down of umbilical cord they held an another ritual called "Baaj Dekhuwa" (Assamese) where they take out the baby to show sun for the first

Table 15.1: List of plants with family, local name and plant parts used

Plant name	*Family*	*Local name*	*Parts used*
Ocimum sanctum	Lamiaceae	Tuloshi	Leaves and apical twig
Vitex negundo	Lamiaceae	Posotia	Leaves
Pogostemon cablin	Lamiaceae	Shukloti	Leaves and apical twig
Leucas aspera	Lamiaceae	Durun bon	Apical twig
Mentha viridis	Lamiaceae	Podina	Leaves and apical twig
Aegle marmelos	Rutaceae	Bel	Fruits and leaves
Citrus lemon	Rutaceae	Nemu	Fruits
Murraya koenigii	Rutaceae	Norosingha	Leaves
Amaranthus viridis	Amaranthaceae	Khutura	Apical twig
Alternanthera sessilis	Ameranthaceae	Matikanduri	Apical twig
Oldenlandia diffusa	Rubiaceae	Bon jaluk	Apical twig
Paederia foetida	Rubiaceae	Vedailota	Leaves and apical twig
Allium sativum	Amaryllidaceae	Nohoru	Bulb
Drymaria cordata	Caryophyllaceae	Laijabori	Whole plant
Psidium guajava	Myrtaceae	Madhuri	Apical twig
Curcuma longa	Zingiberaceae	Halodhi	Rhizome
Piper nigrum	Piperaceae	Jaluk	Fruits
Colocasia esculenta	Arraceae	Kochu	Tender leaves
Euphorbia hirta	Euphorbiaceae	Gakhiroti bon	Apical twig
Eclipta alba	Asteraceae	Kenhraj	Apical twig
Azadirachta indica	Meliaceae	Nim	Leaves
Centella asiatica	Apiaceae	Manimuni	Whole plant
Carica papaya	Caricaceae	Amita	Fruits
Plumbago zeylenica	Plumbaginaceae	Agesita	Leaves
Commelina benghalensis	Commelinaceae	Borkonashimolu	Apical twig
Houttuynia cordata	Saururaceae	Mosondori	Leaves and apical twig
Sida cordifolia	Malvaceae	Sun borolia	Roots
Acorus calamus	Acoraceae	Bos	Rhizome

time. The main purpose of this traditional practice is to improve practice is to improve blood circulation and post-natal recovery (Zumaidar *et al.*, 2019). In the present study, ethnomedicinal knowledge of altogether 28 plants belongs to 19 family and 27 genera used for management of post-natal health were recorded.

The family *Lamiaceae* has highest representation with 4 species followed by *Rutaceae* (3), two species (2 families) and one species (15 families). The different parts of the medicinal plants, viz. apical twig (15), leaves (4), fruit (4), whole plant (2), rhizome (1), bulb(1), root (1) were used. The use of traditional medicinal plants has quantitatively analysed using informants' consensus factor and fidelity level.

Post-natal Health Management

The medicinal plants were used in post-natal health mainly for healing and management of reproductive and child health.

Early Child birth: They used 3 inch of roots of *Sida cordifolia* along with betel nut for three time to give early child birth.

Table 15.2: Data on number of species used against health condition and statistical analysis

Disease category	*No. of informants*	*No. of species*	*Fic*	*No.of informants that use as medicine*	*Fidelity Level (%)*
Early birth	3	2	0.5	3	0.01
Healing practices	67	12	0.83	65	0.010
Pain	63	4	0.95	58	0.01
Regaining of normal uterus	27	6	0.80	19	0.014
Agalactia	43	4	0.92	35	0.012
Edema	59	8	0.87	43	0.013
Menorrhagia	60	8	0.88	43	0.013
Anaemia	12	3	0.81	7	0.017
Common cold	68	3	0.97	65	0.010
Dysentery	45	4	0.93	27	0.016
Milk vomiting	51	1	1	48	0.010
Hiccup	7	1	1	3	0.023
Antihelminthic	33	1	1	15	0.022
Antiallergic	11	1	1	9	0.012

Healing practices: *Colocasia esculenta, Piper nigrum, Houttuynia cordata, Pogostemon cablin, Amaranthus viridis, Leucas aspera, Oldenlandia corymbosa* were used for healing wounds. These were used as vegetables with *Allium sativum* and the fruit of *Piper nigrum. Eclipta alba* and the juice of *Vitex negundo* were most effective healer. The boiled dry fruit juice of *Aegle marmelos* along with spotted snakehead fish (*Channa punctata*) also useful for drying navel of mother.

Used as pain killer: Medicinal plants like *Allium sativum, Alternanthera sessilis, Oldenlandia corymbosa* were used as pain killer. These were used as vegetables, but the paste of *Oldenlandia corymbosa* might be effective in pain and healing.

After 3 days, i.e. after Kochujaal, burned *Allium sativum* has also given to eat as a pain killer. They used *Curcuma longa* as a *chutney* to relieve from pain.

Regaining of reproductive health: *Oldenlandia corymbosa* is most effective in regaining natural state of uterus. It is used as vegetables along with *Paederia foetida, Eclipta alba, Centella asiatica, Murraya koenigii* and a little amount of fruits of *Piper nigrum.*

Agalactia (Gakhirnulua): It is common in case of aged women. *Carica papaya, Euphorbia hirta* and *Piper nigrum, Commelina benghalensis.*

(1) Steam boiled *Euphorbia hirta* was most effective in agalactia.
(2) The mixer of milk and juice of a fistful *Commelina benghalensis* can remove agalactia.
(3) The curry of *Carica papaya* is also most useful in agalactia.

Edema (Ga-ukhoha): It is recognized by the symptoms of swelling of feet and other body parts. To remove edema after birth, there were some prescriptions as follows:

(1) The curry of 3/4 leaves of *Plumbago zeylenica,* one fistful of *Paederia foetida* and *Murraya koenigii* were cooked.
(2) The curry of *Pogostemon cablin* and *Paederia foetida* were used to cure edema.
(3) *Pogostemon cablin* and young leaves of *Colocasia esculenta* were cooked by steam to cure edema.
(4) The steam cooked leaves of *Leucas aspera* and *Pogostemon cablin/Plumbago zeylenica* were also used for edema.
(5) The boiled juice of *Vitex negundo, Pogostemon cablin* and 3/4 leaves of *Plumbago zeylenica* were most effective in edema.
(6) The curry of *Azadirach indica* and 3/4 leaves of *Plumbago zeylenica* were also used.

Menorrhagia (Ga-chola): It is characterized by the uncontrolled bleeding and weakness. Sometimes, it occurs in unexpected birth or birth occurs abnormally, not in appropriate time. Some prescriptions of it are as follows:

(1) The juice mixture of *Ocimum sanctum* (Tuloshi), *Eclipta alba* (Kenhraj), *Psidium guajava* (Madhuri) and fruits of *Piper nigrum* (jaluk). The local practitioner prescribed half cup in twice a day for three days.
(2) The juice mixture of *Aegle marmelos*, root of *uvota bon* (Assamese) and fruits of *Piper nigrum*, half cup for three days.
(3) The juice of *Curcuma longa* along with the juice of *Citrus lemon* is also effective in Menorrhagia.

Anaemia: To increase blood after delivery they prescribed the juice mixture of *Eclipta alba, Ocimum sanctum* and *Psidium guajava* after light food.

Common cold: They used bulb of *Allium sativum* and the rhizome of *Acorus calamus* sewing together to hang on the neck of the baby for curing common cold. To remove fever of the baby, they used the paste of *Drymaria cordata* on their forehead.

Dysentery: To remove dysentery from the baby, they prescribed half spoon of the juice mixture of leaves of *Azadirachta indica*, rhizome of *Acorus calamus* and the bulb of *Allium sativum.* To remove hard faeces of baby, infoemants prescribed half tea spoon of the juice of *Drymaria cordata* and two tea spoonful to mother.

Milk Vomiting (Dudhmur): To remove milk vomiting from the child they prescribed the paste of apical twig of *Ricinus communis* placed on the forehead of the child.

Hiccup: A drop of juice of *Mentha viridis* is most effective in hiccup of baby.

Antihelminthic: The juice of *Mentha viridis* also play a role as antihelminthic agent that can protect the growth of worms.

Antiallergic: The paste of *Mentha viridis* can protect some of the allergies. They used it in case of allergy that is responsible for caterpillar.

Conclusion

Ethno-medicines are the chief sources of primary health care in most of the remote and rural areas of the world. People discovered medicines for their own connection where the medical facilities or physicians cannot reach that place.This study is conducted to list and assess the ethno-medicinal knowledge for management of post-natal health through which a good number of plants have been identified as useful for post-natal health. However, this study is not enough to come to a concrete conclusion of the ultimate remedy for post-natal health care of the study area. There is further scope to undertake detailed research on the active components there in the plants used for care and cure of post-natal conditions. To keep the study on there is a need to conserve the useful plants before extinction due to unscientific exploitation.

REFERENCES

Alexiades, M.N. 1996. "Collecting ethnobotanical data: An introduction to basic concepts and techniques." *Selected guidelines for ethnbotanical research: A field manual* :53-94. The New York Botanical Garden.

Anar, K., Haneel, J. 2015. "Ethnobotancal plants used for post-natal care by traditional practitioners from Kozhikode district, Kerala, India." *Int. J. of Res. In Pharm. and Chem. (IJRPC).* **5**(4):570-581, ISSN 2231-2781.

Jayanta, B., Sarma, J. 2011. "Ethnomedicinal plants used by the people of Golaghat District, Assam, India." *Corpus,* ID 33488237.

Chaturvedi, Archana; Ashok Kumar Tiwari and Ruchi Jakhmola Mani. 2017. "Traditional practices of using various medicinal plants during post-natal care in Chitrakoot district." *Indian Journal of Traditional Knowledge,* **16**(4): 605-613.

Dudi Aishwarya and Dheeraj Singh 2018. "Medicinal plants used during traditional post-natal care practices in Rajasthan, India." *Ethno Med.* **12**(4): 212-220.

K. Anvar and Jazir Haneel, 2015. "Ethnobotanical plants used for post-natal care by traditional practitioners from Kozhikode district, Kerala, India." *IJRPC,* **5**(4):50-581. ISSN :2231-2781.

Kar Peltzer, Nancy Phaswana-Mafuya and Latasha Treger. 2009. "Use of traditional and complementary health practices in prenatal and postnatal delivery in the context of HIV transmission from mother to child (PMTCT) in the Eastern cape, South Africa." *Afr. J. Traditional, Complementary and Alternative Medicines,* **6**(2): 155-162

Karemore, M.N. and J.G. Avari., 2017. "Herbal medicines used during pregnancy, childbirth and postpartum care." *IJPSR* (2017), 8(12): 5326-35.

Konch, Ritamoni; Teron, R. and Tamuli, A. Kr. 2014. *Ethnomedicines for women reproductive health among the Sonowal Kachari tribe of Lakhimpur district, Assam.*

Krippner, S. 2003. *Models of Ethnomedicinal healing*. Presented at Ethnomedicine Conference, Munich, Germany, April 26-27 and October 11-12.

Trotter, R. and Logan, M. 1986. "Informan Consensus : A new approach for identifying potentially effective medicinal plants." In *Plants in Indigenous Medicine and Diet: Biobehavioural Approaches*, Redgrave Publishers, Bedford Hills, New York. 91-112.

Zumaidar; Saudah Saudah and Saida Ranovi E. Harnelly 2019. "Indigenous Knowledge of postnatal mother care using plants by acehnese." *ICONES 2019. Earth Environmental Science*, 364(2019) 012025.

SECTION-IV

Changing Perspectives of Maternal and Child Health and Nutrition Status

16

Lifestyle: Determinant of Maternal and Child Health

Debidas Ghosh, Adrija Tripathy and *Farhin Ara*

1. Introduction

Different attitude, behaviour and practices which we follow on daily basis covering domestic life as well as professional life collectively referred as lifestyle. Lifestyle is directly associated with the state of the health of an individual. The attitudes, practices and behaviours which favour the healthy life known as health friendly lifestyle (Trovato, 2012) and it is the most important part in 21st century. Through lifestyle modification, different non-communicable diseases can be prevented. Hence, these are designated as lifestyle diseases like diabetes, cardiovascular diseases, infertility, obesity, gout etc. By adoption of positive attitude and by developing the healthy lifestyle, significant contributions can be delivered for creating healthy population with special reference to thc maternal and child health. Many governments and non-governmental organizations are now-a-days taking active participation in promoting awareness programme regarding lifestyle modification towards a better and healthy family, society and nation.

Lifestyle and its association with the Health Disorders

Components of the lifestyle and its association with the health disorders in vulnerable groups like pregnant and lactating mothers, adolescent girls and pre-school children groups of the society have been discussed in this chapter.

1.1 Factors Affecting Lifestyle

Internal and external factors responsible to modify lifestyle:

- **Internal Factors**

(a) *Knowledge*—It plays a vital role in lifestyle alteration. Knowledge brings changes in the attitude to adopt healthy practices that finally upgrade the lifestyle as a whole.

(b) *Attitude*—An overall change in attitude is a must step to be taken to change the unhealthy practices. Change in attitude is influenced by the proper knowledge regarding healthy lifestyle.

(c) *Social and lifestyle adoption skill*—In spite of having a clear idea about health friendly practices and unhealthy practices, people sometimes follow the malpractices in their daily routine which cause non-communicable diseases later on. So, adoption of healthy behaviour and the understanding of its social impact may help to alter the lifestyle from unhealthy to healthy mode.

(d) *Psychology*—Psychology plays pivotal role in the adoption of healthy lifestyle. Strong psychological state helps to avoid unhealthy practices that improve the health status.

- **External Factors**

(a) *Media*—Mass-media is one of the important modes of communication. Television, radio, internet etc. are the important sources of information in today's life. Different health shows in television provide scientific information regarding the bad impact of unhealthy work style and/or food style on human health.

(b) *Technology*—Different handy devices for blood sugar measurement, blood pressure determination etc. are easy to use by common people and like this way, technology plays a prime role to assess the health status easily which motivate us to change our lifestyle.

(c) *Economy*—It refers to a specific state of a country or region in terms of the production and consumption of goods and services and the supply of money. Economy plays a very important role in lifestyle modification. Good economical condition of a country helps to minimize the psychological stress of the countrymen in connection with money earning, employment etc. which also drive to follow healthy practices for developing health friendly lifestyle.

(*d*) *Environmental stressor*—Environmental stress like excessive pollution, radiation exposure etc. has direct association with physiological stress generation that ultimately affect the steady state of the human health. Minimization of the pollution by plantation trees, less uses of air conditioners and other sources of radiation exposure should be minimized to check the environmental stress.

(*e*) *Political source*—Political influence is also another important factor for lifestyle modification. Political initiative can make an easy success to any goal related to lifestyle modification by the huge manpower and societal activities.

2. Work Style

There are two major components of lifestyle. One of them is work style which covers pattern of work, duration of work, environment in the working station etc. All are included in work style.

2.1 Types of Work Style and Health Issues

2.1.1 Stressful work style

Stress can be simply defined as body's reaction to any change that needs an adjustment or response. When our body homeostasis is deviated by external or internal factors, then it is designated as stress condition. Stress can be divided in the following ways:

(*a*) *Physical stress*—Any abnormality in steady state like low energy, stomach upset, headache, diarrhea, constipation, nausea and other conditions by physical factors like heat, cold, radiation noise, vibration etc. that hamper the normalcy of human healthcare referred as physical stress.

(*b*) *Emotional stress*—Psychological or mental stress are the outcomes of chronic diseases, anxiety, depression that further affect the normal activities of human health.

(c) *Chemical stress*—Chemical stress occurs when a tissue is damaged due to trauma by chemical substances like chemical pollutants, excess drugs etc. This condition triggers the release of chemicals in cellular environment such as histamine, serotonin, substances P and bradykinin which will alter the cellular environment that ultimately develop health disorder.

Stressful work style is associated with physical health deterioration and also less productivity in work progress. Stress during work may occur by different causes such as excessive work load for daily basis and a fixed target to finish the work regularly (Bhui *et al.*, 2016). Another important cause noted for the stress imposition related to the work when the work demand and work pressure do not complement with the knowledge and ability of the employee and this condition challenge their ability to cope. Environmental factors like high temperature, excessive cold, pollution at work station, excessive light exposure, noise at work station etc. are also another causes for stress imposition on worker. Similarly, poor management in professional field, bad personal management, conflict with higher levels of administration all are responsible for stress imposition that interfere health status.

2.1.2 Long Standing Work Style

The general tendency of human body is to move, as immobility for long term period is beyond the nature of human. Lots of muscular efforts are required to hold the uprights position and it is called as static load or static work. Excessive stress imposition on musculo-skeletal and cardiovascular systems during continuous standing postured work may result discomfort, fatigue and injury (Kaushik and Charpe, 2008) and it may result the following—

- **Slouching**

It refers to the rigidity of the spine specially cervical and thoracic regions. It can cause different health problems including back pain, headache, pulled muscle. Slouching for long period can lead towards skeleton-muscular stress on vertebrate and the discs between the vertebrae.

- **Vericose Vein**

These veins are located in the legs, ankles and feet. Due to the prolonged standing posture, the vein becomes twisted and enlarged (Thomas and Robert, 2015). Gravity pulls the blood downward to the lower part of the body due to prolonged standing. During this phase, the valves present in the vein prevent the blood to flow backward that leads to expansion of veins into balloon to accommodate extra blood.

- **Joint Pain**

Prolonged standing in the same position without any movement for regular basis may reduce the normal lubrication and cushioning of the concerned joint of the knees, hips, ankle and feet resulting in tear (Samad and Shelke, 2016). Pressure and tearing combinely result extreme level of pain and ultimately reduces the ability to work properly.

- **Muscle Fatigue**

Continuous standing sometimes results exhaustion in the muscle that ultimately leads to back pain and swelling in ankles, feet and legs (Krause, 2000).

2.1.3 Continuous Sitting Work Style or Sedentary Work Style

Work pattern in modern era, i.e. m-work to e-work or paper based work to computerized work or paperless work has shifted the nature of work from heavy to sedentary levels. Research revealed that sitting posture in working platform for prolonged period may aggravate the risk of cardio-metabolic disease, obesity, type-2 diabetes, musculo-skeletal disorder and sometimes it leads to certain type of cancer and premature death (Throp *et al.*, 2011). Research also focused that each two hours increment in sitting position, the risk of obesity and diabetes increases by 5 per cent and 7 per cent respectively (Hu *et al.*, 2003). As per WHO, 2013 about 3.2 million people worldwide face premature death each year due to sedentary lifestyle (WHO, 2008). Experiment also showed that people who spend most of their time in sitting position tends to have about 1.4 times greater chance of premature death after 12 years than the persons who sit lesser time at work. Following are the health hazards caused by the continuous sitting posture:

- Report revealed that 53.2 per cent people suffer from lower back pain, 53.5 per cent are having with neck and 51.6 per cent are having with shoulder symptoms among the people involving in sitting posture in work station for more than half of the day.
- As per survey report, occupational sitting is directly associated with hypertension (Dempsey *et al.*, 2018).
- Cardiovascular disease is a remarkable outcome in case of prolonged sitting posture as it interferes insulin secretion that slows down the glucose uptake by skeletal muscle that increases pro-inflammatory cytokines and helps to develop cardiovascular disorder.

3. Food Style

It covers the attitudes and practices of health friendly food intake which are health friendly in specific time and specific amount known as food style.

Different components of food style are:

- Meal frequency/day.
- Nature of meal, i.e. light, moderate, heavy.
- Composition of food in each meal.
- Regular or irregular meal intake on the basis of time.

Food style is of two types:

(a) Healthy food style.
(b) Unhealthy food style.

In healthy food style, the healthy habits and practices regarding food consumption which are helpful for disease prevention and recovery known as healthy food style (Michael, 2015). In contrast, bad habit about food frequency and food selection which are harmful for our health are known as unhealthy food style.

3.1 Type of Food Style and Health Issues

3.1.1 Fast Food Related Food Style

Fast food refers to food products that are prepared and served quickly (Das, 2015). Fast food contains high fat, salt and sugar. Fast food includes burger, French fries, salted food, fried food, carbonated beverages, candies etc.

Fast food consumption at regular basis may result addiction towards those foodstuff. High fat and sugar in fast food develop a vicious cycle that makes people to choose unhealthy food habit due to taste, odour, colour of fast food.

Following are the serious health issues caused by fast food:

High Cholesterol: Fast food contains high fat loaded with calories and trans fat that elevates the bad cholesterol (Bahadoran *et al.*, 2015) and decreases the good cholesterol levels that can create plaque in the artery, lead towards atherosclerosis and ultimately trigger the risk of stroke.

Obesity: Excessive consumption of trans fat and calorie result excessive weight gain (Alter and Eny, 2005) as well as BMI and develop obesity.

High blood pressure: High sodium content leads to the risk of high blood pressure that results chest pain known as angina. Simultaneously, high blood pressure may develop kidney disease.

Headaches and migraine: Processed fast food such as processed meat contains nitrates, nitrites and monosodium glutamate (MSG) which allow excessive blood flow and leads to high pressure and results headaches or migraine attack (Nazari and Eghbali, 2012).

Depression: Fast food contains emulsion, preservative, thickeners, stabilizers and flavour enhancing agents results deterioration in mental state that leads to depression.

Sexual dysfunction: Excessive fast food consumption leads towards the diminution in the sperm count, sperm motility etc. and delayed ovulation, loss of libido which are directly associated with infertility.

3.1.2 Processed Food Related Food Style

Preservatives are natural or synthetic substances that are incorporated in fruits, vegetables, prepared food items, cosmetics to increase the shelf life and enhance the quality by triggering the inhibition and retardation of their acidification, microbial contamination, fermentation and decomposition by food processing industries.

Food preservatives are of two types in broader aspects:

a. *Class I or natural preservatives*: Preservatives that are available from natural sources are considered as natural preservatives. These preservatives are rich in antioxidant property that delays the oxidation and aging process of food item.

Some common examples of natural preservatives are—

Oil: It slows down the oxidation of food when food comes in contact with the air. Thus, it prevents the microorganism to come in contact with food. Oil is used to preserve vegetables in the form of pickle.

Sugar and salt: These natural preservatives are extensively used as preservatives to preserve the meat and vegetable. Salt and sugar absorb the water which is solely responsible for bacterial growth in food.

Lemon juice: Lemon juice contains ascorbic acid and citric acid which prevents the microorganism to spoil the food. Side by side lemon juice is rich in Vitamin C which is a powerful antioxidant. Vitamin C protects the food from oxidation.

Vinegar: Vinegar is extremely acidic in nature as it contains acetic acid. Vinegar is used in pickle and canned food to protect it from microbial growth.

Cloves: It is used as natural preservatives since thousand years. Clove contains high amount of phenolic compound that protects the food from microorganism.

b. *Class II or synthetic preservatives:* Synthetic preservatives are chemical additives that limits the food deterioration which occurs by microorganism. People, consuming food items that contain more than one preservatives are at risk of exposure to multiple chemicals. Example: benzoates, nitrites and nitrates of sodium or potassium, glutamates, glycerides, sorbates, sulfites etc.

   Both natural as well as synthetic preservatives are categorized in 3 types:

Antimicrobials: This type of preservative delays the bacterial, yeast and moulds growth. Example: Benzoates and sorbate are antifungal agent, widely used for preparation of jam, salads, cheese and pickle.

Antioxidants: These types of preservative slow down breakdown of fat or oil in food items. Example: Butylated hydroxytoluene (BHT) and butylated hydroxyanisole (BHA) blocks the systemic chain reactions by conducting chemical reaction with free radical.

Anti-enzymatic preservatives: This type of preservative blocks the enzymatic process. Example: Erythrobic acid and citric acid combinely stops the action of phenolic compounds which are responsible for the brown colour of the fruit and potato surface which are exposed to the nature.

3.1.3 Carbohydrate Enrich Food Style

Excessive consumption of carbohydrate enriched food may cause multiple health deterioration as follows:

Dental cavity: Carbohydrate plays a major role in the decaying of tooth because it acts as a source of energy for the bacteria present in the mouth. These bacteria breakdown sugar and produce high level of acids that remove minerals from teeth. Finally, it increases the sensitivity of the teeth and develops dental cavity.

Diabetes: High carbohydrate rich diet is of high glycemic index that increases blood glucose level. High level of sugar in blood stream increases body's demand for insulin secretion that can contribute to problems with the pancreas to release insulin that may eventually lead to diabetes.

3.1.4 Protein Rich Food Style

Proteins are one of the important building blocks of body as well as it can also serve as a source of fuel which provide as much energy density as carbohydrates. But excessive consumption of protein enriched food is an alarming food style that can cause the following effects on health:

Heart disease: Research revealed that animal protein contributes to a high risk for cardiovascular disease with special reference to the people who eat high animal protein content diet tend to suffer more from heart attacks than people who get protein from plant source. Association of protein intake along with cholesterol elevates the risk of heart attack as the amount of saturated fatty acid content of the food is high and leads towards the development of atherosclerosis.

Osteoporosis: Consumption of protein more than the body's requirement sometimes leads towards the development of osteoporosis as consumption of large amounts of animal protein is associated with calcium loss in the urine that results demineralization of bone and make it fragile.

4. Effect of Lifestyle on Maternal Health

Maternal health is the health of women during pregnancy, childbirth and the postpartum period. Pregnant and/or lactating mothers are one of the vulnerable groups in our society. Pattern of lifestyle is directly related with the state of maternal health status.

4.1 Fast Food Centric Food Style and Maternal Health

4.1.1 Fast Food and Women Infertility

Infertility can be a very distressing condition for the couple. High dietary fat intake through fast food impairs hypothalamic-pituitary-ovarian (HPO) axis and results infertility. Research focused that women who consume fast food in regular basis has the tendency to increase their risk of infertility from 8 per cent to 16 per cent. There are different ways by which fat containing fast food may deteriorate female reproductive function (Denge and Gatfane, 2016).

Fast food has been shown to negatively affect the uterine cycle along with a high chance of an ovulation. Fast foods are energy dense with high amounts of saturated fat, sodium and sugar. A higher concentration of saturated fatty acids in ovarian follicular fluid is directly linked with reduced numbers of mature oocytes. Studies in mice informed that excess dietary fat intake increased lipid content and lipotoxicity resulting in apoptosis in ovarian cells. High intake of fast food is one of the major factors that influence infertility by altering oocyte follicular fluid metabolic markers, called lipoproteins.

The high fat content fast food can cause the polycystic ovary syndrome (PCOS). It is the most common endocrine disorder in women now-a-days. Women with PCOS are generally having with the complications of subfertility, an ovulatory, and hyperandrogenemic conditions and that also increased miscarriage rate which is also directly associated with infertility related complications (Denge and Gatfane, 2016).

4.1.2 Fast Food and Maternal Obesity

High intake of fast food can lead to 'globosity', i.e. global obesity, a new pandemic, which further results diabetes along with cardiovascular disease and coronary heart disease. Fast food consumption and globalization of diet has lead to loss a traditional healthy food practice. Fast foods are responsible for obesity due to its high energy density and it contains high trans fatty acid, excessive refined starch and sugar along with low level of dietary fiber. Multi-factors are responsible for maternal obesity, where fast food habit is one of them. Fast food is the causal factor for increasing maternal obesity at present (Datar *et al.*, 2014).

High gestational weight is associated with consumption of high calorie and high saturated fatty acid dense unhealthy food. During pregnancy, fast food can lead to excessive weight gain that increase the risk of various complications of intrauterine baby like birthing a large baby, preterm labour, gestational diabetes, miscarriage and still birth. The presence of excess fat and simple carbohydrate, the fast food contributes a higher risk for maternal obesity, CVD, diabetes, gout, bone health deterioration type of chronic diseases. Fast food increases the fat in adipose tissue. Leptin is secreted by fat cells (adipocytes) and it maintains the balance between food intake and energy expenditure. Most of the fast foods or junk food, contain heavy amount of sugar. Sugar and fat are directly associated with increased body weights that lead to childhood obesity.

4.1.3 Fast Food and Maternal Diabetes

High amount of fast food eaters mothers suffer from diabetes mellitus. Fast food oriented globosity arises diabetes due to insulin resistance (Sami *et al.*, 2017). Fast foods are high in calories and they contain with low amount of vitamins and minerals, and are usually low in fibre. Fast foods also often contain large amounts of added sugar and are high in saturated fats and trans fats. This can cause them to digest more quickly, which can spike blood sugar levels and increase bad cholesterol levels. High glycaemic index, excess sugar with low dietary fibre containing fast food can overload the body's ability to produce enough insulin, therefore beta cells are exhausted and high blood glucose level is noted.

4.1.4 Fast Food and Maternal Bone Health

Maternal bone health is affected by irregular lifestyle and unbalanced diet. Maternal bone health status is closely related with food pattern (Lim *et al.*, 2018). Nutrients which are responsible for bone mineralization, e.g. calcium and vitamin-D are present in very low amount in fast food. High sugar density in fast food effects the uric acid level in the body. Salt is the one of the key ingredients of fast food. High amount of salt is a big obstacle for strong skeleton of maternal health. So, high salt lose more bone mineral.

High sugar and fat in fast food decreases the bone health status in two ways. Firstly, high saturated fatty acid and sugar blocks the calcium absorption. Secondly, high trans fatty acid in fast food tend to form insoluble 'soaps', which cover the intestine and block calcium absorption from intestine.

4.2 Stressful Work Style and Maternal Health

4.2.1 Oxidative Stress and Maternal Obesity

Adipose tissue is an endocrine and storage tissue necessary for energy homeostasis. It is primarily composed of adipocytes, along with other cells that are fibroblasts, endothelial, immune cells and fibroblastic pre-adipocytes. It also secrets hormones and cytokines such as adipokines or adipocytokines. Adipokines induce the production of reactive oxygen species (ROS) by generating oxidative stress. Excessive adipose tissue resulting from obesity has been identified as a major source of pro-inflammatory cytokines, i.e. tumour necrosis factor-alpha (TNF-α), interleukin (IL)-1β and IL-6. Oxidative damage is higher in obese mother due to depleted antioxidant sources especially antioxidant enzymes such as superoxide dismutase (SOD), glutathione peroxidase, catalase, vitamin E, vitamin C, β-carotene and vitamin A. Activity of SOD in obese individuals is significantly lower compared to the women having normal body weight.

4.2.2 Stress and Maternal Infertility

Oxidative stress influences the entire span of women reproductive life. It has been showed that the age-related diminution in fertility ability is altered by oxidative stress though it plays an important role during pregnancy and normal parturition. The impact of oxidative stress on oocytes and reproductive functions remains unclear. The imbalance between free radical and antioxidants lead to several reproductive diseases such as endometriosis, unexplained infertility and polycystic ovarian syndrome (PCOS). Pregnancy complications including spontaneous abortion, recurrent pregnancy loss in response to oxidative stress. Reactive oxygen species (ROS) are generated as by-products during ovarian physiological metabolism that results oocyte maturation, ovulation, fertilization, implantation, and embryo development, which can ultimately influence pregnancy outcomes. But excessive production of free radical can result impairment in the normal female reproductive pathway such as delayed in the ovulation and other hormonal impairment that directly influence fertility ability of a woman (Natalia *et al.*, 2013).

4.2.3 Stress and Maternal Cardiovascular Disease

About 1 in 16 women within age range 20 are suffering from coronary heart disease which is under the child rearing age. In 21st century, oxidative stress markers have been increasingly adopted in heart failure patients with special reference to the women in child rearing age. Increased ROS production in mother leads to diminution in nitric oxide availability that results vasoconstriction and promoting arterial hypertension. Free radical also negatively influences the myocardial calcium handling that causes arrhythmia. It also boosts up cardiac remodelling by inducing hypertrophic signalling and apoptosis. Finally, excessive ROS promotes atherosclerotic plaque formation (Palinski, 2014).

A variety of experimental studies indicated that excessive ROS generation is implicated in the pathogenesis of heart failure. Reactive oxygen species stimulate myocardial growth and cellular dysfunction followed by activating the signalling kinases and transcription factors. Excessive ROS also stimulates cellular apoptosis signalling kinase-1. Overexpression of this kinase-1 leads to NF-κB-induced cardiac pathological hypertrophy which ultimately interfere the efficiency of heart.

4.2.4 Stressful Work Style and Maternal Osteoporosis

Bone is comprised of three types of cells: osteoclasts, osteoblasts, and osteocytes. There is a tightly-regulated balance between osteoclast-linked removal of old bone and osteoblast-mediated replacement of new bone to maintain skeletal homeostasis. Osteoporosis is a chronic skeletal metabolic disorder characterized by deterioration of bone mineral density and bone mass, resulting in fragile nature of the bone. Though osteoporosis is common in post-menopausal phase among women but in some cases, women develop osteoporosis during pregnancy or breastfeeding stage. Recent studies focused that chronic stress in work station among women has a link with osteoporosis at the post-partum phase. Research showed that mothers suffering from post-natal depression may trigger the risk of osteoporosis by affecting the bone mineral density. The exact mechanism has not been clear but incidence of osteoporosis with physchological stress is influenced by several signalling pathways. Hyperactivity of the hypothalamic-pituitary-adrenocortical (HPA) axis is considered as an important contributor for stress-induced bone loss. It has been noted that blood cortisol levels used to overcome the depressed mental state of patients results osteolysis which leads to low bone mineral density (Salari and Abdollahi, 2014). Simultaneously, stress increases the level of noradrenaline within bone tissue that trigger bone loss and osteoporosis.

5. Effect of Lifestyle on Child Health

Children are always at risk of the communicable as well as non-communication diseases compared to the others as this is one of the vulnerable groups. Modification in lifestyle is an essential component to maintain the health status of the children. But, now a days, the pattern of lifestyle has changed in drastic level and children are attracted towards unhealthy practices which results detrimental effect on their health status.

5.1 Fast Food Centric Food Style and Child Health

5.1.1 Fast Food and Childhood Obesity

As per World Health Organization (WHO), Obesity is defined as abnormal or excessive fat accumulation that presents a risk to health. When the weight gain is more than 20 per cent of age specific height and body weight due to fat deposition known as child obesity. Classification of obesity depending on Body Mass Index (BMI) is presented in Table 16.1 (Nawaryc *et al.*, 2017).

Table 16.1: Classification of the body weight status according to BMI

Classification	*BMI*		
	Children (2-18 yrs) (Percentile)	*Adults (Kg/m^2)*	*Z score*
Underweight	<P5	<8.50	<–1.6
Normal	P5-P84	18.50-24.99	≥–1.6-<1.0
Overweight	P85-P94	25.0-29.9	≥1.0-<1.6
Obese:	≥P95	≥30	
Class I	P95-P98 (Obese<%)	30-34.9	≥1.6-<2.0
Class II	≥P98 (Moderately obese)	35-39.9	≥2.0-<2.5
Class III	>P99 (Severely obese)	≥40	≥2.5

Childhood obesity has reached into epidemic level in both of the developed as well as developing countries. Childhood obesity is a very common problem in recent era. A study has showed that up to 25 per cent of children worldwide consume fast food frequently and very frequently. Apart from fast food consumption, the main reason for childhood obesity is eating too much and exercising too little. Due to the stressful competition among children regarding study and other co-curricular activities, they hardly get time to play in the field. Simultaneously, trend to play indoor games including games in mobile, video game, e-games etc. are another important causes for making the children lazy which also influence the tendency to become obese. Moreover, many families, especially those with two parents working outside the home have greater tendency to make their children habituated with fast food consumption (Almuhanna *et al.*, 2014). Fast food consumption for chronic period may also develop childhood diabetes and it can cause other nuisance afterward. Following reasons are involved in growing the tendency of having fast food and weight gain among child community:

- Busy families cooking less at home and eating outside more.
- Easy access to cheap, high calorie street food, fast food and junk food.
- Bigger food portions both outside and in home.
- Habit of consumption of sweetened drinks that contains huge amounts of sugar.

5.1.2 Fast Food and Benign Hypertension

Hypertension is of two types: (a) Benign hypertension, (b) Malignant hypertension. Term "benign hypertension" is usually slight to moderate severity of hypertension and of long duration. Children suffer from benign hypertension. About 1-3 per cent of children are suffering from benign hypertension worldwide. Fast food and/or fatty food consumption is one of the responsible factors for the development of benign hypertension. Salted fast food contains higher amount of sodium. Chronic consumption of salted fast food may develop hypertension among children. The prevalence of benign hypertension is 3.4 per cent in total population. Globally about 30 per cent boys and 23 per cent girls are suffering from hypertension whereas in Western India about 6.48 per cent children are suffering from hypertension (Buch *et al.*, 2011). Fast food linked overweight is directly proportional to the generation of hypertension among children. Following are the major causes for the benign hypertension (Payaba *et al.*, 2015):

- Fast food linked overweight or obese.
- Having type-2 diabetes or a high fasting blood sugar level due to fast food consumption.
- Having high cholesterol due to fatty food consumption for long time.

- Eating too much salt through fast food like chips.
- Being sedentary or involvement in low physical activity.

5.1.3 Fast Food and Growth Retardation (Stunting)

Growth retardation or stunting is the impaired growth and development that occurs due to the inadequate nutrition or poor nutrition among children. When age-wise height is low due to insufficient nutrition or due to infection known as stunting or growth retardation. Research revealed that excessive consumption of fast food may result in growth stunting. Relation of children with the food is directly related with their growth pattern. Fast food consumption directly affect the release of growth hormone synthesis and along with it, nutrient content of the fast food does not meet the nutritional requirement of the children that leads towards the poor growth and development apart from low immunization status. This phenomenon also affects the pubertal phase among adolescents. Fast food consumption among children is also associated with 'Attention Deficit Disorder' (ADD) among children in their class room as the food additives, artificial colour and the high sodium content of the fast food results huge water retention, interfere mental concentration by decreasing activity of central nervous system which also hamper the physical activity (Arnold *et al.*, 2012).

5.2 Stressful Work Style and Child Health

5.2.1 Excessive Pressure in Study and Mental Retardation

High level of competition in study is directly influenced the mental growth among the children. Fear to the failure in the competition increases the oxidative stress among children that leads towards the physical hazards as well as depression. Low socialization, less time to play, huge study related work pressure make them exhausted. As a result, they do not have any time for the refreshment or amusement resulting mental retardation and ultimately the productivity become less (Raina *et al.*, 2012). Physical and mental rest are most important for resettlement of neural activity at the normal level by synthesizing brain monoamines.

5.2.2 Poor Eyesight due to use of Mobile and Television

Children aged 5-15 years are very much prone to have poor eyesight. Vision plays a vital role in reading. Epidemiological study has shown that 30 per cent children worldwide suffer from blindness before the age of 20 years. Apart from nutritional deficiency, watching television for long time at a close position, use of mobile for long time also affect the eyesight among children. Continuous radiation exposure from the television and mobile may result refractive error and it also trigger the risk of shoulder and neck problem in late life (Mushtaq *et al.*, 2014).

Lifestyle modification can be achieved in positive direction by implementing knowledge, attitude and practices (KAP) package to the community. Knowledge can uproot the misconception, myth and provide proper concept regarding healthy lifestyle. Finally, scientific practices can be achieved by modification of attitude. Thus, several non-communicable diseases can be managed by accepting the healthy practices. Similarly, by sound knowledge about hygiene and sanitation, the healthy attitude and practices are developed among the candidates that also help to challenge the communicable diseases (Fig. 16.1).

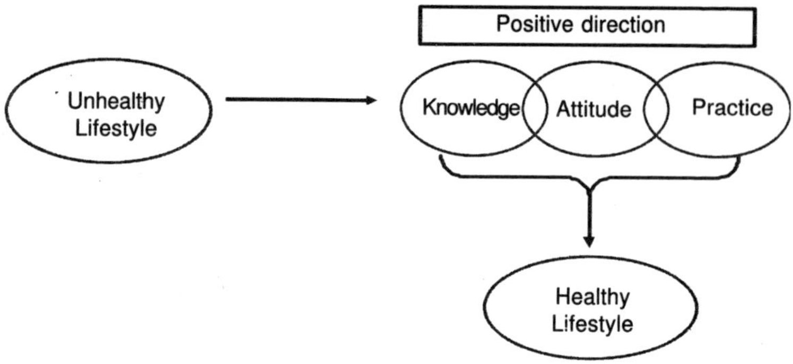

Fig. 16.1: Impact of KAP in lifestyle modification.

6. Spiral Model for KAP for Behavioural Change

Spiral Model for enrichment and positive modification of KAP for creating healthy society and healthy nation where formal and informal education have a great impact.

6.1 Steps that Facilitate to Change Behaviour

Spiral model is advised to change the behaviour about different steps are pre-contemplation, contemplation, preparation, action, maintenance and relapse. If relapsed is noted then reentering the spiral model is essential.

In **Pre-contemplation phase,** a person need information to raise the awareness level about the problem and the possible changes needed to overcome the problem. Nutritional advice to change eating habit is important at this phase. So, it is **knowledge gaining** phase.

Contemplation phase covers the mental conflict about the awareness or knowledge gain in the previous phase and the previous or existing knowledge which he/she has in mind. On the basis of such conflict, the person analyses the advantages and disadvantages for making the changes in dietary practices. This phase helps to **change attitude.**

In **Preparation phase** the person either to move forward or to fall back into contemplation. In this stage, the different inputted **information** help the candidates to proceed forward or reverse direction. In this phase **healthy attitude** is generally imprinted in mind.

Action phase covers the changes achieved by the candidate by such inputted message and help to proceed forward. Here **the attitude is strengthened by the output of**

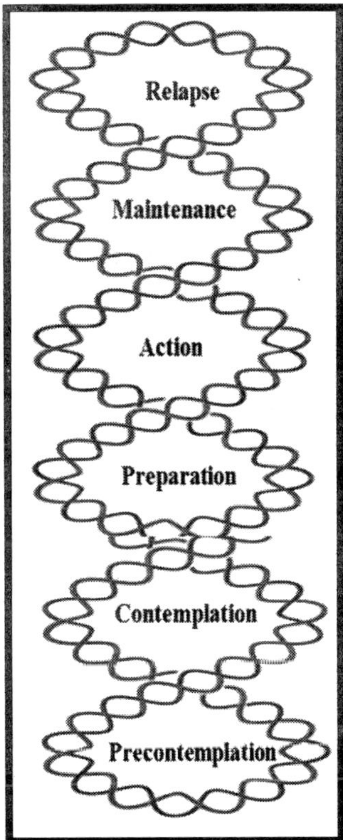

Fig. 16.2: Different phases of spiral mode.

action.

Maintenance phase is the duration where the candidates follow-up the changes in dietary practices on the basis of good results which he/she obtained in respect to previous health status. Strong maintenance prevent relapse and help to grow good **practices.**

If **relapse** occurs then the phases would be restarted from the weak point specific to that candidate.

Conclusion

Lifestyle management has become an essential part of life in every domain. Knowledge regarding healthy lifestyle may act as the key factor to replace the unhealthy practices by healthy one. Implementation of this knowledge to change the attitude is an important part of lifestyle modification through which healthy lifestyle practices can be achieved that ultimately improves the quality of life in all sections especially in the vulnerable sections of our community. Governmental and/or non-governmental organizations may arrange series of seminars or lectures. Through group discussion and mass communication, a positive reflection can be disseminated in the society for practice modification. Formal educational organizations may take an initiative in this aspect by implementation of out-reach services.

REFERENCES

Almuhanna, M.A., Alsaif, M., Alsaadi, M., Almajwal, A. 2014. "Fast food intake and prevalence of obesity in school children in Riyadh City." *Sudan J Paediatr.* **14**: 71-80.

Alter, D.A., Eny, K. 2005. "The relationship between the supply of fast-food chains and cardiovascular outcomes." *Can J Public Health.* **96**: 173-177.

Arnold, L.E., Lofthouse, N., Hurt, E. 2012. "Artificial food colors and attention-deficit/hyperactivity symptoms: Conclusions to dye for." *Neurotherapeutics.* **9**: 599-609.

Bahadoran, Z., Mirmiran, P., Azizi, F. 2015. "Fast food pattern and cardiometabolic disorders: A review of current studies." *Health Promot Perspect.* **5**: 231-240.

Bhui, K., Dinos, S., Miecznikowska, M.G., Jongh, B.D., Stansfeld, S. 2016. "Perceptions of work stress causes and effective interventions in employees working in public, private and non-governmental organisations: a qualitative study." *BJPsych Bull.* **40**: 318-325.

Buch, N., Goyel, J.P., Kumar, N., Parmar, I., Shah, V.B., Charan, J. 2011. "Prevalence of hypertension in school going children of Surat city, Western India." *J Cardiovasc Dis Res.* **2**: 228-232.

Das, J.C. 2015. "Fast food consumption in children: A Review." *Med Clin Rev.* **1**: 1-4.

Datar, A., Nicosia, N., Shier, V. 2014. "Maternal work and children's diet, activity, and obesity." *Soc Sci Med.* **107**: 196-204.

Dempsey, P.C., Larsen, R.N., Dunstan, D.W., Owen, N., Kingwell, B.A. 2018. "Sitting less and moving more implications for hypertension." *Hypertension.* **72**: 1037-1046.

Denge, K., Gattane, R. 2016. "A critical review of association between incompatible diet and infertility with special reference to junk food." *IAMJ.* **4**: 1335-1343.

Hu, F.B., Li, T.Y., Colditz, G.A., Willett, W.C., Manson, J.E. 2003. "Television watching and other sedentary behaviours in relation to risk of obesity and type-2 diabetes mellitus in women." *JAMA.* **289**: 1785-1791.

Kaushik, V., Charpe, N.A. 2008. "Effect of body posture on stress experienced by worker." *Stud Home Comm Sci.* **2**: 1-5.

Krause, N. 2000. "Standing at work and progression of carotid atherosclerosis." *Scand J Work Environ Health.* **26**: 227-236

Lim, H.S., Hwang, H.S., Kang, J., Park, Y.H., Lee, H.H., Kim, T.H. 2018. "Relationship between bone density, eating habit, and nutritional intake in college students." *J Bone Metab.* **25**: 181-186.

Michael, E.J. 2015. "Principles of human nutrition." *Medicine.* **43**: 61-65.

Mushtaq, B., Hamid, M., Shamas, N., Masoodi, M., Munshi, H. 2014. "Effect of television watching on vision of school children in semi-urban area of Kashmir." *Int J Res Med Sci.* **2**: 672-676

Natalia, M., Grindler, and Kelle, H., Moley. 2013. "Maternal obesity, infertility and mitochondrial dysfunction: potential mechanisms emerging from mouse model systems." *Mol Hum Reprod.* **19**: 486–494.

Nawarycz, T., Pytel, K., Drygas, W., Lipman, M.G., Nawarycz, L.O. 2017. "A fuzzy logic approach to measure of weight status and central fatness in adults and adolescents." *Studies in Comput Intell.* **600**: 39-56.

Nazari, F., EghbaliIran, M. 2012. "Migraine and its relationship with dietary habits in women." *J Nurs Midwifery Res.* **17**: 65-71.

Palinski, W. 2014. "Effect of maternal cardiovascular conditions and risk factors on offspring cardiovascular disease." *Circulation,* **129**: 2066-2077.

Payaba, M., Kelishadi, R., Qorbani, M. 2015. "Association of junk food consumption with high blood pressure and obesity in Iranian children and adolescents: the CASPIAN-IV Study." *J Pediatr.* **91**: 196-205.

Raina, S.K, Razdan, S. and Nanda, R. 2012. "Prevalence of mental retardation among children in RS Pura town of Jammu and Kashmir." *Ann Indian Acad Neurol.* **15** : 23-26.

Salari, P., Abdollahi, M. 2014. "The influence of pregnancy and lactation on maternal bone health: A systematic review." *J Family Reprod Health.*

8: 135-148.

Samad, S.A., Shelke, R.D. 2016. "Health effect of prolonged standing at work and its control measures: A review." *Int J Eng Res Gen Sci.* **4**: 527-529.

Sami, W., Ansari, T., Butt, N.S., Hamid, M.R. 2017. "Effect of diet on type 2 diabetes mellitus: A review." *Int J Health Sci (Qassim).* **11**: 65-71.

Thomas, R.W., Robert, B.W. 2015. "Evidence of health risks associated with prolonged standing at work and intervention effectiveness." *Rehabil Nurs.* **40**: 148-165.

Throp, A.A., Owen, N., Neurables, M., Dunstan, D.W. 2011. "Sedentary behaviours and subsequent health outcomes in adults: a systematic review of longitudinal, 1996-2011." *Am J Prev Med.* **41**: 207-215.

Trovato, G.M. 2012. "Behaviour, nutrition and lifestyle in a comprehensive health and disease paradigm: skills and knowledge for a predictive, preventive and personalized medicine." *EPMA J.* **3**: 1-15.

World Health Orgnization. 2008. *Physical inactivity: a global public health problem.* Geneva: World Health Orgnization.

17

Impact of Women Empowerment on Child Health Care Practices and Nutrition

A Study among Oraon Tribe of West Bengal

Chitradip Bhattacherjee and *Subir Biswas*

Introduction

The principle of gender equality is protected and respected in the Constitution of India in Preamble, Fundamental Rights, Fundamental Duties and Directive Principles. The Constitution of India emphasizes equality to women along with empowering the states to adopt measures eradication of discrimination against women. Empowerment can be defined in many ways, however, in women's empowerment, women elaborate and recreate what it is that they can be, do, and accomplish in a circumstance that they previously were denied (Kabeer, 2005), and empowerment clarify accepting and allowing people (women) who are on the outside of the decision-making process into it. "This puts a strong emphasis on participation in political structures and formal decision-making and, in the economic sphere, on the ability to obtain an income that enables participation in economic decision-making" (Rahman, 2013). Women are not just mere participants in the development process, they are agents that can bring forth change when empowered and given the voice.

Despite many international commitments that persuade governments to take action, women are still in a disadvantage. That is why it is very crucial that women be given a voice in decision-making, to further influence policies. Attaining development among all the pillars of sustainable development is unthinkable without empowering women and obtaining gender equality, thereby using the entire potential (Bayeh, 2016). Academic and economic empowerments are the basics to help women to purchase of foods, hygiene products, and medications for their children. Women's control over economic production decisions may be related to food production for home consumption along with providing better health facilities making better child nutritional status for their offspring (Perry 2005; Shroff *et al.*, 2011). Different studies showed previously that sustainable development is impossible without women's empowerment and gender equality. Consequently, it is asserted that gender equality is both a human rights issue and a precondition for, and indicator of; sustainable development (Alvarez, 2013). It is also affirmed that gender discrimination is prevalent across different cultures of the world which needed serious concern to be eliminated for ensuring sustainable development. Furthermore, UN Women (2014) pointed out that to create a sustainable world and to emphasize women's roles in sustaining their families and communities, achieving gender equality is of great importance. On the other hand, if gender equality is not maintained, it will retard the country's development (Stevens, 2010). A study by Parashar (2004), examined the role of mother's empowerment for achieving proper child nutrition and immunization goal and suggested women are to be empowered accordingly along several aspects if they and their children are to be secured for equal access to health care, quality education at all levels. Study also revealed that women's empowerment is a pathway by which a nutrition-sensitive programme can improve child wasting (Heckert *et al.*, 2019). The "Millennium Development Goals" (MDGs) stated eight developmental goals that were set to target for year 2015. These goals focuses on the empowerment of women and children as well as promotion of their health as part in which all the member States have agreed to achieve by the year 2015. A study in Pakistan showed the indicators of women's empowerment, such as the education of the mother and employment status had a negative relationship with child malnutrition (Shafiq *et al.*, 2019). A study by Chatterjee and Dubey (2018) also shows three dimensions of women autonomy—decision making, exposure to domestic violence and financial independence have significant association with long-term nutritional status in rural India justifying women empowerment as clearly emerging key variable to tackle malnutrition problem.

Materials and Methods

Present research had been conducted among four districts of West Bengal, India, viz. Jalpaiguri, Howrah, Hooghly and North 24 Parganas. Total 200 Oraon families having one boy and one girl child below 6 years of age were selected for the present research from rural, urban and peri-urban areas through stratified random sampling method as per the availability of research participants within inclusion criteria. Total 400 Oraon children (200 of each sex) and their parents were selected as the participants for the present research. From those selected families general demographic data and socio-economic data were collected by interview method from parents. Along with that, standard anthropometric measurements were collected from children like height, weight, arm-circumference and head-circumference with caring information like place of birth, exclusive breast feeding practice, immunization status and disease treatment facilities and cross verified from relevant documents where available such as vaccination card, birth certificate. The anthropometric measurements were first classified in respect of WHO 2007 standardized reference values by means of height-for-age, weight-for-age, weight-for-height, arm-circumference-for-age and head-circumference-for-age. The collected information and nutritional statuses were later tabulated in Microsoft excel 2007 and statistically analyzed in IBM SPSS 24.0 to find out the possible outcome from the study at 0.05 significance level. The work has been approved by the Institutional Ethics Committee of West Bengal State University.

Results and Discussions

The present study deals with four intensive observations: relations between mother's education and child care practices, relation between mother's occupation and child care practices, relation between mother's education and child health statuses and relations between mother's occupation and child health statuses.

(1) Total percentage of mother having primary education was found 36 per cent whereas without schooling was 53 per cent and only 11 per cent mother found having secondary or higher education. But the result showed that

49.9 per cent Oraon mothers have fixed occupational orientation as they mostly work as tea gardens labourer, daily labourer or contractual staff, whereas 50.5 per cent Oraon mothers found to be non-working or house wife (Table 17.1).

Table 17.1: Mother's Education and Occupation

Mother's Education		*Mother's Occupation*	
Category	*No (%)*	*Category*	*No (%)*
Can sign only	106 (53%)	House wife	101 (50.5%)
Primary	72 (36%)		
Secondary or Higher	22 (11%)	Working (daily labour, tea garden worker etc.)	99 (49.5%)
Total	200	Total	200

(2) Child caring practices by mother's education: The results in Table 17. 2 show that mothers having primary and

Table 17.2: Child Care Practices by Mother's Education

Category	*Variables*	*Can Sign (%) only*	*Primary (%)*	*Secondary (%)*	*Total*	*Chi-square Value*	*p-value*
Place of Birth	Home	128 (60.4)	46 (31.9)	6 (13.6)	180	47.864	<0.001*
	Hospital	73 (34.4)	87 (60.4)	33 (75)	193		
	Nursing home	11 (5.2)	11 (7.6)	5 (11.4)	27		
Exclusive Breast Feeding	Yes	209 (98.6)	142 (98.6)	44 (100)	5	0.626	0.731
	No	3 (1.4)	2 (1.4)	0	395		
Immunization Status	Full	189 (89.2)	139 (96.5)	44 (100)	372	10.889	0.004*
	Partial	23 (10.8)	5 (1.3)	0	28		
Disease Treatment Facilities	Registered Doctor	11 (5.2)	110 (76.4)	44 (100)	165	249.794	<0.001*
	Quack Doctor	201 (94.8)	34 (23.6)	0	235		

* p-value less than 0.05; difference is statistically significant.

secondary education have a high rate (68% and 86.4%) of institutional delivery rather than mothers who can only sign and mostly avail home delivery practices (60.4%). The difference found statistically significant. Exclusive breast feeding was found almost equal (98.6%, 98.6% and 100%) and do not have any significant differences between mother's education. When dealing with immunization status, the data showed mothers having primary and secondary education are more careful about complete immunization dozes (96.5% and 100%) compared to mothers who can sign only (89.2%). The difference also found statistically significant. Disease treatment facilities towards children are also a major step towards child caring. It was observed that only 5.2 per cent mothers who can sign takes their children to registered doctors for treatment where the rate is very high among primary (76.4%) and secondary level (100%) educated mothers. The difference is highly significant statistically (Table 17.1).

(3) **Child caring practices by mother's occupations**: Two major occupational groups were identified for data analysis: House wives and Working mothers. The data showed that about 59.4 per cent house wives availing home delivery facilities whereas only 30.3 per cent working mothers having delivery at home and 69.7 per cent availing institutional delivery. The difference is highly significant at $p<0.05$ level. When dealing with exclusive breast feeding practices, it was found satisfactory among both house wives (98.5%) and working mothers (99%) resulting no statistically significant differences between them. Immunization process also showed quite satisfactory among both occupations where 90.6 per cent and 95.5 per cent children were given full immunization dozes having no statistical difference between them. But when dealing with disease treatment facilities, it was observed that only 9.7 per cent house wife mothers taking their children to registered medical practitioners where among working mothers 90.3 per cent children getting treatment from registered doctors. The difference of chi-square test is significant at $p<0.05$ level (Table 17.3).

Table 17.3: Child Care Practices by Mother's Occupation

Category	*Variables*	*House Wife (%)*	*Working (%)*	*Total*	*Chi-square Value*	*p-value*
Place of Birth	Home	120 (59.4)	60 (30.3)	180	36.835	<0.001*
	Hospital	68 (33.7)	125 (63.13)	193		
	Nursing home	14 (6.9)	13 (6.57)	27		
Exclusive Breast Feeding	Yes	199 (98.5)	196 (99)	395	0.183	0.509
	No	3 (1.5)	2 (1)	5		
Immunization Status	Full	183 (90.6)	189 (95.5)	372	3.629	0.077
	Partial	19 (9.4)	9 (4.5)	28		
Disease Treatment Facilities	Regis-tered	16 (9.7)	149 (90.3)	165	187.053	<0.001*
	Quack Doctor	186 (92.1)	49 (24.7)	235		

* p-value less than 0.05; difference is statistically significant.

(4) Nutritional status of children by mother's education: Child nutritional status was analyzed in respect of WHO 2006 standardized reference values by means of Height-for-age, weight-for-age, weight-for-height, arm-circumference-for-age and head-circumference-for-age statuses. Collected anthropometric measurements were compared with WHO reference data to find out level of malnutrition among children under study. Result showed that height-for-age status among children are quite different between mothers' education, i.e. children from mother who can sign only having 48.1 per cent stunted children whereas among primary and secondary educated mother it is less (27.1% and 22.7%). The result showed statistically significant difference among them at $p<0.05$ level. In case of weight-for-age, weight-for-height, arm-circumference-for-age and head-circumference-for-age there are also differences regarding mothers' educational qualifications but those differences are not statistically significant (Table 17.4).

Table 17.4: Child Health Status by Mother's Education

Nutritional Indicators	*Variables*	*Can Sign (%) only*	*Primary (%)*	*Secondary (%)*	*Total*	*Chi-square Value*	*p-value*
Height-for-age	Normal	110 (51.9)	105 (72.9)	34 (77.3)	249	20.887	<0.001*
	Stunted	102 (48.1)	39 (27.1)	10 (22.7)	151		
Weight-for-age	Normal	124 (58.5)	84 (58.3)	32 (72.7)	240	3.338	0.188
	Under weight	88 (41.5)	60 (41.7)	12 (27.3)	160		
Weight-for-height	Normal	164 (77.4)	112 (77.8)	37 (84.1)	313	3.308	0.508
	Wasted	40 (18.9)	27 (18.8)	4 (9.1)	71		
	Obese	8 (3.8)	5 (3.5)	3 (6.8)	16		
Arm-circumference-for-age	Normal	123 (58)	94 (65.3)	32 (72.7)	249	4.232	0.120
	Wasted	89 (42)	50 (34.7)	12 (27.3)	151		
Head-circumference-for-age	Normal (52)	119 (57.6)	83 (61.4)	27	229	0.421	0.810
	Microcephally	93 (43.9)	61 (42.4)	17 (38.6)	171		

*p-value less than 0.05; difference is statistically significant.

(5) Nutritional status of children by mother's occupation: The nutritional status of children in respect of mother's occupation is also very important part to understand the impact of women empowerment towards their children. Study showed that in case of height-for-age status children of working mother showing 75.8 per cent normal and 24.2 per cent stunted, whereas among children of housewife, it is 49 per cent normal and 51 per cent stunted. The difference is statistically significant at $p<0.05$ level. Other nutritional statuses also showed some differences among children between working and housewife mother, but those are not statistically significant (Table 17.5).

Table 17.5: Child Health Status by Mother's Occupation

Nutritional Indicators	*Variables*	*House Wife (%)*	*Working (%)*	*Total*	*Chi-square Value*	*p-value*
Height-for-age	Normal	99 (49)	150 (75.8)	249	30.442	<0.001*
	Stunted	103 (51)	48 (24.2)	151		
Weight-for-age	Normal	121 (59.9)	119 (60.1)	240	0.002	0.524
	Under-weight	81 (40.1)	79 (39.9)	160		
Weight-for-height	Normal	256 (77.2)	157 (79.3)	313	0.340	0.844
	Wasted	37 (18.3)	34 (47.9)	71		
	Obese	9 (4.5)	7 (3.5)	16		
Arm-circum-ference-for-age	Normal	118 (58.4)	131 (66.2)	249	2.553	0.067
	Wasted	84 (41.6)	67 (33.8)	151		
Head-circum-ference-for-age	Normal	113 (55.9)	116 (58.6)	229	0.286	0.332
	Micro-cephally	89 (44.1)	82 (41.4)	171		

*p-value less than 0.05; difference is statistically significant.

Conclusion

The Ministry of Women and Child Development (2015), Government of India has implemented several policies for ensuring equal access to education for women and girls and also to maintain women's health which includes both nutrition and health services to be adopted and special attention to be given to the needs of women and the girl at all stages of the life cycle. The present research was based on first hand data to understand if various policies undertaken by governmental and non-governmental organizations for women empowerments so far have positive impact on Oraon women and children's health and care facilities and to which extent it is important. The results from different objectives of the study reveal the fact that mostly the educational qualification and occupation of the mother clearly plays significant role in child care practices and nutritional statuses. Along with that, it is also clearly evident from the result that children from higher educated mother and working mother showed less percentage of long term malnourishment than others. Thus, it is very clear from the present study that women empowerment is necessary for better nurturing of the children for healthy future.

Furthermore to bring absolute women empowerment among Oraon tribes under study steps are still pending and to be taken care of by respected authorities.

Acknowledgements

The present study is a part of Post doctoral research of first author entitled "A Socio-Cultural Study of Gender Role and Attitude towards Child Health Care among the Oraon Tribes of West Bengal" funded by Indian Council of Social Science Research [F. No. 3-3/2017-18/PDF/GEN of 2017-18]. Authors are thankful to funding authority and all the study participants who helped in data collection for the present research. Author also acknowledges West Bengal State University for providing institutional support for the present research.

REFERENCES

Alvarez, M. 2013. *From Unheard Screams to Powerful Voices: A Case Study of Women's Political Empowerment in the Philippines*. Graduate School of International Studies, Seoul National University.

Bayeh, E. 2016. "The role of empowering women and achieving gender equality to the sustainable development of Ethiopia." *Pacific Science Review B: Humanities and Social Sciences*, 2(1): 37-42.

Chatterjee, P., and Dubey, A. 2018. "The Role of Women's Empowerment on Child Nutrition in India." *SSRN Electronic Journal*. doi: 10.2139/ssrn.3144587

Heckert, J., Olney, D., Ruel, M. 2019. "Is women's empowerment a pathway to improving child nutrition outcomes in a nutrition-sensitive agriculture program?: Evidence from a randomized controlled trial in Burkina Faso." *Social Science and Medicine*, **233**: 93-102. doi: 10.1016/j.socscimed.2019.05.016

Kabeer, N. 2005. "Gender equality and women's empowerment: A critical analysis of the third millennium development goal 1." *Gender and Development*, **13**(1): 13-24.

Ministry of Women and Child Development. 2015. NATIONAL POLICY FOR THE EMPOWERMENT OF WOMEN (2001). Retrieved 4 September 2019, from https://wcd.nic.in/womendevelopment/national-policy-women-empowerment

Parasar, S. 2004. *A Multidimensional Approach to Women's Empowerment and its Links to the Nutritional Status and Immunization of Children in India.* Available at: http://www.allacademic.com/meta/p109193_index.html. accessed 12 June, 2019.

Perry, D. 2005. "Wolof Women, Economic Liberalization, and the Crisis of Masculinity in Rural Senegal." *Ethnology*, **44**(3): 207. doi: 10.2307/3774056.

Rahman, M. 2013. "Women's Empowerment: Concept and Beyond." *Global Journal of Human Social Science*, **13**(6):8-13.

Shafiq, A., Hussain, A., Asif, M., Hwang, J., Jameel, A., and Kanwel, S. 2019. "The Effect of 'Women's Empowerment' on Child Nutritional Status in Pakistan." *International Journal of Environmental Research and Public Health*, **16**(22): 4499. doi: 10.3390/ijerph16224499.

Shroff, M., Griffiths, P., Suchindran, C., Nagalla, B., Vazir, S., and Bentley, M. 2011. "Does maternal autonomy influence feeding practices and infant growth in rural India? *Social Science and Medicine*." **73**(3), 447-455. doi: 10.1016/j.socscimed.2011.05.040

Stevens, C. 2010. *Are Women the Key to Sustainable Development?* Available at: https://www.bu.edu/pardee/files/2010/04/UNsdkp003fsingle.pdf, accessed 14 June, 2019.

18

Sexual Dimorphism in Linear Growth among 3-12 year Old Bengalee Children

Pikli Khanra, Soma Pal and *Kaushik Bose*

Introduction

Post-natal linear growth can be described in terms of three distinct phases: the nutrition-dependent infancy phase, the growth-hormone-dependent childhood phase and puberty, with the additional growth during adolescent which is driven by sex steroids (Karlberg, 1989). Worldwide, most of the studies regarding linear growth among children estimated retarded linear growth among children of under five years of age (Nuruddin *et al.*, 2009; Wang *et al.*, 2009; Meshram *et al.*, 2011; Meshram *et al.*, 2012; Nguyen *et al.*, 2014; Motbainor *et al.*, 2015; Aguayo *et al.*, 2016; Gunardi *et al.*, 2017; Mahapatra *et al.*, 2019). Furthermore, previously, numerous studies have assessed the association between leg length or body proportions and quality of living environment of populations. Leitch (1951) was probably the first medical researcher to propose that a ratio of leg length to total stature could be a good indicator of nutritional history and general health in the early life of an individual. Leitch found that improved nutrition during infancy and childhood did indeed result in a greater increase in leg length than in total height or weight. She also reported that longer-legged children were also less susceptible to bronchitis, which was then a scourge of poorly fed children. Later, several studies support Leitch's findings and hypotheses (Thomas and Duncan, 1954; Wolanski, 1979; Tanner *et al.*, 1982; Buschang *et al.*, 1986; Dickinson *et al.*, 1990; Gurri and Dickinson, 1990; Murguia *et al.*, 1990; Wolanski *et al.*, 1993; Siniarska, 1995; Wolanski, 1995; Jantz and Jantz, 1999).

Numerous previous studies (Norgan, 1998; Frisancho *et al.*, 2001; Dangour *et al.* 2001; Dangour *et al.*, 2002; Bogin *et al.*, 2001; Bogin *et al.*, 2002; Smith *et al.*, 2002, Smith *et al.*, 2003; Bogin and Varela-Silva, 2003; Bogin and Rios, 2003; Gunnell *et al.*, 2003; Ferrie *et al.*, 2006; Frisancho, 2007; Li *et al.*, 2007; Dasgupta *et al.*, 2008; Floyd, 2008; Kim *et al.*, 2008; Malina *et al.*, 2008; Whitley *et al.*, 2008) have also been strongly agreed with the hypotheses that human body proportions are sensitive indicators of the quality of the environment for growth during infancy, childhood, and juvenile years of development, the time of life during which the lower limbs grow at a faster rate than the upper limbs. Frisancho *et al.* (2001) noted that leg length of Mexican Americans aged 2-17 years old was significantly associated with socio-economic status of their families. Children from better-off families had significantly longer legs, but equal trunk length, compared with boys and girls from poorer families. Another study (Dangour, 2001) has reported similar findings among two tribes of Amerindian children living in Guyana. Bogin *et al.*, (2002) found even greater plasticity [phenotypic properties of the human body change in response to external (environmental) factors] in the children of Maya families emigrating from Guatemala to the United States of America. A recent study (Nowak-Szczepanska and Koziel, 2016) has observed sexual dimorphisms in the longitudinal growth of the relative length of particular segments of upper limb (forearm length) and lower limb (knee height) among Polish adolescents. They proposed that relatively longer forearms, particularly in relation to the trunk in girls, could have evolved as an adaptation to more efficient infant carrying and protection during breastfeeding.

Different lower limb body segments such as subischial leg length was assessed by Gunnell *et al.* (2003), Ferrie *et al.* (2006), Wadsworth *et al.* (2002), and Li *et al.* (2007) and relative subischial leg length was studied by Floyd *et al.* (2008) and sitting height ratio was used by Frisancho *et al.*(2001); Malina *et al.* (2008); Dasgupta *et al.* (2008) and Bogin *et al.* (2002) to evaluate how long leg and body proportion ratios are good indicators of the quality of the environment and of the plasticity of the human body. Similarly, iliac height was studied by Whitley *et al.* (2008) and Kim *et al.* (2008); knee height was studied by Dixon *et al.* (2008) and knee height ratio were studied by Floyd *et al.* (2008) to support the same extent. In contrast to previous studies, Schooling *et al.*

(2008a, b); Padez *et al.* (2009) and Kinra *et al.* (2011) found complications in the relationship between leg length, health, socio-economic-status, and better environments for growth in their studies among Chinese people aged 50 years and above, Mozambique adolescents and Indian adolescents, respectively.

Human leg length, however, it is measured, trunk length and their proportions [e.g., relative leg length or the sitting height ratio (sitting height/height×100)] are associated with epidemiological risk of several diseases and syndromes. The research also reports that leg length, rather than trunk length, is a better predictor of adult-onset disease, such as coronary heart disease (CHD), and atherosclerosis. Relatively shorter legs and shorter stature due to relatively shorter legs may increase the risk for overweight, coronary heart disease and diabetes (Smith *et al.*, 2001; Lawlor *et al.*, 2002, 2003, 2004; Langenberg *et al.*, 2005, Ferrie *et al.*, 2006, Tiling *et al.*, 2006). These proportions are also associated with liver dysfunction (Fraser *et al.*, 2008) and some kind of cancers (Gunnell *et al.*, 2001).

During the last two decades, several researchers have investigated growth pattern of children and adolescents of India across the country (Mitra *et al.*, 2002; Busi *et al.*, 2003; Busi and Rao, 2003; Busi *et al.*, 2004; Khalil and Khan, 2004; Bose *et al.*, 2005; Rao *et al.*, 2005; Rao *et al.*, 2006; Medhi *et al.*, 2006; Sharma *et al.*, 2007; Chakraborty *et al.*, 2008; Rao *et al.*, 2009; Kaur *et al.*, 2012; Qamra *et al.*, 2012; Verma, 2012; Kolekar and Sawant, 2013; Patil *et al.*, 2013; Basu *et al.*, 2014; Talwar and Airi, 2015; Ahirwar and Gautam, 2015; Kharri and Rao, 2015a, 2015b; Patil *et al.*, 2015; Aditi [Mukherjee] *et al.*, 2016; Kuiti *et al.*, 2017; Pal and Bose, 2017; Bharathi *et al.*, 2017; Thakur and Gautam, 2017; Dutta and Sengupta, 2019; Neeta Devi, 2019; Longkumar, 2019). A detailed literature search reported inadequate data regarding sexual dimorphism of linear growth in terms of height acromion (Pal and Bose, 2017), sitting height (Pal and Bose, 2017), and subischial leg length (Bose *et al.*, 2005, Pal and Bose, 2017) among children of Bengalee ethnicity. Hence, our study was undertaken to assess sexual dimorphism in linear growth pattern in height, height acromion, sitting height, knee height and SLL among Bengalee children aged from 3 to 12 years old of Purba Medinipur District of West Bengal, India.

Materials and Methods

The cross-sectional study was undertaken among children aged from 3 to 12 years from Desopran Block (also known as Contai-II) and Haldia Municipality of Purba Medinipur District, West Bengal, India. The Purba Medinipur District (also known as East Midnapore District) has a long coastal line of 65.5 kilometres. The major rivers such as Haldia, Rupnarayan, Rasulpur, Bagui and Keleghai flow from north to south or south-east direction of the district. The study area of present investigation was situated across the riverside of Haldia and Rasulpur.

Three colonies, namely Calcutta Port Trust (CPT), Indian Oil Corporation (IOC) and Haldia Riverside Estate Limited (HREL) and Rairarchak village of Township area were selected from Haldia Municipality. Similarly, Kultalia, Sikdarchak and Uttar Amtalia villages of Amtalia Gram Panchayat from Contai-II Block were selected on the basis of opportunity sampling method for data collection of present investigation. The villagers were selected due to convenience. All children present at the time of measurement were included in our study. The participants were selected using opportunity sampling method. Data were collected through door to door visit. The Purba Medinipur district has a population of 50,95,875 which include 5,87,654 children under age of 0-6 years as per census of India (Census of India, 2011). Objectives of the study were clearly stated to the guardians of the children and verbal consent was taken before the measuring children. Necessary administrative approval was taken from Haldia Municipality and Contai-II Community Development Block and ethical clearance was obtained from Vidyasagar University before the commencement of the study. Present investigation was undertaken in accordance with the ethical guidelines for human experiments, as laid down by the Helsinki Declaration of 2000 (Touitou *et al.*, 2004).

A total of 1242 children aged from 3 to 2 years old were enrolled (614 boys; and 628 girls) for the present investigation. Date of birth of children was collected from the birth certificate or child health card. Further, it was verified by parents (especially by mother) of children. The exact age of the children was calculated

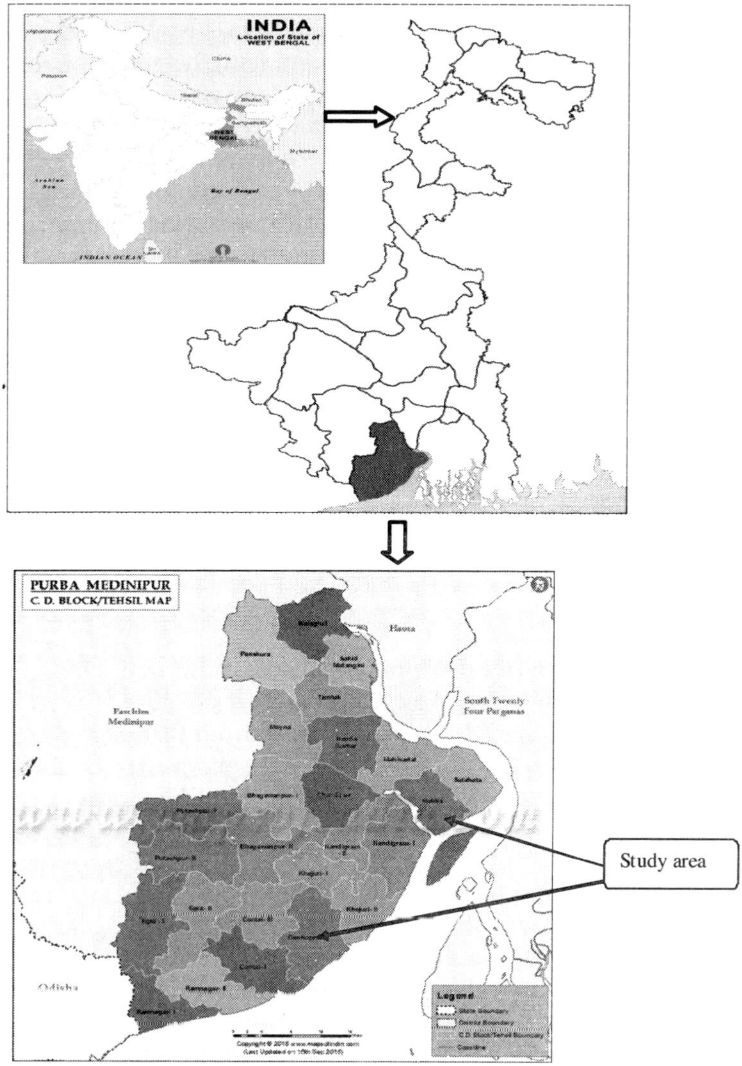

Fig. 18.1: Location of study area in Purba Medinipur District, West Bengal and India.

by subtracting the date of birth from date of survey. Data was collected by first author (PK) during the period from December 2014 to April 2016. All participants belonged to Bengalee ethnicity. Anthropometric variables, namely height (cm), height acromion (cm), sitting height (cm), and knee height (cm) were measured by following standard procedures (Lohman *et al.*, 1988) and data was recorded as per standardized reference manual (WHO, 1995). Subischial leg length (SLL) was derived by deducting sitting height (cm.) from height (cm.). Same calibrated measuring equipment was used for collecting anthropometric measures for all participants to reduce error.

Data was analysed using Statistical Package for Social Sciences (SPSS, version 16.0). Descriptive statistics (mean and standard deviation) was calculated for quantitative variables. Independent sample t-tests were executed to observe the age specific sex differences in anthropometric variables. One-way analysis of variance (ANOVA -F test) tests were performed to study the significant age variations in mean anthropometric values for both sexes.

Results

Table 18.1 represents the descriptive statistics (mean and standard deviation), t-test and One-Way ANOVA (F) test values of height (cm) of the participants. Results of t-test showed that there were no significant sex differences in mean height except at 4 ($t = -2.01$ and $p<0.05$) and 9 ($t = 2.29$ and $p<0.05$) years. Significant age variations were found in mean height of both sexes ($F = 258.11$, $p<0.001$ for boys and $F = 200.21$, $p<0.001$ for girls). Descriptive statistics (mean and standard deviation), t-test and One-Way ANOVA (F) test values of height acromion (cm) and sitting height are presented in Table 18.2. Results of t-test revealed that significant sex differences in mean height acromion were found at age of 3 ($t = -2.40$, $p<0.05$), 4 ($t = -2.32$, $p<0.05$) and 9 ($t = 2.11$, $p<0.05$) years. Significant age differences in mean height acromion was also observed for both sexes (boys: $F = 229.22$, $p<0.001$ and girls:

Table 18.1: Descriptive statistics (mean and standard deviation), t-test and F-test values of height (cm)

Age (Years)	*n#*		*Height (cm)*				*t*
			Boys		*Girls*		
	Boys	*Girls*	*Mean*	*SD*	*Mean*	*SD*	
3	61	61	99.75	5.37	100.82	7.21	-0.93
4	62	61	101.70	6.42	104.22	7.45	**-2.01***
5	60	66	109.43	5.91	108.17	6.24	0.92
6	63	62	113.44	5.06	112.34	4.92	1.23
7	61	61	115.94	5.69	115.20	6.13	0.69
8	61	63	122.22	6.84	120.84	7.71	1.06
9	60	62	126.99	8.21	123.52	8.49	**2.29***
10	61	68	131.37	8.72	129.96	8.82	0.91
11	63	63	136.72	9.37	135.39	9.55	0.79
12	62	61	142.30	7.53	142.68	8.69	-0.26
Total (age combined)	614	628	120.03	15.42	119.40	15.03	0.738
	F = 258.11*** (for boys)				**F = 200.21***** (for girls)		

\# Present sample size is used for subsequent analysis;
* means significance at the level of p<0.05; and
*** means significance at the level of p<0.001.

Table 18.2: Descriptive statistics (mean and standard deviation), t-test and F-test values of height acromion (cm) and sitting height (cm)

Age (years)	*Height acromion (cm)*					*Sitting height (cm)*				
	Boys		*Girls*		*t*	*Boys*		*Girls*		*t*
	Mean	*SD*	*Mean*	*SD*		*Mean*	*SD*	*Mean*	*SD*	
3	75.07	6.03	77.94	7.12	**-2.40***	52.35	4.67	54.73	5.35	**-2.62***
4	77.76	6.36	80.72	7.74	**-2.32***	54.39	4.36	56.69	4.89	**-2.76****
5	85.35	6.14	84.86	7.30	0.40	58.40	4.19	58.14	3.37	0.39
6	89.16	4.67	88.83	5.21	0.46	61.48	3.43	59.67	3.09	**3.09****
7	91.80	5.82	90.99	7.89	0.65	61.31	4.17	60.98	4.85	0.40
8	97.79	6.75	96.24	8.21	1.15	63.86	3.96	62.15	4.46	**2.26***
9	101.87	7.97	98.68	8.69	**2.11***	66.15	4.10	64.02	4.98	**2.59***
10	105.83	8.31	104.16	9.34	1.07	67.81	4.67	66.01	5.27	**2.05***
11	110.22	9.26	109.21	9.77	0.59	69.28	4.99	68.76	5.62	0.56
12	114.58	7.06	114.87	7.71	-0.22	71.57	3.99	72.01	5.00	-0.54
Total(age combined)	95.00	14.51	94.60	14.44	0.477	62.68	7.36	62.34	7.00	0.832
F = 229.22*** (boys)			**F = 145.15***** (girls)			**F=134.70***** (boys)			**F=81.70***** (girls)	

* means significance at the level of p<0.05; ** means significance at the level of p<0.01; and *** means significance at the level of p<0.001.

F = 145.15, p<0.001). Significant sex differences were found in all age group except 5, 7, 11 and 12 years. Age differences in mean sitting height were also statistically significant for both sexes (boys: F = 134.70, p<0.001 and girls: F = 81.70, p<0.001). Descriptive statistics (mean and standard deviation), t-test and One-Way ANOVA (F) test values of knee height (cm) and SLL (cm) are shown in Table 18.3. Significant sex differences in mean knee height were found at the age of 4 (t = -2.25, p<0.05) and 9 (t = 2.71, p<0.01) years. Results of t-test also revealed that there were no significant sex differences in mean SLL. Results of One-Way Analysis of Variance (ANOVA) test (F test) revealed that significant age differences were observed in mean knee height (boys: F = 169.77, p<0.001 and girls: F = 103.76, p<0.001) and SLL (boys: F = 172.25, p<0.001 and girls: F = 140.19, p<0.001) in both sexes. With increasing age, all linear measurements showed gradual increment among both sexes except in sitting height and SLL for boys. No significant sexual differences in all linear measurements was

Table 18.3: Descriptive statistics (mean and standard deviation), t-test and F-test values of knee height (cm) and subischial leg length (cm)

Age (years)	*Knee Height (cm)*					*Subischial leg length (cm)*				
	Boys		*Girls*		*t*	*Boys*		*Girls*		*t*
	Mean	*SD*	*Mean*	*SD*		*Mean*	*SD*	*Mean*	*SD*	
3	27.59	2.28	28.31	3.25	-1.41	47.41	4.54	46.09	4.72	1.57
4	28.28	2.69	29.62	3.79	**-2.25***	47.32	4.63	47.53	5.21	-0.24
5	31.08	2.23	30.92	3.23	0.32	51.03	4.11	50.04	5.30	1.17
6	32.57	2.04	32.83	3.16	-0.55	51.96	4.12	52.67	4.70	-0.90
7	33.67	2.55	33.61	2.95	0.12	54.63	4.21	54.22	4.92	0.50
8	35.91	3.11	34.97	3.52	1.57	58.36	4.59	58.69	5.52	-0.36
9	37.76	3.52	35.97	3.80	**2.71****	60.84	6.24	59.50	6.74	1.14
10	39.11	4.01	38.11	4.46	1.33	63.56	5.30	63.96	6.41	-0.38
11	40.76	3.88	40.96	4.07	-0.29	67.44	6.02	66.63	5.23	0.80
12	42.28	3.65	42.42	3.70	-0.21	70.73	4.95	70.67	6.11	0.06
Total (age combined)	34.92	5.74	34.80	5.71	0.363	57.35	9.23	57.05	9.58	0.599
F = 169.77*** (boys)			**F = 103.76***** (girls)			F=**172.25***** (boys)			**F= 140.19***** (girls)	

* means significance at the level of p<0.05; ** means significance at the level of p<0.01; and *** means significance at the level of p<0.001.

observed in total (age combined). Boys had significantly longer sitting height than girls counterpart at 6, 8, 9 and 10 years.

Discussion

Anthropometric variations in body forms and proportions can be better interpreted through proper understanding of growth pattern and differential growth rate of the children. The accurate knowledge of growth and development helps to understand and monitor the morbidity pattern and nutritional status of an individual and of the community. Growth studies are also helpful either for improving the health condition of human population or for administering any health intervention programme (Qamra *et al.*, 2012).

The aim of the present study was to understand the linear growth profile among Bengalee children aged from 3 to 12 years. Figure 18.2 presents the comparison of mean height (cm.) among studied children with other studies. Bengalee children

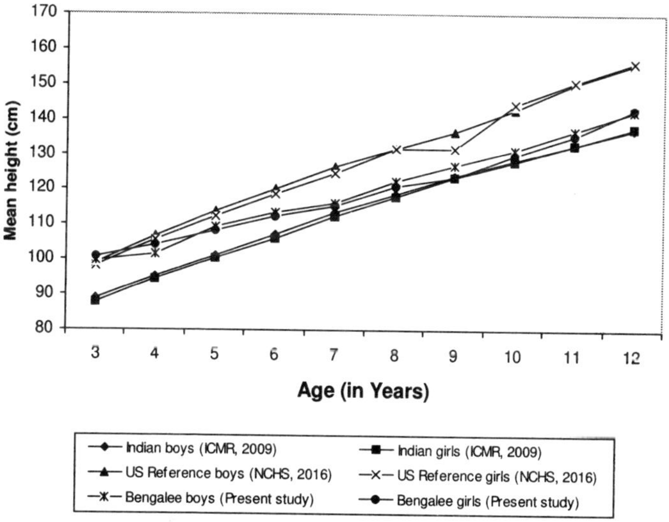

Fig. 18.2: Comparison of mean height (cm.) among studied children with other studies.

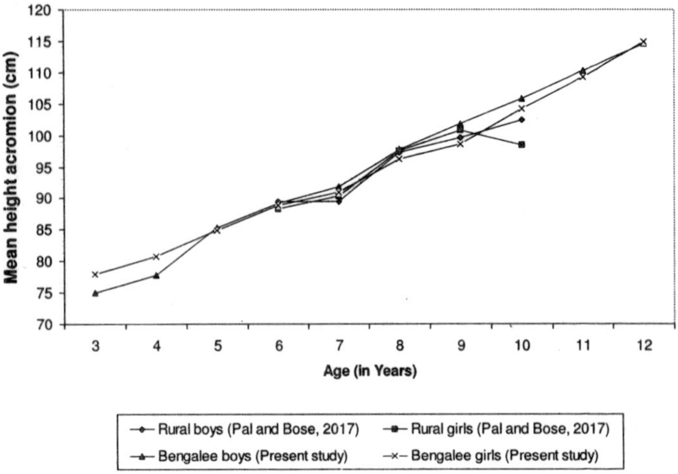

Fig. 18.3: Comparison of mean height acromion (cm.) among studied children with other studies.

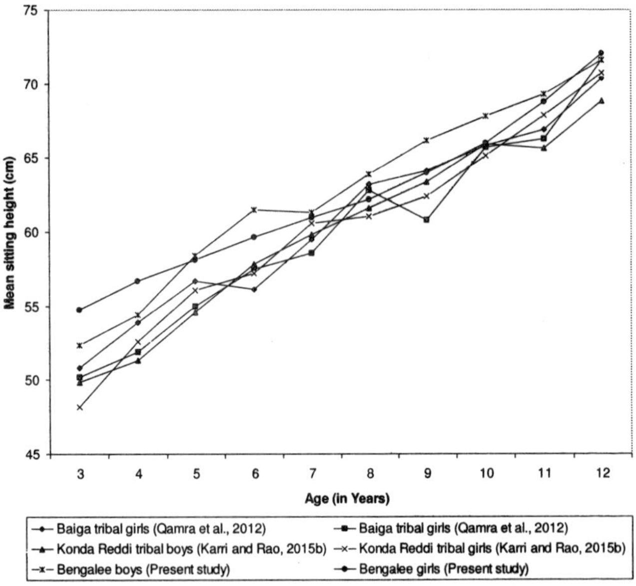

Fig. 18.4: Comparison of mean sitting height (cm.) among studied children with other studies.

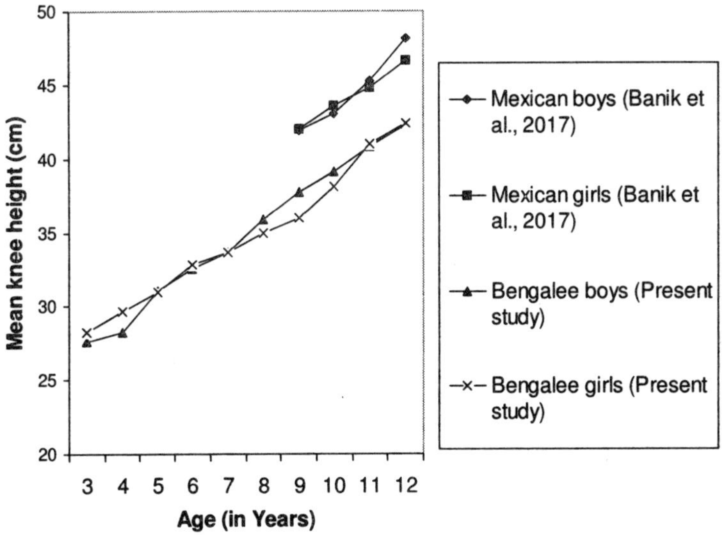

Fig. 18.5: Comparison of mean knee height (cm.) among studied children with other studies.

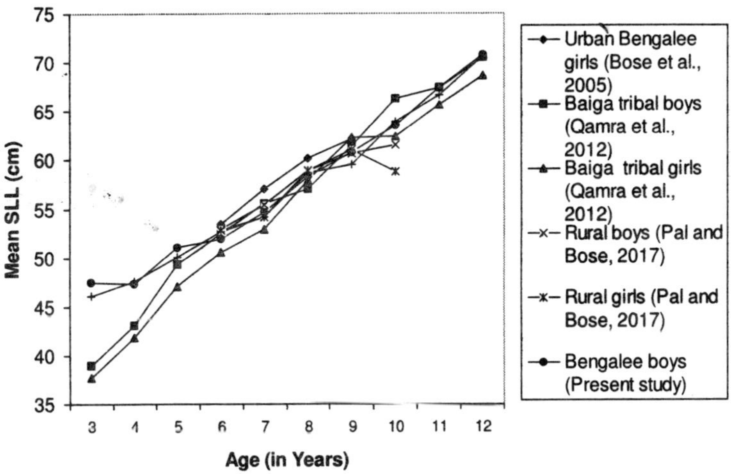

Fig. 18.6: Comparison of mean subischial leg length (cm.) among studied children with other studies.

were relatively shorter than United States reference values (NCHS, 2016) in all age groups except at 3 years. It was also observed that

Bengalee children were taller than Indian rural children (ICMR, 2009) except at 9 years for girls. Comparison of mean height acromion is shown in Figure 18.3. Bengalee boys had lower height acromion value in the age group 3 and 4 years but with increasing age there was evidence of catch up growth potential. Rural children (Pal and Bose, 2017) of Hooghly District, West Bengal had similar mean height acromion at the age group 6, 7, 8 and 9 years. Figure 18.4 displays the comparison of mean sitting height among studied children with other studies. Bengalee children had relatively longer sitting height than Baiga (Verma, 2012) and Konda Reddi (Patil *et al.*, 2015) tribal children of India. Figure 18.5 shows the comparison of mean knee height of studied children with other studies. Bengalee children had relatively shorter mean knee height when compared to Mexican children (Banik *et al.*, 2017) of Merida, Yucatan. Comparisons of mean SLL among studied children with other studies are presented in Figure 18.6. At the age groups 3, 4, and 5 years Bengalee children had longer subischial leg length than Baiga (Qamra *et al.*, 2012) tribal children. In contrast, at the age group 6, 7, 8 and 9 years urban Bengalee girls (Bose *et al.*, 2005) had longer SLL than rural children (Pal and Bose, 2017); Baiga tribal children (Qamra *et al.*, 2012) and present studied children.

Conclusion

In our study, we assessed the linear growth patterns of Bengalee children and compared our findings with other studies. Sexual dimorphism in height and knee height was observed significantly at 4 and 9 years. Height acromion had significant differences at 3, 4 and 9 years among the studied children. Sitting height also demonstrated significant sex dimorphism at 3, 4, 6, 8, 9 and 10 years. In earlier years of growth and development such as at 3 and 4 years, Bengalee girls had significantly longer linear growth. However, later at 12 years, both sexes had similar growth pattern. Our children were taller than Indian rural children studied by Indian Council of Medical Research (ICMR, 2009) but shorter than NCHS reference value (NCHS, 2016). Bengalee children of Purba Medinipur had relative longer linear growth measurements than various tribal children of India. Further studies, preferably londgitudinal, are required to better understand the linear growth patterns of Bengalee children. Ethnic variation in sexual dimorphism in linear growth is of immense value in the study of human population variation.

Acknowledgements

All participants and their parents are sincerely acknowledged for their kind cooperation during data collection. Block Development Officer of Desopran Block and Chairperson of Haldia Municipality are also gratefully acknowledged for giving their permissions. The University Grants Commission is also acknowledged for financial support to one of the author (SP) in the form of UGC-NET SRF (Ref No.: 590/(NET-DEC. 2013). Dr. Raja Chakraborty is gratefully acknowledged for his valuable inputs before and during the course of data collection.

REFERENCES

Aditi (Mu kherjee), P., Dinda, A,, Adak, D,K. "Physical growth among pre-adolescent Muria children (6-10 years) of Bastar district, Chhatisgarh: Bio-cultural perspectives." *Hum Bio Rev*. 2016; **5**(4): 388-404.

Aguayo, V.M., Nair, R., Badgaiyan, N., Krishna, V. "Determinants of stunting and poor linear growth in children under 2 years of age in India: an in depth analysis of Maharashtra's comprehensive nutrition survey." *Mater Child Nutr.* 2016; **12**(suppl.):121-140. http://doi.org/10.1111/mcn.12259.

Ahirwar, A., Gautam, R.K. "Growth pattern among Bharia boys—A tribe of Patalkot, Chhindwara (MP), India." *Hum Bio Rev.*2015; **4**(3): 221-235.

Banik, S.D., Salehabadi, S.M., Dickinson, F. "Preece-Baines Model 1 to Estimate height and knee height Growth in boys and girls from Merida, Mexico." *Food Nutr Bull.* 2017; **38**(2): 182-195. http://doi.org/10.1177/0379572117700270.

Basu, D., Islam, G., Gogoi, R., Dey, S., Deori, J. "Child's growth and nutritional status in two communities—Mishing tribe and Kaibarta caste of Assam, India." *Int J SociolAnthropol.*2014; **6**(2): 59-69. http://doi.org/10.5897/IJSA2013.0494.

Bharthi, K., Ghritlahre, M., Das, S., Bose, K. "Nutritional status among children and adolescents aged 6-18 years of Kolam tribe of Andhra Pradesh, India." *Anthropol Rev.*2017; **80**(2): 153-163. http://doi.org/10.1515/anre-2017-0010.

Bogin, B., Kapell, M., Varela-Silva, M.I., Orden, A.B., Smith, P.K., Loucky, J. "How Genetic Are Human Body Proportions?" In: Dasgupta P, Hauspie R. eds. *Perspectives in Human Growth, Development and Maturation.* Springer, Dordrecht; 2001: 205-221. https://doi.org/10.1007/978-94-015-9801-9_17.

Bogin, B., Rios L. "Rapid morphological change in living humans: implications for modern human origins." *Com BiochemPhysiol Part A:*

Mol Integr Physiol. 2003; **136**(1):71-84. https://doi.org/10.1016/S1095-6433(02)00294-5.

Bogin, B., Smith, P., Orden, A.B., Varela-Silva, M.I., Loucky, J. "Rapid change in height and body proportions of Maya American children." *Am J Hum Bio*. 2002; **14**(6): 753-761. https://doi.org/10.1002/ajhb.10092.

Bogin, B., Varela-Silva, M.I. "Anthropometric variation and health: a biocultural model of human growth." *J Child Health*.2003; **1**(2): 149-172. https://doi.org/10.3109/713610278.

Bose, K., Bhattacharya, S., Basu, K., Ghosh, S., Mukhopadhyay, A., Bhadra, M. "Age trends in anthropometric characteristics among 6-9 years old Bengalee Hindu school girls of Kolkata, India." *AnthropAnz*.2005; **63**(4): 439-448. http://www.jstor.org/stable/29542690.

Buschang, P.H., Malina, R.M., Little, B.B. "Linear growth of Zapotec school children: growth status and yearly velocity for leg length and sitting height." *Ann Hum Bio*. 1986; **13**(3): 225-234. https://doi.org/10.1080/03014468600008391.

Busi, B.R., Rao, B.D., Rao, V.L.N. "Growth progression in physical and physiological variables among Jalaris of Visakhapatnam district, Andhra Pradesh." *Anthropol*. 2003; **5**(4): 269-282. https://doi.org/10.1080/09720073.2003.11890819.

Busi, B.R., Rao, B.D. "Growth Progression in Physical and Physiological Variables Among Relli's of Visakhapatnam District of Andhra Pradesh." *J Hum Ecol*. 2003; **14**(2): 101-111. https://doi.org/10.1080/09709274.2003.11905605.

Busi, B.R., Rao B.D., Rao, V.L.N. "Growth progression in physical and physiological variables among Yata's of Visakhapatnam district, Andhra Pradesh." *Anthropol*. 2004; **6**(1): 239-246. http://doi.org/10.1080/09720073.2004.11890860.

Chakraborty, U., Dutta, C.S., Dutta, G., Ghosh, T. "A comparative study of physical growth and nutritional status in Santal children of Ghatsila and Bolpur." In: Kaushik Bose guest (ed._ *Health and Nutritional Problems of Indigenous Population : Tribes and Tribals*. Kamla-Raj Enterprises, New Delhi; 2008; (spl2): 79-86.

Dangour, A.D., Schilg, S., Hulse, J.A., Cole, T.J. "Sitting height and subischial leg length centile curves for boys and girls from Southeast England." *Ann Hum Bio*. 2002; **29**(3): 290-305. https://doi.org/10.1080/03014460110085331.

Dangour, A.D. "Growth of upper- and lower-body segments in Patamona and Wapishana Amerindian children (cross-sectional data)." *Ann Hum Bio*. 2001; **28**(6): 649-663. https://doi.org/10.1080/03014460110047982.

Dasgupta, P., Saha, R., Nubé, M. "Changes in body size, shape and nutritional status of middle-class Bengali boys of Kolkata, India, 1982–2002." *Econ Hum Bio*. 2008; **6**(1): 75-94. https://doi.org/10.1016/jehb.2007.05.001.

Dickinson, F., Cervera, M., Murguia, R., Uc, L. "Growth, nutritional status and environmental change in Yucatan, Mexico." *Stud Hum Ecol*. 1990; **9**: 135-149.

Dixon, B., Darlow, B., Prickett, T. "How useful is knemometry in measuring neonatal growth?" *J Paediatr Child Health.* 2008; **44**(7-8): 444-448. https://doi.org/10.1111/j.1440-1754.2008.01328.x.

Dutta, D., Sengupta, S. "Physical growth and nutritional status among the children of Northeast India." In: Sengupta S., Dutta D. (eds.) *Growth and nutritional status: perspectives from Northeast India.* Gyan Publishing House, Daryaganj, New Delhi; 2019: 37-47.

Ferrie, J.E., Langenberg, C., Shipley, M.J., Marmot, M.G. "Birth weight, components of height and coronary heart disease: evidence from the Whitehall II study." *Int J Eepidemiol.* 2006; **35**(6):1 532-1542. https://doi.org/10.1093/ije/dyl184.

Floyd, B. "Intergenerational gains in relative knee height as compared to gains in relative leg length within Taiwanese families." *Am J Hum Bio.*2008; **20**(4): 462-464. https://doi.org/10.1002/ajhb.20768.

Fraser, A., Ebrahim, S., Smith, G.D., Lawlor, D.A. "The associations between height components (leg and trunk length) and adult levels of liver enzymes." *J Epidemiol Community Health.* 2008; **62**(1): 48-53. http://dx.doi.org/10.1136jech.2006.053181.

Frisancho, A.R., Guilding, N., Tanner, S. "Growth of leg length is reflected in socio-economic differences." *Acta Med Auxaolog.* 2001; **33**: 47-50.

Frisancho, A.R. "Relative leg length as a biological marker to trace the developmental history of individuals and populations: growth delay and increased body fat." *Am J Hum Bio.* 2007; **19**(5): 703-710. https://doi.org/10.1002/ajhb.20676.

Fryar, C.D., Gu, Q., Ogden, C.L., Flegal, K.M. "Anthropometric data for children and adults: United States, 2011-2014." *National Centre for Health Statictics, Vita Health Stat* 3(39). 2016.

Gunardi, H., Soedjatmiko, S., Sekartini, R., *et al.* "Association between parental socio-demographic factors and declined linear growth of young children in Jakarta." *Med J Indonesia.* 2017; **26**(4): 286-292. https://doi.org/10.13181/mji.v26i4.1819.

Gunnell, D., Okasha, M., Davey Smith, G., Oliver, S.E., Sandhu, J., Holly, J.M.P. "Height, leg length, and cancer risk: a systematic review." *Epidemiol Rev.* 2001; **23**(2): 313-342.

Gunnell, D., Whitley, E., Upton, M.N., McConnachie, A., Smith, G.D., Watt, G.C.M. "Associations of height, leg length, and lung function with cardiovascular risk factors in the Midspan Family Study." *J Epidemiol Community Health.* 2003; 57(2):141-146. http://dx.doi.org/10.1136/jech.57.2.141.

Gurri, F.D., Dickinson, F. "Effects of socio-economic, ecological, and demographic conditions on the development of the extremities and the trunk: a case study with adult females from Chiapas." *J Hum Ecol.* 1990; **1**(2): 125-138.

https://en.wikipedia.org/wiki/Purba_Medinipur_district accessed June 20, 2019.

https://www.census2011.co.in/census/district/19-purba-medinipur.html accessed on June 21, 2019.

https://www.mapsofindia.com/maps/westbengal/tehsil/purba-medinipur.html accessed 21st July, 2019.

Indian Council of Medical Research (ICMR). "Nutrient Requirement and Recommended Dietary Allowances for Indians: A Report of the Expert Group of the Indian Council of Medical Research." ICMR 2009; India.

Jantz, L.M., Jantz, R.L. "Secular change in long bone length and proportion in the United States, 1800-1970." *Am J Phys Anthropol.* 1999; **110**(1):57-67. https://doi.org/10.1002/(SICI)1096-8644(199909)110:1<57::AID-JPA5>3.0.CO;2-1.

Karlberg, J. "On the construction of the infancy-childhood-puberty growth standard." *Acta Paediatr.* 1989; **78**(s356): 26-37. https://doi.org/10.1111/j.1651-2227.1989.tb11237.x.

Karri, B., Rao, V.L.N. "Growth pattern among Kolam children and adolescents aged 0-18 years: 10 anthropometric measurements." *Int J Res.*2015a; **2**(7): 102-108.

Karri, B., Rao, V.L.N. "Growth pattern among Konda Reddi children and adolescents aged 0 to 18 years." *Int J Res Advent Tech.*2015b; **3**(11): 46-58.

Kaur, N., Uppal, M., Sidhu, S. "Physical Growth Status of Affluent Arora Children of Amritsar." *Hum Bio Rev*. 2012; **1**(3): 268-281.

Khalil, S., Khan, Z. "A study of physical growth and nutritional status of rural school going children of Aligarh." *Ind J Prevent Soc Med.* 2004; **35**(3-4): 90-98.

Kim, J.M., Stewart, R., Shin, I.S., Kim, S.W., Yang, S.J., Yoon, J.S. "Associations between head circumference, leg length and dementia in a Korean population." *Int J Geriatr Psychiatry.* 2008; **23**(1): 41-48. https://doi.org/10.1002/gps.1833.

Kinra, S., Sarma, K.R., Hards, M., Smith, G.D., Ben-Shlomo, Y. "Is relative leg length a biomarker of childhood nutrition? Long-term follow-up of the Hyderabad Nutrition Trial." *Int J Epidemiol.*2009; **40**(4): 1022-1029. https://doi.org/10.1093/ije/dyr074.

Kolekar, S.M., Sawant, S.U. "A Comparative study of physical growth in Urban and rural school children from 5 to 13 years of age." *Int J Recent Trends Sci Tech.* 2013; **6**(2): 89-93.

Kuiti, B.K., Dash, I., Jana, M., Pratihar, S., Bose, K. "Growth Pattern of School Going Children of Medinipur Districts of West Bengal, India." *J Life Sci.* 2017; **9**(1): 18-27. https://doi.org/10.1080/09751270.2017.1343706.

Langenberg, C., Hardy, R., Breeze, E., Kuh, D., Wadsworth, M.E. "Influence of short stature on the change in pulse pressure, systolic and diastolic blood pressure from age 36 to 53 years: an analysis using multilevel models." *Int J Epidemiol.* 2005; **34**(4): 905-913. https://doi.org/10.1093/ije/dyi071.

Lawlor, D., Ebrahim, S., Smith, G.D. "The association between components of adult height and Type II diabetes and insulin resistance: British Women's Heart and Health Study." *Diabetologia.* 2002; 45(8): 1097-1106. https://doi.org/10.1007/s00125-002-0887-5.

Lawlor, D.A., Davey, Smith, G., Ebrahim, S. "Association between leg length and offspring birthweight: partial explanation for the trans-generational association between birthweight and cardiovascular disease: findings from the British Women's Heart and Health Study." *Paediatr Perinatal Epidemiol.* 2003; **17**(2): 148-155. https://doi.org/10.1046/j.1365-3016.2003.00479.x.

Lawlor, D.A., Taylor, M., Davey, Smith, G., Gunnell, D., Ebrahim, S. "Associations of components of adult height with coronary heart disease in postmenopausal women: the British women's heart and health study." *Heart.* 2004; **90**(7): 745-749. http://dx.doi.org/10.1136/hrt.2003.019950.

Leitch, I. "Growth and health." *Br J Nutr.* 1951; 5:142-151 [reprinted *Intern J Epidemiol.* 2001; **30**(2): 212-216].

Li, L., Dangour, A.D., Power, C. "Early life influences on adult leg and trunk length in the 1958 British birth cohort." *Am J Hum Bio.* 2007; **19**(6): 836-843. https://doi.org/10.1002/ajhb.20649.

Lohman, T.G., Roche, A.F., Martorell, R. *Anthropometric standardization reference manual.* Chicago, IL, USA; Human Kinetics Books: 1988.

Longkumar, T. "Growth, nutrition, and physical activity: an anthropological study among the Ao Naga children from Nagaland, Northeast India." In: Sengupta S., Dutta D. eds. *Growth and nutritional status: perspectives from Northeast India.* Gyan Publishing House, Daryaganj, New Delhi; 2019: 195-205.

Mahapatra, B., Dey, J., Pal, S., Bose, K. "Prevalence of Undernutrition among Santal Preschool Children of Two Districts of West Bengal, India." *Hum Bio Rev.* 2019; **8**(2): 179-196.

Malina, R.M., Peña Reyes, M.E., Little, B.B. "Secular change in the growth status of urban and rural school children aged 6-13 years in Oaxaca, southern Mexico." *Ann Hum Bio.* 2008; **35**(5): 475-489. https://doi.org/10.1080/03014460802243844.

Medhi, G.K., Barua, A.A., Mahanta, J. "Growth and nutritional status of school age children (6-14 years) of tea garden worker of Assam." *J Hum Ecol.* 2006; **19**(2): 83-85. https://doi.org/10.1080/09709274.2006.11905860.

Meshram II, Arlappa, N., Balakrishna, N., *et al.* "Prevalence and determinants of undernutrition and its trends among pre-school tribal children of Maharashtra State, India." *J Trop Pediatr.* 2011; **58**(2): 125-132. https://doi.org/10.1093/tropej/fmr035.

Meshram II, Arlappa N., Balakrishna, N., Rao, K.M., Laxmaiah, A., Brahmam, G.N.V. "Trends in the prevalence of undernutrition, nutrient and food intake and predictors of undernutrition among under five year tribal children in India." *Asia Pac J Clin Nutr.* 2012; **21**(4): 568-576. http://doi.org/10.6133/apjcn.

Mitra, M., Kumar, P.V., Ghosh, R., Bharati, P. "Growth pattern of the Kamars– a primitive tribe of Chhattisgarh, India." *Coll Antropol.*2002; **26**(2): 485-499.

Motbainor, A., Worku, A., Kumie, A. "Stunting is associated with food diversity while wasting with food insecurity among underfive children in East and West Gojjam Zones of Amhara Region, Ethiopia." *Plos One*. 2015; **10**(8):e0133542. http://doi.org/1371/journal.pone.0133542.

Murguía, R., Dickinson, F., Cervera, M., Uc, L. "Socio-economic activities, ecology and somatic differences in Yucatan, Mexico." *Stud Hum Ecol.* 1990; **9**(1): 111-134.

Neeta Devi, R.K. "Growth pattern and nutritional status among the urban Meitei girls of Imphal Valley, Manipur." In: Sengupta S., Dutta D. eds. *Growth and nutritional status: perspectives from Northeast India.* Gyan Publishing House, Daryaganj, New Delhi; 2019: 147-162.

Nguyen, P.H., Saha, K.K., Ali, D., *et al.* "Maternal mental health is associated with child undernutrition and illness in Bangladesh, Vietnam and Ethiopia." *Pub Health Nutr.* 2014; **17**(6): 1318-1327. https://doi.org/10.1017/S1368980013001043.

Norgan, N.G. "Body-proportion differences." In: Ulijaszek S.J., Johnston F.E., Preece, M.A., eds. *Cambridge encyclopedia of human growth and development.* Cambridge University Press; 1998: 378-379.

Nowak-Szczepanska, N., Koziel, S. "Sexual dimorphism in growth in the relative length of the forearm and relative knee height during adolescence." *Am J Phys Anthropol.* 2016; **161**(2): 276-282. https://doi.org/10.1002/ajpa.23028.

Nuruddin, R., Lim, M.K., Hadden, W.C., Azam, I. "Comparison of estimates of undernutrition for pre-school rural Pakistani children based on the WHO standard and the National Center for Health Statistics (NCHS) reference." *Pub Health Nutr.*2009; **12**(5): 716-722. https://doi.org/10.1017/S1368980008002383.

Padez, C., Varela, Silva, M.I., Bogin, B. "Height and relative leg length as indicators of the quality of the environment among Mozambican juveniles and adolescents." *Am J Hum Bio.*2009; **21**(2): 200-209. https://doi.org/10.1002/ajhb.20854.

Pal, S., Bose, K. "Anthropometric characteristics of rural primary school children of Hooghly District." *Hum Bio Rev.* 2017; **6**(1): 30-46.

Patil, S.S., Patil, S.R., Durgawale, P.M., Kakade, S.V., Abhishek, K. "Study of physical growth standards of adolescents (10-15 years) from Karad, Maharashtra." *Int J Collaborative Res Int Med Public Health.* 2013; **5**(1): 10-18.

Patil, S.S., Patil, S.R., Durgawale, P.M., Kakade, S.V. "Study of Physical Growth Standards of Adolescents in the Age Group of 10 to 15 Years from Satara District of Maharashtra, India." *J Krishna Inst Med Sci.* 2015; **4**(4): 42-56.

Qamra, S., Shrivastava, P., Roy, J. "Growth Profile of Baiga Children—A Primitive Tribe of District Dindori of Madhya Pradesh, India." *Coll Antropol.* 2012; **36**(3): 929-936.

Rao, V.L.N., Busi, B.R., Rao, C.S., Bharathi, K. "Patterns of growth among Savaras of Srikakulam district, Andhra Pradesh." *South Asian Anthrpol.* 2009; **9**(1): 21-30.

Rao, V.L.N., Rao, B.D., Rao, C.S., Bharathi, K., Busi, B.R. "Physical Growth among Gadaba Tribal Population of Vizianagaram District, Andhra Pradesh." *South Asian Anthropol.*2006; **6**(2): 175-184.

Rao, V.L.N., Rao, B.D., Rao, C.S., Busi, B.R. "Patterns of growth and physiological variables among Khond tribal population of Visakhapatnam district, Andhra Pradesh." *Anthropol.* 2005; **7**(4): 237-245. https://doi/10.1080/09720073.2005.11890915.

Schooling, C.M., Jiang, C.Q., Heys, M., *et al.* "Are height and leg length universal markers of childhood conditions? The Guangzhou Biobank cohort study." *J Epidemiol Community Health.* 2008a; **62**(7): 607-614. http://dx.doi/org/10.1136/jech.2007.065003.

Schooling, C.M., Jiang, C.Q., Heys, M., *et al.* "Is leg length a biomarker of childhood conditions in older Chinese women? The Guangzhou Biobank Cohort Study." *J Epidemiol Community Health.* 2008b; **62**(2): 160-166. https://dx.doi.org/10.1136/jech.2006.058917.

Sharma, A., Sharma, K., Mathur, K.P. "Growth pattern and prevalence of obesity in affluent school children of Delhi." *Pub Health Nutr.* 2007; **10**(5): 485-491. https://doi.org/10.1017/S1368980007223894.

Siniarska, A. "Family environment and body build in adults of Yucatan Mexico." *Am J Phys Anthropol (Suppl).* 1995; **20**: 196.

Smith, G.D., Greenwood, R., Gunnell, D., Sweetnam, P., Yarnell, J., Elwood, P. "Leg length, insulin resistance, and coronary heart disease risk: the Caerphilly Study." *J Epidemiol Community Health.* 2001; **55**(12): 867-872. http://dx.doi.org/10.1136/jech.55.12.867.

Smith, P.K., Bogin, B., Varela-Silva, M.I., Loucky, J. "Economic and anthropological assessments of the health of children in Maya immigrant families in the US." *Econ Hum Bio.* 2003; **1**(2): 145-160. https://doi.org/10.1016/S1570-677X(02)00032-1.

Smith, P.K., Bogin, B., Varela-Silva, M.I., Orden, B., Loucky, J. "Does immigration help or harm children's health? The Mayan case." *Soc Sci Quart.* 2002; **83**(4): 994-1002. https://doi.org/10.1111/1540-6237.00128.

Talwar, I., Airi, P. "Physical Growth and Nutritional Status of Children aged 6-8 years of Panchkula city (Haryana), India." *Hum Bio Rev.* 2015; **4**(1): 1-26.

Tanner, J.M., Hayashi, T., Preece, M.A., Cameron, N. "Increase in length of leg relative to trunk in Japanese children and adults from 1957 to 1977: comparison with British and with Japanese Americans." *Ann Hum Bio.* 1982; **9**(5): 411-423. https://doi.org/10.1080/03014468200005951.

Thakur, R., Gautam, R.K. "Pre- and post-pubertal growth difference among boys and girls of 5-18 years of age: A cross-sectional study among central Indian Population." *Hum Bio Rev.* 2017; **6**(2): 164-187.

Thomson, A.M., Duncan, D.L. "The diagnosis of malnutrition in man." *NutrAbstr Rev.* 1954; **24**(1): 1-18.

Tilling, K., Lawlor, D.A., Davey Smith, G., Chambless, L., Szklo, M. "The relation between components of adult height and intimal-medial thickness in middle age: the Atherosclerosis Risk in Communities Study." *Am J Epidemiol.* 2006; **164**(2): 136-142. https://doi.org/10.1093/aje/kwj184.

Touitou, Y., Portaluppi, F., Smolensky, M.H., Rensing, L. "Ethical principles and standards for the conduct of human and animal biological rhythm research." *Chronobiol Int.* 2004; **21**(1): 161-170. https://doi.org/10.1081/CBI-120030045.

Verma, D.K. "Pattern of growth in height and weight among Gadaba boys and girls of Bastar District, Chhattisgarh (India)." *Int J Sociol Anthropol.* 2012; **4**(4): 147-154. http://doi.org/10.5897/IJSA11.149.

Wadsworth, M.E., Hardy, R.J., Paul, A.A., Marshall, S.F., Cole, T.J. "Leg and trunk length at 43 years in relation to childhood health, diet and family circumstances; evidence from the 1946 national birth cohort." *Int J Eepidemiol.* 2002; **31**(2): 383-390. https://doi.org/10.1093/ije/31.2.383.

Wang, X., Höjer, B., Guo, S., Luo, S., Zhou, W., Wang, Y. "Stunting and 'overweight' in the WHO Child Growth Standards–malnutrition among children in a poor area of China." *Pub Health Nutr.* 2009; **12**(11): 1991-1998. https://doi.org/10.1017/S1368980009990796.

Whitley, E., Gunnell, D., Davey Smith, G., Holly, J.M., Martin, R.M. "Childhood circumstances and anthropometry: the Boyd Orr cohort." *Ann Hum Bio.* 2008; **35**(5): 518-534. https://doi.org/10.1080/03014460802294250.

Wolanski, N., Dickinson, F., Siniarska, A. "Biological traits and living conditions of Maya Indian and non-Maya girls from Merida, Mexico." *Int J Anthropol.* 1993; **8**(4): 233-246. https://doi.org/10.1007/BF02442158.

Wolanski, N. "Household and family as environment for child growth. Cross cultural studies in Poland, Japan, South Korea and Mexico." In: Wright S.D., Meeker D.E., Griffore R., (eds.) *Human ecology: progress through integrative perspectives.* Bar Harbor, ME, USA: The Society for Human Ecology; 1995: 140-152.

Wolanski, N. "Parent-offspring similarity in body size and proportions." *Stud Hum Ecol.* 1979; **3**:7-26.

World Health Organization. *Physical Status: The use and interpretation of anthropometry.* Technical Report Series no. 854.WHO 1995; Geneva.

19

Nutritional Status by Composite Index for Anthropometric Failure

A Study among Urban Bengali Adolescents in Howrah District, West Bengal, India

Swastika Roy and *Jyoti Ratan Ghosh*

Introduction

Health is a prerequisite for human development and is an essential component for the well-being of the mankind. The health problems of any community are influenced by interplay of various factors including biological, social, economic and political ones. The common beliefs, customs, practices related to health and disease in turn influence the health seeking behaviour of the community (Gopalan, 2008). Undernutrition continues to the principal cause of ill-health and premature mortality and morbidity among children living in developing countries (Nandy *et al.*, 2005). As today's children are the citizen of tomorrow's world, their survival, protection and development are prerequisite for the future development of humanity (Bakhetia and Jain, 2007). It has been estimated that approximately 70 per cent of the world's malnourished children live in Asia (Khor, 2005). Undernutrition in children can manifest itself in several ways and is most commonly assessed through the measurement of weight and height. A child can be too short for his or her age (stunted), can have low weight for his or her height (wasted), or can have low weight for his or her age (underweight). A child who is underweight can also be stunted or wasted or both (Ghai *et al.*, 2006). The phenomenon of malnourished girl child is more important in the context of her role as a mother, who being a stunted mother give birth to a stunted child and the circle rotates (Khan and Raza, 2014). According to National Family Health Survey-3 (NFHS-3), the prevalence of stunting, wasting, and underweight among under-3 children in West Bengal was 41.8 per cent, 19.2 per cent and 37.6 per cent respectively. In developing countries, children and adults are vulnerable to malnutrition because of low dietary intakes, infectious diseases, lack of appropriate care, and inequitable distribution of food within the household (Khan and Raza, 2014). The prevalence of undernutrition during childhood is considered to have highly detrimental effects on health in those children who survive to adulthood (WHO, 1995).

The three most widely used conventional anthropometric indices of nutritional status in children are stunting, wasting and underweight (WHO, 1995). However, studies demonstrated that these conventional indices can only be used for the categorization of children into the general categories of undernutrition and do not provide the opportunity to determine the overall prevalence of undernutrition (Mandal and Bose, 2009; Sen *et al.*, 2011). This is because of the overlapping of the children into multiple categories and thus these indices were unable to provide a comprehensive estimate of the number of undernourished children in a population (Svedberg, 2000; Bose and Mandal, 2010). In order to overcome this limitation, Svedberg (2000) proposed the construction of an aggregate indicator for anthropometric failure in terms of composite index of anthropometric failure (CIAF), which incorporates all undernourished children, be they wasted and/or stunted and/or underweight. The original model, proposed by Svedberg (Svedberg, 2000), comprised six sub-groups of anthropometric failure (i.e. Group A to F) to which Nandy *et al.* (2005) supplemented one more sub-group (i.e. Group Y) and recommended its use in preference to the conventional measures of undernutrition. The objective of the present study was to assess the prevalence of undernutrition by CIAF among urban adolescents of Howrah District, West Bengal, India.

Materials and Methods

The present cross-sectional study was carried out among school going adolescents of Howrah District, West Bengal, India. A total of 510 (Boys=258; Girls=252) adolescents aged between 10-17 years were measured. Assents and informed consent was obtained from each participant and their parents before the study. Information on ethnicity, age and gender was collected on a pre-tested schedule. The ages were recorded as reported by School's ID and also verified from schools registered. The anthropometric measurements recorded were height and weight following the standard techniques of Lohman *et al.* (1988). Height of the children was recorded with the help of an anthropometer to the nearest 0.1 cm. The weight of the children was recorded with minimum clothing using a portable weighing machine to the nearest 0.5 kg. Three most commonly used indicators of undernutrition, i.e. stunting, wasting and underweight were used to evaluate the nutritional status of the subjects and along with these CIAF was also used to evaluate the nutritional status for the total children (WHO, 1995; Svedberg, 2000; Nandy *et al.*, 2005). Internationally accepted National Centre for Health Statistics (NCHS) (Hamill *et al.*, 1979; WHO, 1983) for age and sex specific ≤2 z scores were used to define stunting, wasting and underweight.

For assessing the CIAF, Svedberg's (2000) model of six groups including no failure; wasting only; wasting and underweight; wasting, stunting and underweight; stunting and underweight; and lastly stunting only children was considered. Along with Svedberg's model, an additional subgroup, i.e. underweight only, proposed by Nandy *et al.* (2005), was also used for CIAF. These groups are presented in Table 19.1. However, the CIAF excludes all children belongs to group A, i.e. those who were not in anthropometric failure and considered all children who have

Table 19.1: Classification of the composite index of anthropometric failure (CIAF)*

Groups	*Description*	*Wasting*	*Stunting*	*Underweight*
A	No failure	No	No	No
B	Wasting only	Yes	No	No
C	Wasting and underweight	Yes	No	Yes
D	Wasting, stunting and underweight	Yes	Yes	Yes
E	Stunting and underweight	No	Yes	Yes
F	Stunting only	No	Yes	No
Y	Underweight only	No	No	Yes

* Based on Nandy *et al.*, 2005.

wasting, stunting and/or are underweight (i.e., groups B to F and Y).

The statistical analysis was carried out using SPSS for Windows (Version 20). The descriptive statistics includes mean, standard deviation and frequency distribution. Chi-square and t-test analysis were also performed. A p-value of less than 0.05 was considered as significant.

Results

Mean and standard deviation of anthropometric variables are presented in Table 19.2. The mean height and weight for boys were 153.58 (±12.08) cm and 48.81 (±13.25) kg, respectively. On the other hand, the mean height and weight for girls were 144.37 (±8.09) cm and 42.93 (±12.12) kg, respectively. Comparison of anthropometric variables between boys and girls revealed significantly ($p<0.05$) higher mean height and weight in boys compared to girls. Prevalence of undernutrition among the studied population is presented in Table 19.3. The overall prevalence of stunted and underweight adolescents in the studied population were 29.01 per cent (boys 14% and girls 44.4%) and 12.7 per cent (boys 11.2% and 14.3%), respectively. According to the WHO, 1983 the range for weight by stature for boys was up to 145 cm and for girls it was up to 137 cm. In this study only 72 boys were within 145 cm among the total boys and for girls only 52 were within 137 cm among the total girls. However, it was observed that none of the boys were wasted. But, in girls 5.76 per cent were wasted. Moreover, there was significant ($p<0.05$) sex differences in the prevalence of stunting, wasting and underweight.

Interestingly, CIAF showed a higher prevalence of undernutrition compared with other three indicators, i.e. stunting, wasting and underweight in both boys and girls. The proportions of adolescents in each of subgroups of anthropometric failure among the studied population are presented in Table 19.4. It was observed that, out of six subgroups of CIAF, the overall prevalence stunted only (Group F) was 23.49 per cent (boys 9.68% and girls 37.3%), followed by group E (containing, who are stunted and underweight) with 5.5 per cent (boys 4.26% and girls 6.74%), group C (containing, who are wasted and underweight) with 0.79 per cent (only in girls) and group D (containing, who are wasted, stunted and under weight) with 0.39 per cent (only in girls). However, only underweight (i.e., group Y) account for 6.65 per cent (boys 6.97% and girls 6.34%). There was significant ($p<0.05$) sex differences between no failure and CIAF.

Table 19.2: Mean and standard deviation of anthropometric variables

Variables	*Boys*		*Girls*		*t**
	Mean	*SD*	*Mean*	*SD*	
Height (cm)	153.58	12.08	144.37	8.09	10.23
Weight (kg)	48.81	13.25	42.93	12.12	5.25

*Height, $p<0.05$; Weight, $p<0.05$

Table 19.3: Prevalence of undernutrition among the studied populations

Nutritional Status	*Boys*		*Girls*		*Total*	
	N	*%*	*N*	*%*	*N*	*%*
Stunted	36	14.0	112	44.4	148	29.01
Wasted	0	0	3	5.76	3	5.76
Underweight	29	11.2	36	14.3	65.0	12.7

$\chi^2 = 10.19$, $p<0.05$;
* The Percentage of wasted girls was calculated among 52 girls.

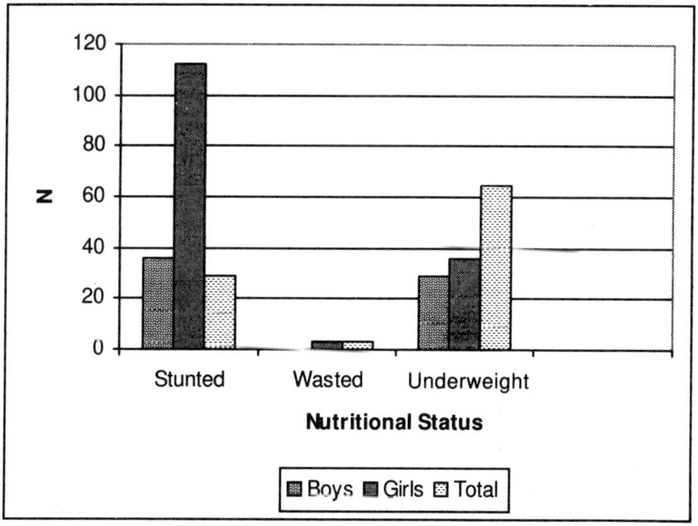

Fig. 19.1: Undernutrition among the studied populations.

Table 19.4: Anthropometric failure among the studied populations

Groups		*Boys*		*Girls*	
		N	*%*	*N*	*%*
Anthropometric failure	A (no failure)	204	79.06	122	48.41
	B (wasting only)	0	0	0	0
	C (wasting and underweight)	0	0	2	0.79
	D (wasting, stunting and underweight)	0	0	1	0.39
	E (stunting and underweight)	11	4.26	17	6.74
	F (stunting only)	25	9.68	94	37.3
	Y (underweight only)	18	6.97	16	6.34
	Total (CIAF, B-Y)	54	20.93	130	51.58

$\chi^2 = 64.81$, $p < 0.05$.

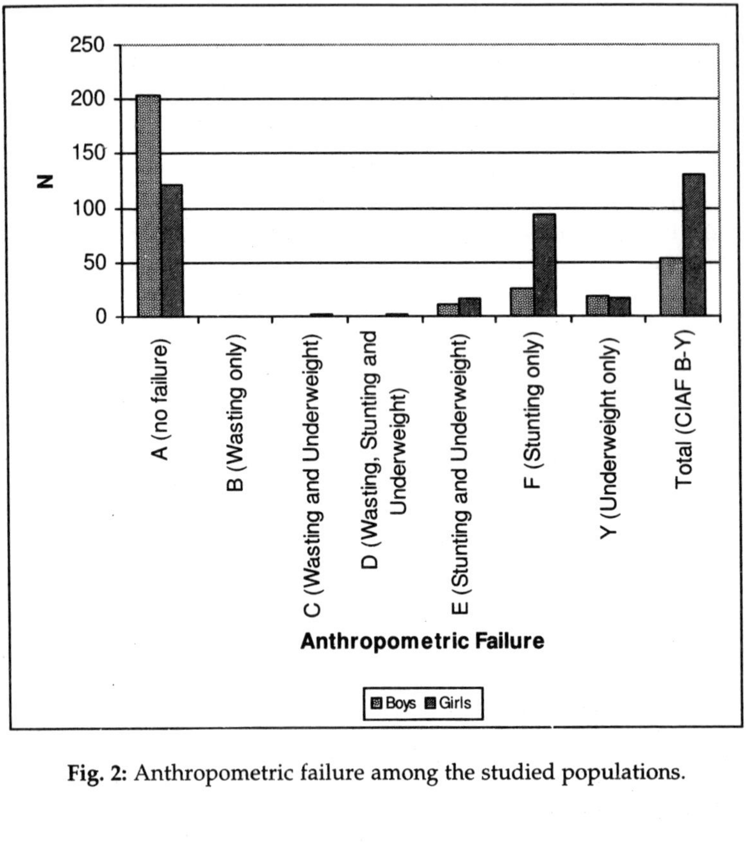

Fig. 2: Anthropometric failure among the studied populations.

Discussion

The CIAF gives a near complete picture of undernutrition and also helps in prioritizing undernourished children, as multiple anthropometric failures were related with greater childhood morbidity (Nandy *et al.*, 2005). Conventional indicators of undernutrition, namely stunting, wasting and underweight independently provide important information on different aspects of chronic or acute undernutrition. Results derived from conventional indicator are also valuable for clinicians and fieldworkers, who need to respond differently to different types of undernutrition. On the other hand, from a policy and planning perspective, understanding the overall prevalence of undernutrition is very important for resource allocation. For this purpose, the CIAF is the only indicator at present to measure overall prevalence of undernutrition. Moreover, the CIAF takes into account the differences among the conventional indicators, and thus more sensitive indicator of changes in undernutrition (Nandy and Miranda, 2008).

In view of this, the present investigation was undertaken to evaluate the levels of stunting, wasting and underweight especially to assess the overall prevalence of undernutrition by using CIAF among urban adolescents of Howrah District, West Bengal, India. The result revealed that the overall prevalence of stunted and underweight adolescence in the studied populations was 29.01 per cent and 12.7 per cent, but it was also revealed that none of the boys were wasted and interestingly, for girls the prevalence of wasted was 5.76. This was in corroboration with other studies (Mandal *et al.*, 2015). Comparison of the prevalence of stunting and underweight in adolescents revealed lower prevalence of stunting and underweight in girls compared to the boys. Similar higher prevalence of stunting and underweight in girls compared to boys was also observed by Medhi *et al.* (2006) in 6-14 years children of Assam. However, the overall prevalence of stunting and underweight was higher among Assam children (Medhi *et al.*, 2006) compared to the present study. It is well established that these conventional indices reflect distinct biological processes and only give ideas about the general categories of undernutrition. Moreover, due to its overlapping into multiple categories, these indices were not useful to determine the overall prevalence of undernutrition for anthropometric failures (Svedberg, 2000; Nandy *et al.*, 2005; Sen *et al.*, 2011). Thus, CIAF, as an aggregated single anthropometric measure has become a better option to understand the overall prevalence of undernutrition in children for policy and monitoring.

In the present study, along with conventional indices, CIAF was also used to measure nutritional status and the result revealed higher incidence of undernutrition by CIAF compared to the conventional measures both in boys and girls. The CIAF indicated that 20.93 per cent boys and 51.58 per cent girls of the studied populations had single and/or multiple anthropometric failures, but the conventional indices demonstrated that 14.0 per cent boys and 44.4 per cent girls (overall 29.01%) were stunted, only 5.76 per cent girls were wasted and 11.2 per cent boys and 14.3 per cent (overall 12.7%) girls were underweight.

Though, CIAF is a relatively recent development, a number of studies (Nandy *et al.*, 2005; Mandal and Bose, 2009; Sen *et al.*, 2011; Shit *et al.*, 2012; Dasgupta *et al.*, 2014) has applied CIAF to understand the overall prevalence of undernutrition. Most of the studies (Mandal and Bose, 2009; Shit *et al.*, 2012; Dasgupta *et al.*, 2014), which has been done in preschool children also observed very high prevalence of undernutrition by CIAF. However, very few studies (Sen *et al.*, 2011; Thakur and Gautam, 2015) have been done in school going children and adolescent. In a recent study, Sen *et al.* (2011) also observed very high prevalence (57.6%) of undernutrition by CIAF in school going children of North Bengal. In conclusion, the result of the present study revealed that the overall prevalence of undernutrition by CIAF was higher in urban adolescent girls than boys. Moreover, CIAF could be a better indicator of nutritional stress as compared to the traditional measures of stunting, wasting and underweight. The potential advantage of the CIAF may be that it can highlight the seriousness and severity of overall undernutrition, i.e. the actual load of undernutrition in a population. However, one of the limitations of the present study is the small sample size. Further studies are needed among a larger sample for effective planning of nutritional intervention programmes.

Acknowledgements

The authors are grateful to the all participants. The authors are also grateful to the Department of Anthropology, Visva-Bharati for providing all the facilities for conducting this research.

REFERENCES

Bakhetia, P., Jain, R. 2007. "Anthropometric profile and physical performance of rural school girls." *Anthropologist.* **9**: 139-141.

Bose, K., Mandal, G.C. 2010. "Proposed new anthropometric indices of childhood undernutrition." *Mal J Nutr.* **16**: 131-136.

Das, S., Bose, K. 2011. "Assessment of nutritional status by anthropometric indices in Santal tribal children." *J Life Sci,* **3**: 81-85.

Dasgupta, A., Parthasarathi, R., Prabhakar, V.R., Biswas, R., Geethanjali, A. 2014. "Assessment of undernutrition with composite index of anthropometric failure (CIAF) among under-five children in a rural area of West Bengal." *Ind J Comm Health.* **26**: 132-138.

Ghai, O.P., Gupta, P., Paul, V.K. 2006. "Ghai essential paediatrics, adolescent health and development." *Paediatrics.* **6**: 66.

Gopalan, C. 2008. "The current national nutrition scene: Areas of Concern." *NFI Bulletin.***29**: 1-8.

Hamill, P.V., Drizd, T.A., Johnson, C.L., Reed, R.B., Roche, A.F., Moore, W.M. 1979. "Physical growth: national center for health statistics percentiles." *Am J ClinNutr.* **32**: 607-629.

International Institute for Population Sciences (IIPS) and Macro International. 2007. National Family Health Survey (NFHS-3). Mumbai, India: IIPS.

Khan, R.E.A., Raza, M.A. 2014. "Nutritional status of children in Bangladesh: measuring composite index of anthropometric failure (CIAF) and its determinants." *Pak J CommerSoc Sci.* **8**: 11-23.

Khor, G.L. 2005. "Micronutrient status and intervention programs in Malaysia." *Food Nutr Bull.* **26**: S281-S285.

Lohman, T.G., Roche, A.F., Martorell, R. 1988. *Anthropometric standardization reference manual.* Chicago: Human Kinetics Books.

Mandal, G.C., Bose, K. 2009. "Assessment of overall prevalence of undernutrition using composite index of anthropometric failure (CIAF) among preschool children of West Bengal, India." *Iran J Pediatr.* **19**: 237-243.

Mandal, S., Ram Prabhakar, V., Pal, J., Pasthasarathi, Biswas, R. 2014. "An assessment of nutritional status of children aged 0-14 years in a slum area of Kolkata." *International Journal of Medicine and Public Health*-2.

Medhi, G.K., Barua, A., Mohanta, P. 2006. "Growth and nutritional status of school age children (6-14 years) of tea garden worker of Assam." *J. hum. Ecol.* **19**(2): 83-85.

Mondal, T., Mondal, S., Biswas, M. 2015. "An assessment of nutritional status of children of Government aided primary school of West Bengal." *International Journal of Elementary Education.* **4**(3): 41-45.

Nandy, S., Irving, M., Gordon, D., Subramanian, S.V., Smith, G.D. 2005. "Poverty, child undernutrition and morbidity: new evidence from India." *Bull World Health Organ.* **83**: 210–216.

Nandy, S., Miranda, J.J. 2008. "Overlooking undernutrition? Using a composite index of anthropometric failure to assess how underweight misses and misleads the assessment of undernutrition in young children." *Soc Sci Med.* **66**: 1963-1966.

Sen, J., Dey, S., Mondal, N. 2011. "Conventional nutritional indices and composite index of anthropometric failure: which seems more appropriate for assessing undernutrition among children? A cross-sectional study among school children of the Bengalee Muslim population of North Bengal, India." *IJPH.* **8**: 172-185.

Shit, S., Taraphdar, P., Mukhopadhyay, D.K., Sinhababu, A., Biswas, A.B. 2012. "Assessment of nutritional status by composite index for anthropometric failure: a study among slum children in Bankura, West Bengal." *Indian J Public Health.* **56**: 305-307.

Svedberg, P. 2000. *Poverty and undernutrition: Theory, measurement, and policy.* Oxford India. New Delhi.

Thakur, R., Gautam, R.K. 2015. "Nutritional status among boys and girls of a central Indian Town (Sagar)." *Anthropological Review.* **78**: 197–212.

World Health Organization. 1983. Measuring change in nutritional status. Guidelines for assessing the nutritional impact of supplementary feeding programs for vulnerable groups. Geneva.

World Health Organization. 1995. The use and interpretation of anthropometry – report of WHO expert committee. *WHO Tech Rep Series 854.* Geneva.

20

Nutritional Profile among Under Graduate Girls of Coimbatore

Chhandika Roy

Introduction

The WHO (Nelson, 2014) defines 'Adolescents' as people in the age group of 10-19 and 'Youth' as the 15-24 year age group. While some describe adolescence is the period between 12 to 21 years (Mahan *et al.*, 2012) or ages of 13 and 20 (Roth, 2011), 12-19 years (Kaur *et al.*, 2009). The term Adolescent comes from Latin word 'Adolescence' meaning to grow up showing the special characters of adolescence (Kar *et al.*, 2015). Adolescence is the phase of change from childhood to adulthood (Singh *et al.*, 2012) which is portrayed by accelerated physical, hormonal and emotional changes (Srilakshmi, 2011; Mahan *et al.*, 2012; Joshi, 2015). There are around 1.2 billion of adolescents (Kar *et al.*, 2015). According to WHO (2018), there are 1.1 million deaths every year due to premature death, illness, and injury among adolescents. Deaths due to HIV related diseases are not getting low in this age group (WHO, 2020). India is home for 275 million adolescents that is 22.5 per cent of total population 1220 million people (Swaminathan, 2013). Adolescence is one of the most exciting and challenging stage in human development with tremendous physiologic, psychological and cognitive fluctuations. Puberty is one of the major changes in adolescent life in which a child becomes capable of sexual reproduction (Mahan *et al.*, 2012). Adolescents experience high levels of stress, depression, anxiety, moodiness and it is more during examination days, adequate nutrition and proper nutrition knowledge helps them to overcome such conditions (Tiwari and

Yegammai, 2011). In developing country like India, 70-80 per cent of adolescents are suffering from nutritional deficiency conditions, poor resistance to diseases and improper growth for their age (Kaur *et al.*, 2009; Mehta, 2014), girls are more at risk among developing countries like India where they are married at an early age, early pregnancy (Singh *et al.*, 2012; Kar *et al.*, 2015). During adolescence, nutrient requirements increases due to growth spurt, 20 per cent of final adult height and 50 per cent of adult weight are attained, bone mass increases by 45 per cent and bone remodelling occur and soft tissues, organs and red blood cell mass increases in size (Gluseppina, 2000; Singh *et al.*, 2012). Nutritional assessment works upon few parameters, dietary behaviour, physical anthropometry, clinical history and examinations and biochemical examination (Supriya, 2017).

Nutritional deficiencies may lead to dangerous consequences, mainly in rural adolescent girls (Singh *et al.*, 2012). If their nutritional needs are not met, they are likely to give birth to undernourished children, thus carrying undernutrition to next generation (Shivaramakrishnan *et al.*, 2011). In developing countries, factors associated with undernutrition of adolescents are: poor household economic condition, periodic food-shortage, child-labour (marker of household income-poverty), burden of disease, poor knowledge about long-term consequences of under-nutrition of adolescents, quantity and quality of food, and access to health and nutrition services (Alam *et al.*, 2010; Singh *et al.*, 2012). According to NFHS-4 (2015-16), nutritional status of 15-49 years women is 28.4 per cent are categorized as BMI below normal (<18.5) and 20.9 per cent are overweight or obese (>25.0) in Tamil Nadu. Adolescence is a heterogeneous group and thus various factors influence one's health. Adolescence constitutes one among the nutritionally vulnerable group, so they deserve proper

Table 20.1: Recommended Dietary Allowance for adolescence (female)

Nutrients	*13-15 yr*	*16-18 yr*
Energy (Kcal)	2100	2100
Proteins (gms)	65	63
Calcium (Mg)	600	500
Iron (Mg)	28	30

Source: NIN 2017 (RDA, 2010).

attention to grow healthy and be healthy beautiful woman in future. Their nutritional needs should be taken care as they are the future mothers (Dietary Guidelines for Indians, 2011).

In view of the foregoing discussion, the present micro level investigation was undertaken with an objective to assess nutritional profile and dietary intake among the adolescent girls.

Materials and Methods

Avinashilingam Institute for Home Science and Higher Education for Women (Deemed University) situated in Coimbatore city was selected for the present investigation. It was selected due to easy accessibility and co-operation extended by the University authority. A total of 100 Under Graduate girls of adolescent 17-21 years were included randomly for the present investigation. Among these 100 adolescent girls, five girls were randomly selected for dietary survey, to assess the nutrient intake for three days with the use of food weighment survey. A questionnaire was prepared for collecting the information regarding the socio-economic background, lifestyle pattern, dietary habits, and health status and morbidity pattern of the selected population. Anthropometry is the way to measure body dimensions and total composition of the human body which consist of muscle mass, fat reserves and vital part of nutrition assessment (Mahan *et al.,* 2012; Joshi, 2016; Srilakhsmi, 2016; Supriya, 2017). Assessment of nutritional status of the population is an important step in formulation of public health strategy to stop malnutrition from the society (Bamji *et al.,* 2009). The nutritional status of respondents was assessed by various parameters such as anthropometric measurements (height, weight, body mass index, waist circumference and hips circumference, waist-hip ratio), clinical observation (clinical signs and symptoms, diet survey, illness and treatment) and biochemical estimation. The adiposity measure of Body Mass Index (BMI=weight/height^2, kg/m^2), Waist-Hip-Ratio (WHR=WC/HC) have been calculated using standard equations. The cut off used for calculating BMI were according to Asia-Pacific (BMI) based on BMI proposed by Lim *et al.* (2017) 18·5 kg/m^2 underweight; 18·5–22.9 kg/m^2 Normal; 23–24.9 kg/m^2 increased risk or overweight; and ≥25 kg/m^2 or higher high risk or obese (Roy *et al.,* 2020). The cut offs used for WHR were classified as low

(WHR ≤ 0.80), moderate (WHR 0.81-0.85) and high risk (WHR >0.85). Haemoglobin (hb) was estimated by Sahli's haemoglobinmeter method (Bent, 2005; Anand and Anuradha, 2019) and compared with the standard values by WHO criteria to find out the anaemic status of the selected subjects (Anand and Anuradha, 2019). Based on WHO criteria haemoglobin (gm/dl) grading is <7.00 gm/dl is severe anaemic, 7.00-9.9 gm/dl is moderate anaemic, 10.00-11.90 gm/dl is mild anaemic, >12 gm/dl is normal. The application form explaining the experimental design and protocols used in the research study was submitted to the Institutional Human Ethics Committee (IHEC) Ethics Clearance of Avinashilingam Institute for Home Science and Higher Education for Women, Coimbatore was obtained for the smooth conduct of the study. The raw data collected were consolidated and statistical methods like mean, standard deviation were used at necessary places for further analysis. Nutrient analysis was done with the help of Nutritive value of Indian Foods book by NIN.

Results and Discussion

The study entitled "A Study on Nutritional Profile among the Under Graduate Girls of Coimbatore" was carried out to assess the nutritional profile of Adolescent girls, who are very important section of our society. Adolescents aged between 10-19 years account for more than one-fifth of the world's population. In India, this age group forms 21.4 per cent of total population (Prabhakaran, 2003), 243 million adolescents dwell in India (UNICEF, 2011). Unfortunately, adolescent girls are a neglected sector of the population of our country. The results observed by household and dietary survey of the selected subjects (N=100) revealed that: Majority of the adolescent girls selected for the study belongs to nuclear family, low income group and follow Hinduism. All the respondents were unmarried and studying in under graduate courses. A study by Haboubi and Shaikh (2019) found that better economic environment favours better expression of genetic potential for growth. Another study by Singh *et al.* (2014) revealed contemporary findings that morbidities among adolescents were more due to nutrition and personal hygiene.

The height and weight of the selected subjects was found to be less than the standard height for all age groups, i.e. for 17 years

(152.83±4.17 cm), 18 years (156.39±5.57 cm), 19 years (156.82±7.35 cm), 20 years (156.09±6.81 cm), 21 years (154.86±10.78 cm) respectively and weight for all age group, i.e. 17 years (40.75±4.60 kg), 18 years (47.61±8.41 kg), 19 years (51.42±9.61), 20 years (50.96±12.10), 21 years (49.14±16.60), respectively. Among the 100 selected subjects, 41 per cent of the selected subjects were underweight, 35 per cent normal, 11 per cent overweight, 13 per cent were in the category of obese. In contrast to our study, Singh *et al.* (2012) reported that 50 per cent as normal BMI, 27 per cent below normal and 16 per cent were at the risk of obesity among rural adolescents. The findings of Kaur *et al.* (2009) among adolescents in a senior secondary school reported that 68 per cent had normal BMI. Singh *et al.* (2012) reported, 57 per cent were under normal BMI, whereas 26.6 per cent were underweight found in a community based study. One out of six adolescents aged 10-19 years was overweight (WHO, 2018). Similar findings were found by Deshmukh *et al.* (2006) that, 53.8 per cent of the adolescents were thin, 44 per cent were normal and 2.2 per cent were overweight. The difference was statistically significant (<8th standard) and lower economic status. Undernutrition is common among adolescents (Singh *et al.*, 2012; Kumar, 2012) (Kaur *et al.*, 2009). There is a positive association between eating pattern and BMI. Finding revealed that 57 per cent adolescent had normal BMI. In our study, 54 per cent of the subjects belong to 0.80 cm or below which is a normal waist to hip ratio, whereas 26 per cent belongs to 0.81-0.85 cm that is moderate health risks and 20 per cent of the subjects were 0.85 cm or more which determines high health risks. Poor eating habits and early accessibility of mobile phones are predictors of malnutrition among school going adolescent girls in

Table 20.2: Measurement of height among the selected adolescents

Age in years	*Number*	*Height*	*ICMR standards**
		Mean + S.D	
17	6	152.83 + 4.17	160.2
18	18	156.39 + 5.57	161.1
19	46	156.82 + 7.35	160.7
20	23	156.09 + 6.81	160.7
21	7	154.86 + 10.78	160.7

* ICMR standards (2010).

Table 20.3: Measurement of weight among the adolescents population

Age in years	*Number*	*Weight* *Mean + S.D*	*ICMR standards**
17	27	40.75 + 4.60	52.8
18	20	47.61 + 8.41	53.8
19	33	51.42 + 9.61	53.8
20	14	50.96 + 12.10	54.8
21	6	49.14 + 16.60	54.8

* ICMR standards (2010).

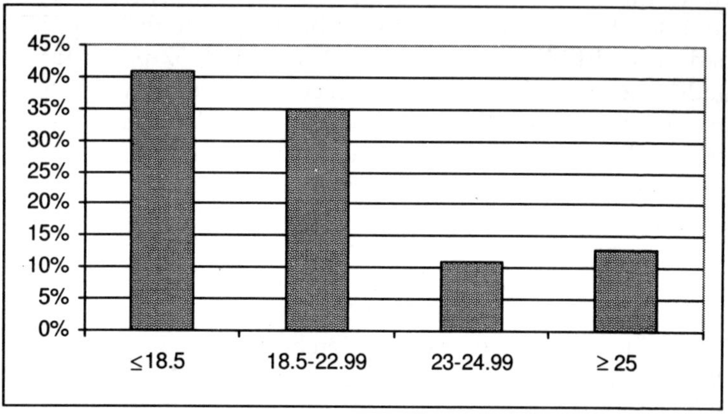

Fig. 20.1: BMI of the selected respondents.

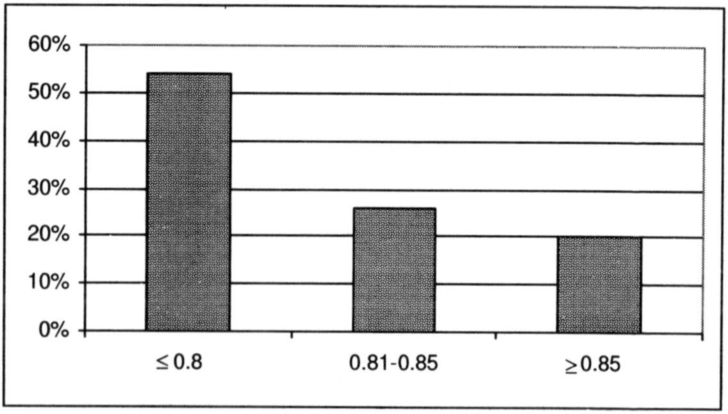

Fig. 20.2: WHR of the selected population.

Table 20.4: Consumption of foods

Food groups	*Daily*	*Alternate days*	*Weekly*	*Monthly*	*Occasionally*
Consumption of Cereals*					
Rice	100	—	—	—	—
Wheat and wheat products	9	18	52	8	8
Ragi	—	6	14	20	51
Consumption of pulses*					
Bengal gram	9	39	28	9	10
Green gram	8	22	47	6	10
Peas	8	21	38	21	11
Red gram	6	15	30	22	22
Black gram	4	23	35	10	23
Consumption of leafy vegetables*					
Agathi	1	10	31	30	24
Amaranth	—	12	19	21	35
Ponnakanni	4	24	39	13	17
Drumsticks leaves	—	4	27	30	31
Other Leafy Vegetables	3	12	29	33	19
Consumption of other vegetables*					
Beans	10	39	34	10	6
Bitter gourd	—	11	31	12	34
Brinjal	4	31	39	13	13
Cucumber	3	19	26	26	29
Drumstick	4	22	42	15	15
Ladysfinger	4	31	38	13	11
Pumpkin	—	23	27	15	33
Plantain flower	3	11	11	13	54
Consumption of roots and tubers*					
Potato	19	38	32	3	8
Carrot	12	30	41	3	11
Beetroot	2	21	51	11	12
Yam	1	10	29	19	29
Onion	100	—	—	—	—
Consumption of fruits*					
Apple	5	10	28	17	39
Banana	35	26	19	9	10
Dates fresh	12	20	18	15	31
Grapes	9	17	24	21	26
Guava	7	13	16	31	29
Sweet lemon	4	19	16	24	30
Papaya	6	10	33	14	29
Pine apple	6	12	19	18	29
Consumption of milk and milk products*					
Milk	68	12	4	5	4
Curd	38	26	17	3	10
Butter milk	15	14	29	8	19
Butter	—	8	27	16	28
Ghee	10	10	23	15	27

*Multiple responses.

Ethiopia, a study by Kahssay *et al.* (2020). A global study on adolescence physical activity indicates that they do not meet the present physical activity norms (Guthold *et al.*, 2020) hence they must be encouraged to participate in physical activities (Mikaelsson *et al.*, 2018; Dore *et al.*, 2020).

From the study it was found that, more than half of the adolescent girls were (57%) vegetarian and most of them (53%) consumes three meals a day, followed by two meals (28%), (14%) less than two meals in a day and 5 per cent consumes more than three meals a day. Breakfast was skipped by more than half (52% of the adolescents girls, whereas few skip lunch and dinner and 39% never skip meals, meal skipping is a common habit among adolescents (Mahan *et al.*, 2012).

Regarding consumption of various foods from food groups 100 per cent consume rice daily among other cereals, consumption of leafy vegetables, other vegetables, fruits, milk and milk products were found to be lower than pulses and roots and tubers. Consumption of processed foods was found to be more consumed occasionally.

Most of the girl attained puberty at 11-13 years of age (57%), 93 per cent of the selected subjects have their menstrual cycle regular, whereas 7 per cent gets irregular periods.

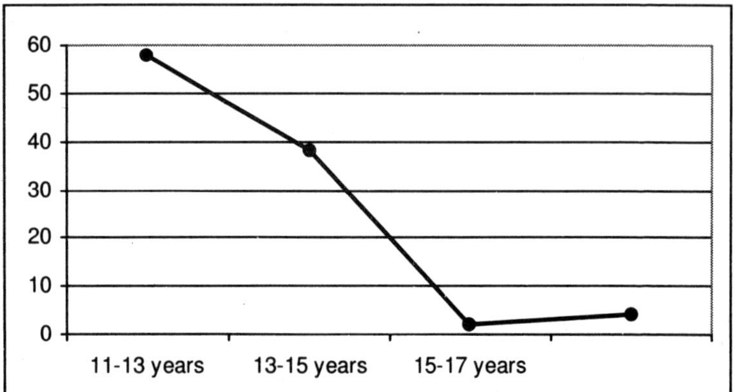

Fig. 20.3: Age at menarche of the selected subjects.

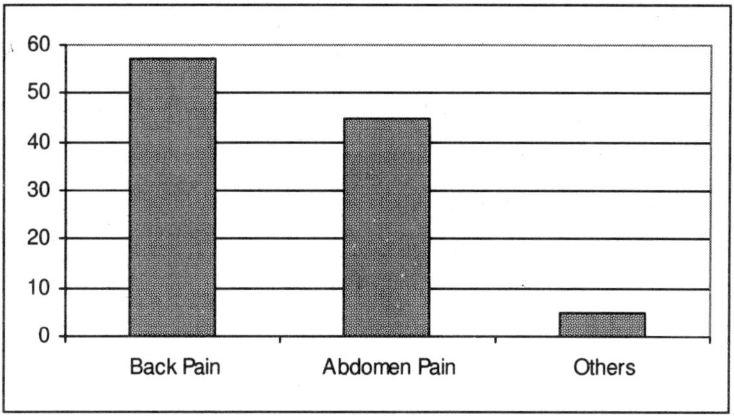

Fig. 20.4: Problems faced during menstruation.

It was found that 65 per cent have menstruation for 3-5 days, (30%) 5-7 days, less than 3 days (5%), more than 7 days (1%). Fifty per cent of the adolescents girls suffer from back pain during menstrual cycle, 45 per cent suffer from abdomen pain and 5 per from other problems.

Among adolescent girls, 68 per cent faced the problem of hair loss, 6 per cent has dental carries, 2 per cent has bleeding gums, 3 per cent has other problems and only one per cent has pale eyes which indicates anaemic.

Table 20.5: Clinical signs of the selected adolescence girls

Clinical signs	*Number*	*Percentage*
Pale eyes	1	1
Bleeding gums	2	2
Dental carries	6	6
Hair loss	68	68
Others	3	3

From the selected subjects, 21 per cent have some PCOS symptoms such as irregular periods (9%), excess hair growth (9%), cyst (3%) and 79 per cent do not have any symptoms of PCOD. Biochemical parameters analysis revealed that 72 per cent of the adolescent girls were non-anaemic whereas, 21 per cent were mild anaemic, 7 per cent were moderate anaemic. According to WHO factsheet (2018), Iron deficiency anaemia was the second leading cause for death to adolescents. A study by Ali *et al.* (2016) observed that anaemia is the most common nutritional problem in the adolescent girls seen in 53.30 per cent followed by thinness in 35.70 per cent whereas a study by Pattnaik *et al.* (2013) found that 75.6 per cent girls were mild anaemic, (Veena and Kowsalya, 2012) clinical symptoms among adolescents girls were there with sub-clinical signs of anaemia. Another study showed that the nutritional status of the Scheduled Caste adolescent was very poor, underweight, anaemic and many deficiency signs were present, further intake of most of the foods and nutrients were also lower than the RDA (Kumari and Singh, 2007). Overweight is associated with low haemoglobin levels in adolescent girls (Bagni *et al.*, 2013). National Nutrition Mission aims at 50 per cent reduction in prevalence of anaemia among 15-49 years women within 2012 to 2030 (ICMR, 2019).

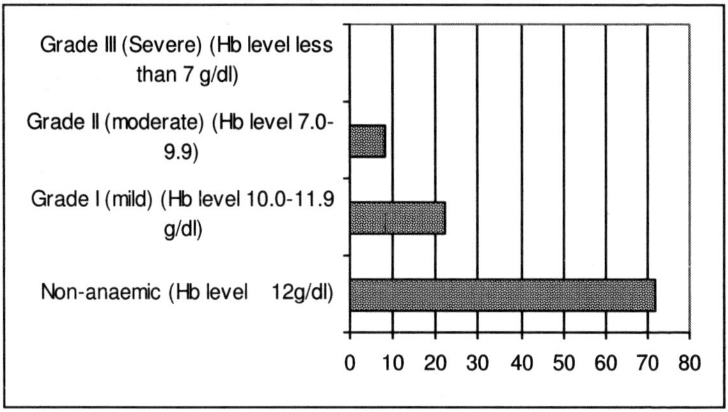

Fig. 20.5: Hb levels of the selected adolescent girls.

Regarding the morbidity pattern, 19 per cent has skin infections, 7 per cent has urinary tract infection, 8 per cent has eye infection followed by 6 per cent ear infection. 33 per cent of the adolescent girls suffered from cold and cough few days back and it was common than other illness, followed by fever and vomiting.

Among the adolescent girls consumption of cereals (+9.0), pulses (+22.3), fats and oils (+27.5), sugar and jaggery (+25) was found to be more than other food groups. Requirement of calcium is more in adolescents (Dietary Guidelines for Indians, 2011). The mean nutrient intake of the adolescent girls was found to be inadequate in the sense of iron, calcium, beta carotene and ascorbic acid. Similar findings were seen in Kodaliven *et al.* (2002) adolescent girls consume energy more than RDA, whereas the intake of micronutrients such as vitamin A and riboflavin were comparatively less (Roy and Subramanian 2017) which is similar to our study. Aberoumand (2011) proved that protein intake was more than energy, and intake of trace elements should be in concern to avoid deficiency in future. Insufficient quantity of vitamins and other micronutrients intake was seen among adolescent soccer players (Noronha *et al.*, 2020). A study supports that there is low evidence on nutrition education and macronutrient supplementation among adolescents (Salam *et al.*, 2019).

Table 20.6: Mean food intake of adolescents

Food groups	*RDA**	*Mean food intake*	
		Actual intake	*% Excess/ deficit*
Cereals (g)	330	360	+9.0
Pulses (g)	60	73.4	+22.3
Green leafy vegetables (g)	100	78.7	-21.3
Roots and tubers (g)	100	123	+23
Other vegetables (g)	200	130	-35
Fruits (g)	100	52.5	-47.5
Milk and milk products (ml)	500	320	-36
Fats and oils (ml)	40	51	+27.5
Sugar and jaggery (g)	20	25	+25

*ICMR (2010).

Table 20.7: Mean nutrient intake of adolescent girls

Nutrients	*RDA**	*Mean nutrient intake*	
		Actual intake	*% Excess/ deficit*
Energy (kcal)	2440	2872	+17.2
Protein (g)	55.5	67.83	+22.21
Fat (g)	35	51.62	+47.48
Iron (mg)	26	16.35	-37.11
Calcium (mg)	800	714	-10.75
Beta-carotene (mcg)	4800	2670.3	-44.36
Thiamine (mg)	1.0	1.20	+20
Riboflavin (mg)	1.2	1.50	+25
Nicotinic acid (mg)	14	17.23	+23.07
Pyridoxine (mg)	2.0	2.1	+5
Ascorbic acid (mg)	40	32.57	-18.57

Conclusion

Adolescents are a crucial segment of our society. This phase of life is vital since these years are formative period in the life of an individual as major changes occur, e.g. physical, psychological and behavioural changes. During this period, their nutrients requirements also increases. If these nutritional needs are not met deficiencies may results. Adolescent girls are more vulnerable than boys mostly in developing countries. Young girls are married at an early age and enter in reproductive phase at a young age. The existence of different ill habits and disorder lifestyle indicate a need to educate and create awareness among the adolescents on healthy lifestyle and good food habits. Thus, developing good and healthy eating habits in adolescence are bridge to good health in later age.

Acknowledgements

The author expresses her reverential gratitude to the higher authorities of Avinashilingam Institute for Home Science and Higher Education for Women, Deemed University, Coimbatore for providing the help needed for smooth conduct of the study. The investigators also express deepest sense of gratitude to the study population for their kind co-operation.

REFERENCES

Aberoumand Ali. 2011. "Assessment of dietary intake and nutritional status of students in the Ramin University of Iran." *Indian J of Nutr Diet.* **48**: 478-482.

Alam, N., Roy, S.K., Ahmed, T., Ahmed, A.M. 2010. "Nutritional status, dietary intake, and relevant knowledge of adolescent girls in rural Bangladesh." *J Health Popul Nutr.* **28**: 86-94. DOI:org/10.3329/jhpn.v28i1.4527.

Ali, D., Fazili, A., Shah, R.J., Rafiq, M.M. 2016. "A study on the prevalence of nutritional problems of school going adolescent girls of Kashmir Valley with special focus on anemia." *Int J Cur Rev.* **8**: 6-12.

Anand, D., Anuradha, R.K. 2019. "Prevalence of anaemia among adolescent girls: a cross-sectional study." *Int J Health Sci Res.* **9**: 27-31.

Bagni, U.V., Luiz, R.R., Da Veiga, G.V. 2013. "Overweight is associated with low hemoglobin levels in adolescent girls." *Obes Res Clin Pract.* **7**: 218-229. DOI:10.1016/j.orcp.2011.12.004.

Bamji, S., Kamala Krishnaswamy, Brahman, G.N.V. 2009. *Text book of Human Nutrition,* 3rd eds. Oxford and IBH Publication Company Pvt. Ltd., p. 151.

Deshmukh, P.R., Gupta, S.S., Bharambe, M.S., Dongre, A.R., Maliye, C., Kaur, S., Garg, B.S. 2006. "Nutritional Status of Adolescents in Rural Wardah." *Indian J of Pediatr.* **73**: 139-141.

Dietary Guidelines for Indians: A Manual. 2011. Guideline 5. National Institute of Nutrition, Indian Council of Medical Research. NIN, Hyderabad. 34.

Doré, I., Sylvester, B., Sabiston, C., Sylvestre, M.P., O'Loughlin, J., Brunet, J., Be'langer, M. 2020. "Mechanisms underpinning the association between physical activity and mental health in adolescence: a 6-year study." *Int J Behav Nutr Phys Act.* 17. DOI:org/10.1186/s12966-020-0911-5.

Gluseppina, D. 2000. "Nutrition in adolescents." *Pediat Rev.* **21**: 32-33.

Guthold, R., Stevens, G.A., Riley, L.M., Bull, F.C. 2020. "Global trends in insufficient physical activity among adolescents: a pooled analysis of 298 population-based surveys with 1.6 million participants." *Lancet Child Adolesc Health.* **4**: 23-35p. DOI:org/10.1016/ S2352-4642(19) 30323-2.

Haboubi, G.J., Shaikh, R.B. 2009. "A Comparision of the Nutritional Status of Adolescents from Selected Schools of South India and UAE: A Cross-sectional Study." *Indian J Community Med.* **34**:108-111. DOI: 10.4103/0970-0218.51230.

Indian Council of Medical Research. 2019. Release of India State-Level Malnutrition Paper, Press release. https://www.icmr.nic.in/sites/default/files/press_realease_files/India_State_Level_Malnurition_Paper_Release.pdf.

Joshi, S.A. 2016. "Balanced diet and nutrition during normal life cycle." *Nutrition and dietetics.* 4th eds.pp. 179 and **434**.

Kahssay, M., Mohamed, L., Gebre, A. 2020. "Nutritional status of school going adolescent girls in Awash town, Afar Region, Ethiopia." *J Environ Public Health.* https://doi.org/10.1155/2020/7367139.

Kar, A.K., Choudhury, A., Singh, A.P. 2015. "Understanding normal development of adolescent sexuality: A bumpy ride." *J Hum Reprod Sci.* **8**: 70-74. DOI: 10.4103/0974-1208.158594.

Kaur, L., Kaur, G., Mala, D., Gohlan, D. 2009. "Association between BMI and eating pattern: study among adolescents." *Nurs Midwifery Res J.* **5**: 38-44p.

Lim, J.U., Lee, J.H., Kim, J.S., Hwang, Y.I., Kim, T.H., Lim, S.Y., Yoo, K.H., Jung, K.S., Kim, Y.K., Rhee, C.K. 2017. "Comparison of World Health Organization and Asia-Pacific body mass index classifications in COPD patients." *Int J Chron Obstruct Pulmon Dis.* **12**: 2465–2475. DOI:org/10.2147/COPD.S141295.

Mahan, L.K., Stump, S.E., Raymond, J.L. 2012. *Nutrition in Adolescence. Krause's Food, Nutrition and Diet Therapy,* 13th eds. Published by the Curtis Center, Independence Sq. West, Philadelphia Pennsylvania.

Mehta, J.S. 2014. *Nutrition of Adolescents, Basic Nutrition Management,* Avishkar Publishers. p. 93.

Mikaelsson, K., Rutberg, S., Lindqvist, A.K., Michaelson, P. 2019. "Physically inactive adolescents' experiences of engaging in physical activity." *Eur J Physiother.* 22. DOI: org/10.1080/21679169.2019.1567808

National Family Health Survey-4 (2015-16). *State Fact Sheet Tamil Nadu.* International Institute for Population Science. http://rchiips.org/NFHS/pdf/NFHS4/TN_FactSheet.pdf

National Institute of Nutrition. 2017. *Recommended Dietary Allowance (2010) of nutrients for adolescents in 24 hours.* Nutrition needs of Adolescence, Nutrition Information Communication and Education (NICE) Portal. http://vikaspedia.in/health/women-health/adolescent-health-1/management-of-adolescent-health/nutritional-needs-of-adolescents-and-anaemia.

Nelson, B.D. 2014. *Essential Clinical Global Health,* Wiley Blackwell. UK.

Noronha, D.C., Santos, M.I.A.F., Santos, A.A., Corrente, L.Z., Fernandes, R.K.N., Barreto, A.C.A., Santos, R.G.J., Santos, R.S., Gomes, L.P.S., Nascimento, M.V.S. 2020. "Nutrition knowledge is correlated with a better dietary intake in adolescent soccer players: a cross-sectional study." *J Nutr Metab.* DOI:org/10.1155/2020/3519781.

Parvizy, S., Ahmadi, F. 2009. "A qualitative study on adolescence, health and family." *Ment Health Fam Med. PMC.* **6**: 163-172.

Pattnaik, S., Patnaik, L., Kumar, A., Sahu, T. 2013. "Prevalence of Anemia among adolescent girls in a rural area of Odisha and its epidemiological correlates." *Indian J Matern Child Health.* **15:** 1-11.

Prabhakaran, S. 2003. "Nutritional status of adolescent girls residing in a university hostel." *Indian J Nutr Diet.* **40**: 238-273.

Ravindra, K.R. 2012. *Nutrition for Women,* Sports Publication, 1st eds. pp. 27 and 76.

Roth, R.A. 2011. *Diet during Childhood and Adolescence, Nutrition and Diet Therapy.* 10th eds. p. 257.

Roy, C., Mondal, N., Singh, H.V. 2020. "Anthropometric measurements and its indication towards health among post-menopausal women of Mishing community, Lakhimpur district, Assam." *Human Biol.* **9**: 183-200.

Roy, C., Subramanian, A. 2017. "Nutritional and Health {rofile of 17-21 Years to-be Mothers." *Int J Sci Nat.* **8**: 409-413.

Salam, R.A., Das, J.K., Ahmed, W., Irfan, O., Sheikh, S.S., Bhutta, Z.A. 2019. "Effects of preventive nutrition interventions among adolescents on health and nutritional status in low and middle income countries: a systematic review and meta-analysis." *Nutrients.* 12. doi:10.3390/nu12010049

Shivaramakrishna, H.R., Deepa, A.V., Sarithareddy, M. 2011. "Nutritional status of Adolescent Girls in Rural Area of Kolar District—A Cross-Sectional Study." *Al Ameen J of Medical Science.* **4**: 243-246.

Singh, J.P., Kariwal, P., Gupta, S.B., Singh, A.K., Imtiaz, D. 2014. "Assessment of nutritional status among adolescents: a hospital based cross-sectional study." *Int J of Res in Medi Sci.* **2**: 620-624. DOI: 10.5455/2320-6012.ijrms20140547.

Singh, S., Kansal, S., Kumar, A. 2012. "Assessment of nutritional status of adolescent girls in rural area of district Varanasi." *Indian J Res.* **6**: 30-34. www.anvikshikijournal.com.

Srilakshmi, B. 2011. *Nutritional and Food requirements of Adolescents, Dietetics.* 6th eds, New Age International Publishers. pp. 106-107.

Supriya, V. 2017. *Assesment of nutritional Status. Clinical Nutrition and Dietetics Manual for Nurses,* Jaypee Publishers. p. 217.

Swaminathan, N. 2008. *Adolescent Health Problems, Health Action.* p. 13.

Tiwari, R., Yegammai, C. 2011. "Impact of nutrition education and positive therapy on stress and anxiety in school going adolescents." *Indian J of Nutr Diet.* **48**: 469-477.

United Nations International Children's Education Fund. 2019. Adolescence A Age of Opportunity, Press Release. http://unicef.in/Uploads/Publications/Resources/pub_doc118.pdf

United Nations International Children's Education Fund. 2019. Child and adolescent health and well-being, Adolescent health and well-being. https://www.unicef.org/health/adolescent-health-and-well-being.

Veena, K.A., Kowsalya, S. 2012." Prevalence of Micronutrients Deficiency Signs and Symptoms among Adolescents of Ramanathapuram District." *J of Pharm Biomed Sci.* **18**: 1-3.

Venkaiah, K, Damayanti, K., Nayak, M.U., Vijayarafhavan, K. 2002. "Diet and nutritional status of rural adolescents in India." *Eur J Clin Nutr.* **56**: 1119-1125.

World Health Organization. 2000. Young people's health—a challenge for society. Report of a Study Group on Young People and Health for All by the Year (2000), *Technical Report Series, No 731.* Geneva: World Health Organization; 1986. who.int/iris/bitstream/handle/10665/

41720WHO_TRS_731.pdf;jsessionid=F3A91191373CAE26D623787457B69CC0?sequence=1

World Health Organization. 2018. Fact sheets, Adolescents: health risks and solutions. https://www.who.int/news-room/fact-sheets/detail/adolescents-health-risks-and-solutions.

World Health Organization. 2020. The changing world of adolescent sexual and reproductive health and rights, Newsroom. Departmental News. https://www.who.int/news-room/detail/03-02-2020-the-changing-world-of-adolescent-sexual-and-reproductive-health-and-rights.

SECTION-V

Recent Trends and Developments in Maternal and Child Healthcare

21

Maternal and Child Healthcare in the Era of Mobile Applications

Shreyasi Roy and *Jaydip Sen*

Introduction

Mobile phones were introduced in 1973 with the sole purpose of making and receiving calls. However, with the advancement in technology and availability of several features such as camera, internet, wi-fi, global positioning systems (GPS), sound recorders, large memories, high-resolution screens and many more, the usage of mobile phones has evolved. According to the latest *Trai Telecom Subscription Data* (dated 31st May, 2019), India's telecommunication network has the world's second largest telephone users with about 1.183 billion subscribers. This group is attributed to both fixed as well as mobile phone users. Additionally, the aforementioned source also revealed that India has the world's second-largest Internet user-base with 460.24 million broadband internet subscribers.

Mobile Phone as an Aid to Health Care Management

With the rapid improvements in technology, mobile phones were found boost digital transformation in health care management. The introduction of mobile computing devices (such as PDAs: personal digital assistants, smart phones, android phones and tablets) has greatly impacted the health care management by assimilating both computing and communication features in a single device that can be held in a hand or stored in a pocket. As the use of such devices increases, it is highly expected that mobile phone users will also be able to regularly check their health status at any time and place (Kim *et al.*, 2014). Studies in rural India reported that most of the respondents were willing to receive health-related information on their mobile phones (DeSouza *et al.*, 2014; Sankaranarayanan and Sallach, 2014). The health-related information could be achieved through several ways. One is "medical and clinical apps" that assist with answering clinical practice and other questions at the point of care exist such as drug reference guides, medical calculators, clinical guidelines and other decision support aids, textbooks, and literature search portal. Several apps have also been designed to conduct medical examinations such as hearing or vision tests and several surgical procedures. Second is through personalized messages related to health. Tele-consultation through e-mail has proved to be another great aid in diagnosis, referral, treatment and follow-up of patients in several areas in India (Deodhar, 2002). Recently, medical consultation is also done through *Whatsapp*.

Mobile Phones Among Pregnant Women of India

A recent study in Tamil Nadu (Jayasaalen *et al.*, 2018) revealed that the women in the middle class and lower middle class families use smart phone and its applications more frequently during their pregnancy period for various reasons in comparison to the women in the upper middle class and higher income women. Study by Hazra *et al.* (2018) revealed that mobile phone messaging to husbands improve maternal and child health behaviour in India. A study by Sharma *et al.* (2011) revealed that text messaging was more effective than pamphlets in improving knowledge, attitude and practices of mothers. Studies have also proved that mobile phones' messaging is a great revolution to a sound antenatal care (Pai *et al.*, 2013; Bangal *et al.*, 2017; Indira *et al.*, 2017).

Apart from messaging, mobile phones have several apps installed that aim at reducing maternal and child health issues. Most of these are launched by Government of India or other institutions, such as:

(i) CycleBeads® is a mobile application that basically cites Standard Days Method™ (SDM) using first day of menstrual cycle. SDM is designated as a modern method of family planning used by women to prevent pregnancy or plan a pregnancy by tracking their menstrual cycle. This app is being used by women of several countries like Egypt, Ghana, Jordan, Kenya, Nigeria, Rwanda including India and is available in several languages like English, French, Spanish, Arabic, Turkish and Hindi. A study based on market-testing this app (Haile *et al.*, 2018) disclosed that women preferred this app as it is simple, cost-effective and easy to use. Additionally, many women are considering it safer compared to other family planning methods, especially hormonal methods.

(ii) CycleTel Family Advice (CFA) was an SMS-based service designed to improve knowledge of fertility and family planning. It was developed by the Institute for Reproductive Health (IRH) at Georgetown University (IRH) with support from the United States Agency for International Development (USAID) through the Fertility Awareness for Community Transformation (FACT) project and from the United Nations Foundation through the Innovation Working Group Catalytic mHealth grants programme. It was implemented in March 2015.

(iii) MOTHER application, a part of the *National Mobile Governance Initiative,* designed to deliver personalized messages to pregnant and lactating women through their mobile phones. This app basically provides the generic alerts (both in the form of text and audio) regarding antenatal, post-natal and child care based on the last menstrual period date of the women.

(iv) MIRA channel (also called Women Mobile Lifeline Channel) is an integrated mobile phone channel that was launched by *ZMQ Development*, a Technology for Development based social enterprise on 8th March, 2012 (International Women's Day). Apart from India, this channel has also been implemented in other low-resource countries such as Afghanistan and Uganda. Through several sub-channels (such as Pre-natal care, Child immunization, Newborn care, Family planning and Adolescent health issues), this channel delivers information to women interactively in order to build their knowledge and create awareness on critical health issues.

(v) Kilkari (a Hindi term literally meaning "baby's gurgle") mobile service gets transpired as an automated call yielding weekly, time-appropriate, 72 audio messages based on pregnancy, childbirth and child care from the second trimester of pregnancy until the child is one year old. This information is delivered only when a pregnant women and her husband or other family member subscribes to this service. This informative mobile service was launched in Jharkhand, Odisha, Uttar Pradesh, Uttarakhand and high priority districts (HDPs) of Madhya Pradesh and Rajasthan.

(vi) Under a partnership forged between the Bihar government, Bill and Melinda Gates Foundation (BMGF) and BBC Media Action (India), the project 'Mobile Kunji' has been implemented in eight districts of Bihar. This project is portrayed as an audio-visual aid basically designed for over 2 lakh community health workers (CHWs) of Bihar. By 'audio-visual', it means it is an amalgamation of both Interactive Voice Response (IVR)-based mobile service and a printed deck of cards on a ring. The Kunji cards have been designed to look like a mobile phone with illustrations supporting arguments and key messages. Each card has a unique toll-free short code that corresponds to a specific audio message in the IVR service. The short code which when dialled by the CHW from his/her mobile phone, takes the listener (or the audience) to free audio recording (delivered by a fictional doctor character named Dr. Anita) that further elaborates the health message that the particular card carries.

(vii) With the collaborative efforts of NEEDS (an Indian NGO) and SIMAVI (a Dutch NGO), a software application named Mobile for mothers (Mfm) was conceptualized and implemented between 2011 and 2015 in few blocks (like Litipara and Deoghar) of Jharkhand state of India. It was implemented to reinforce the role of CHWs in improving maternal health outcomes by delivering maternal health education messages among others through dramas and dance, and programmes geared at increasing male involvement in maternal health care (Ilozumba *et al.*, 2018a, 2018b).

(viii) 'Aarogyam' was an innovative initiative launched in Uttar Pradesh in 2008 with an aim to provide health care services to citizens at their door steps for ensuring safe motherhood and child survival components of Reproductive and Child Health (RCH). It prepares a complete health data base with respect to target group, that is, pregnant/lactating mothers and children in immunization age group. Once the data is uploaded into Aarogyam software, automated calls are periodically generated to provide information on child immunization, antenatal and post-natal, safe delivery and pulse polio campaign through use of Integrated Voice Recording System (IVRS) and telecommunication technology.

(ix) The mobile Mitra (mMitra) initiative was introduced by a Mumbai-based non-profit organization dealing in Advancing Reducing Mortality and Morbidity of Mothers, children and Neonates (ARMAAN). It aimed at providing free mobile voice call service that sends timed and targeted preventive care information weekly or biweekly to the subscribers' phones.

(x) Another application ImTeCHO (Innovative mobile-phone Technology for Community Health Operators) has been developed to yield various technology-based job aids to facilitate scheduling of home visits, screening for complications, counselling during home visits, and supportive supervision by Accredited Social Health Activists (ASHAs) and Primary Health Centre (PHC) staffs (Modi *et al.*, 2015, 2017, 2019). The application was launched in Gujarat.

(xi) Mobile Academy is a free 240 minutes audio training course designed to boost up the knowledge base of ASHAs regarding maternal and child health. This application offers cost-effective, flexible, and more convenient as well as more efficient training opportunities to ASHAs. The application was launched in Jharkhand, Madhya Pradesh, Rajasthan and Uttarakhand (Uttaranchal) in the first phase.

(xii) Developed in collaboration between Maternity Foundation, University of Copenhagen and University of Southern Denmark, the Safe Delivery App was launched at national level in India on December 2017. It is a smartphone application that empowers skilled birth attendants with direct and access to evidence-based and up-to-date guidelines. The instruction videos are based on international guidelines of WHO (World Health Organization), ALSO (International Advanced Life Support in Obstetrics), FIGO (The International Federation of Gynaecology and Obstetrics), RCOG (The Royal College of Obstetricians and Gynaecologists), and ACOG (The American Congress of Obstetricians and Gynaecologists). The application aims to improve the quality of emergency obstetric and neonatal care and thereby strengthen health care workers' skills and quality of care primarily in developing countries including India.

(xiii) Another safe delivery mobile application named LaQshya (as a Labour Room Quality Improvement Initiative) was launched by the Ministry of Health and Family Welfare (MoH&FW), Government of India on the occasion of Universal Health Coverage Day of 2017. The application was developed for health workers having in view to improve quality of care in intra-partum and immediate postpartum care taking place in the labour room and maternity operation theatres. Moreover, the application has designs on managing normal and complicated deliveries in the peripheral areas.

(xiv) The Android Tablet app for the Simplified Gestation Age Score (T-SGAS) was developed by the team at Research Triangle Institute (RTI). This application was developed to have early identification of preterm neonates in cases where gestation age is unknown (Patel *et al.*, 2019). It displays de-identified photographs of skin, breasts, and genitalia across a range of GAs and line drawings of infant posture, each of which is delineated with a score. The user is trained to choose the photograph or line drawing that most closely matches the newborn being evaluated, and the app determines the neonate's GA category (preterm or term) from the cumulative score. This application is supposed to be a great aid in cases where ultrasound is unavailable or restricted (Patel *et al.*, 2019).

(xv) MAMA (Mobile Alliance for Maternal Action) was launched on Mother's Day 2011 by former U.S. Secretary of State Hillary Clinton as an innovative public-private partnership between the Johnson and Johnson, USAID, the UN Foundation, the mHealth Alliance, and Baby Centre. Additionally, this programme was developed in collaboration with the White House Office of Science and Technology Policy and the U.S. Department of State. This programme aims to deliver free vital stage-based culturally-sensitive health-related messages to new and expectant mothers at least 2-3 times per week through mobile phone technology. This programme was implemented in four countries of Bangladesh, India, South Africa and Nigeria.

(xvi) ReMiND (Reducing Maternal and Newborn Death) project in April 2011 came up with increased and sustainable improvements in maternal, newborn and child survival in the state of Uttar Pradesh. Through this project, Catholic Relief Services (CRS) and Dimagi are using CommCare to help ASHAs counsel and evaluate women and their newborns for danger signs before, during and after pregnancy. Software such as the ASHA app and Sangini app came in the limelight during this project. The first app is a phone-based counselling job aid to support the ASHA to mobilize the beneficiary to access health services whereas the second app helps the ASHA supervisor (also called Sanginis) to have access on the performance of the ASHAs.

(xvii) In 2015, ICDS Systems Strengthening and Nutrition Improvement Programme (ISSNIP) integrated ICDS across 57 districts in seven States/Union Territories (UTs) of India with an at-scale mHealth intervention called Common Application Software (CAS) which is installed on smart mobile phones and with accompanying multi-level data dashboards (Nimmagadda *et al.*, 2019). According to the latest Press Information Bureau of Delhi (dated on 28th December, 2018), this application has expanded and rolled out across 64 districts in nine states/ UTs of India such as Andhra Pradesh (10 districts), Bihar (6 districts), Chhattisgarh (7 districts), Jharkhand

(7 districts), Madhya Pradesh (16 districts), Rajasthan (9 districts), Uttar Pradesh (6 districts), Dadra and Nagar Haveli (1 district) and Daman and Diu (2 districts).

(xviii) Suyojana (in rural Karnataka) is a mobile-based application that improves the decision-making process in maternal and child care activities undertaken by Auxiliary Nurse Midwives (ANMs). It empowers ANMs to effectively carry out activities as basic as registration of pregnant women to more advanced intervention like routine immunization, identifying medical complications and providing referrals.

(xix) mLabor is a CommCare Mobile Partograph and labour ward management app that was initially developed by Dimagi to build on paper partograph. Owing to the presence of several barriers of paper partograph, the digital counterpart was developed aiming to reduce partograph's barriers (Schweers *et al.*, 2016). The later application possessed more efficiency, more error reduction and more usability in comparison to the non-digital version.

(xx) As a mobile-based interactive multimedia learning app for ASHAs, m-sakhi (sakhi means "a friend" in Hindi) was launched. It is an all-in-one job aid and electronic medical record system that replaces multiple paper-based tools and helps health workers gain access to the most up-to-date training and information in easy-to-understand, convenient formats that work for them. The Manthan Project initially developed this app on the open-source CommCare platform using Java-enabled, keypad-based mobile phones. Later on, this was modified for touch-phones using an open-source Android platform.

(xxi) Mobile-based helpline on sexual and reproductive health (SRH) is another appreciative mode of family planning. A non-randomized controlled trial conducted in Maharashtra (Kulathinal *et al.*, 2019) revealed that the intervention building upon a mobile helpline on SRH was associated with the increased use of reversible contraception compared with the control area.

(xxii) 'Khushi baby' is a mobile app for CHWs that interfaces with a digital necklace worn by child via Near Field

Communication (NFC). In this method, an electronic copy of all information of a child's medical and immunization records is stored on a pendant of a necklace (or worn on a black thread). The CHWs scan the pendant using this app to transfer vaccination data that automatically gets uploaded to the cloud. This mainly reduces the burden of paperwork, loss of any medical record and irregular vaccination.

(xxiii) iCHRcloud (Integrated Child Health Record Cloud) is a web- and mobile-based child health imprints for Smart health care. This application is based on HL7 protocol enabling integration with hospital's HIS/EMR system. It provides Java (Enterprise Service Bus and Hibernate) based web portal for doctors and mobile application for parents, enhancing doctor-parent engagement. It leverages highchart to automate chart preparation and provides access of data *via* Push Notification (GCM: Google Cloud Messaging and APNS: Apple Push Notification Service) to parents on iOS and Android mobile platforms.

(xxiv) ShishuPoshan, another mobile-based fitness application was developed with the collaboration of Mumbai Breastfeeding Promotion Committee (MBPC), Breastfeeding Promotion Network of India (BPNI) Maharashtra, Department of Community Medicine-Seth G.S. Medical College and KEM Hospital of Mumbai and TATA Consultancy Services (TCS). Launched on World Breastfeeding Week of 2016, the application yields scientific guidance regarding breastfeeding and baby's nutrition to new mothers (Bhate *et al.*, 2019). Additionally, the application also claims to answer and address various issues regarding baby's nutrition. The application is available in three languages, namely English, Hindi and Marathi.

(xxv) Another application named "mHealth based Preterm Home care Program" (mHealthPHCP), also known as NeoRaksha mobile health application was developed to monitor parent-infant interaction and inspect development and follow-up of preterms thereby diminishing mortalities, morbidities, and disabilities linked with prematurity (Nayak *et al.*, 2019).

Several apps are found to be available in Google Play that are used by Indian mothers and/or expectant mothers and are most often given positive reviews. Few of them are as follows:

(a) MomJunction is an app that possesses personalized pregnancy calendar, weight gain calculator, contraction timer and an important section named 'Mom Community' where a user can get connected with other users (pregnant lady or others) to get a view of their pregnancy experience.
(b) Parentlane app is an app-based social platform for baby care and parenting. It aids to track baby development score, baby feeding process and many more. Moreover, this app is gifted with other important features such as tutorial videos on parenting tips, nutritious baby food recipes, vaccination chart, reminders and due alerts for newborn baby etc. This app is available in ten Indian languages including Hindi.
(c) Parentune Parent app provides tried and tested tips on pregnancy, baby care, parenting support and solutions validated by fellow parents and vetted by experts, doctors and nutritionists. Apart from pregnancy-related queries, the app also helps to discover reliable child care products and perfect child growth tracker tips, videos for child's every stage. Provision for live-chat is also available where the user can get their solutions instantly.
(d) Babygogo app is another pregnancy and parenting app that provides topic-related albums, articles and videos. The app helps to track baby growth as per age. The app also aids to set reminders for busy parents and also include features for storing medical reports.
(e) 'Mylo: Pregnancy and Baby Companion' is an app that mothers can have access to several queries. This app is personalized for every stage, i.e., how to get pregnant, care during pregnancy and after delivery.
(f) GyOb is another app that provides pregnancy-related information. The app also carries the Electronic Medical Data that include path lab reports, prescriptions in chronological order and medical history besides the programmed medical procedures.

(g) Momspresso (formerly, mycity4kids) is a platform providing finely brewed content that answers all parenting questions.
(h) 'Healofy: Indian women' is an app for all ages. This is all-rounder guidance for every issue faced by a woman in her life. For an expectant mother and new mothers, this app is very helpful for providing tips on pregnancy diet, breastfeeding, baby care and parenting.
(i) 'Happy Pregnancy App' provides scientific and useful information on several topics based on pregnancy and child care with illustrative images and videos. This app is available in both Hindi and English languages.
(j) Another smartphone application named 'Preterm Care: Do not Harm' was launched in July-August 2019 in both android (as AIIMS WHOCC PTC) and iOS platforms (as Preterm Care). Developed by the team at All India Institute of Medical Sciences, WHO collaborating center (AIIMS WHOCC), the app gives an opportunity for users to learn and practice skills related to clinical procedures and use of essential equipment at partnering institutions.

Last but not the least, smart phones have equipped themselves with a high-quality optical system and a coaxial light source that drive us to use them even for fundoscopy. Moreover, this gives ease of handling while capturing images, cost-effectiveness, greater portability and safer light source that reduces retinal irradiance (Lord *et al.*, 2010; Kim *et al.*, 2012; Fung *et al.*, 2014). The last few years have observed the use of smartphone-based screening system for retinopathy of imaging among neonates (Vinekar *et al.*, 2014; Goyal *et al.*, 2019; Lekha *et al.*, 2019).

Conclusion

The digital revolution has affected virtually every aspect of our lives, and health is no exception. India has also been seen to embrace the digital world in terms of health care management. Mobile applications play an increasingly important role in supporting maternal and child health care in India. It could be conjectured that mobile applications with improved efficiency, time-saving, 24/7 access, cost-reduction, higher productivity, faster decision making process and multiple features would be developed more for maternal and child health care in the near future.

REFERENCES

Aarogyam. Available online at: https://oneworld.net.in/focus-area/knowledge-and-research/aarogyam-an-ict-based-approach-for-improving-reproductive-and-child-health accessed on 12th December, 2019.

Bangal, V., Borawake, S., Gavhane, S., Aher, K. 2017. "Use of mobile phone for improvement in maternal health: A randomized control trial." *Int J Reprod Contracept Obstet Gynecol.* **6**(12): 5458–5463.

Bhate, K., Gangal, P., Shanbhag, S., Solanki, M., Sable, P., Shinde, S.R., Bhavsar, K., Vishwakarma, K., Kimbahune, S.M. 2019. "ShishuPoshan application: ICT to solve issues of high social importance by scaled behavior change", 2019. 11th International Conference on Communication Systems and Networks (COMSNETS), Bengaluru, India.

Deodhar, J. 2002. "Telemedicine by email—experience in neonatal care at a primary care facility in rural India." *J Telemed Telecare.* **8**: S20-S21.

DeSouza, S.I., Rashmi, M.R., Vasanthi, A.P., Joseph, S.M., Rodrigues, R. 2014. "Mobile phones: the next step towards healthcare delivery in rural India?" *PLoS One.* **9**(8): e104895.

Fung, T.H., Smith, L.M., Patel, C.K. 2014. "Contemporary imaging of retinopathy of prematurity." *Infant.* **10**: 143–146.

Goyal, A., Gopalakrishnan, M., Anantharaman, G., Chandrashekharan, D.P., Thachil, T., Sharma, A. 2019. "Smartphone guided wide-field imaging for retinopathy of prematurity in neonatal intensive care unit—a Smart ROP (SROP) initiative." *Indian J Ophthalmol.* **67**(6): 840-845.

Haile, L.T., Fultz, H.M., Simmons, R.G., Shelus, V. 2018. "Market-testing a smartphone application for family planning: assessing potential of the CycleBeads app in seven countries through digital monitoring." *Mhealth.* 4: 27.

Hazra, A., Khan, M.E., Mondal, S.K. 2018. "Mobile Phone Messaging to Husbands to Improve Maternal and Child Health Behavior in India." *J Health Commun.* **23**(6): 542-549.

ICDS-CAS. Available online at: https://icds-wcd.nic.in/nnm/NNM-Web-Contents/LEFT-MENU/ICT-RTM/ICDS-CAS Username Management Guidelines English.pdf accessed on 10th December 2019.

Ilozumba, O., Dieleman, M., Kraamwinkel, N., Van Belle, S., Chaudoury, M., Broerse, J.E.W. 2018a. "I am not telling. The mobile is telling: Factors influencing the outcomes of a community health worker mHealth intervention in India." *PLoS ONE* **13**(3): e0194927.

Ilozumba O., Van Belle S., Dieleman M., Liem L., Choudhury M., Broerse, J.E.W. 2018b. "The Effect of a Community Health Worker Utilized Mobile Health Application on Maternal Health Knowledge and Behavior: A Quasi-Experimental Study." *Front Public Health.* **6**: 133.

Indira, E., Thomas, P.E., Hari, M. 2017. "Mobile Text Messages—A Silent Revolution for a Sound Antenatal care." *Indian J Public Health Res Dev.* **8**(4): 563-569.

Jayaseelan, R., Pichandy, C., Rushandramani, D. 2015. "Usage of Smartphone Apps by Women on their Maternal Life." *Res J Sci Technol.* **7**(3): 158-164.

Khushi baby. Available online at: https://www.thebetterindia.com/61540/khushi-baby-vaccination-immunization-history/ accessed on 10th December, 2019.

Kim, D.Y., Delori, F., Mukai, S. 2012. "Smartphone photography safety." *Ophthalmol.* **119**(10): 2200-2201.

Kim, H.S., Lee, K.H., Kim, H., Kim, J.H. 2014. "Using mobile phones in healthcare management for the elderly." *Maturitas.* **79**(4): 381-388.

Kulathinal, S., Joseph, B., Säävälä, M. 2019. "Mobile Helpline and Reversible Contraception: Lessons From a Controlled Before-and-After Study in Rural India." *JMIR Mhealth Uhealth.* **7**(8): e12672.

Lekha, T., Ramesh, S., Sharma, A., Abinaya, G. 2019. "MII RetCam assisted smartphone based fundus imaging for retinopathy of prematurity." *Indian J Ophthalmol.* **67**(6): 834-839.

Lord, R.K., Shah, V.A., San Filippo, A.N., Krishna, R. 2010. "Novel uses of smartphones in ophthalmology. *Ophthalmol.* **117**(6): 1274-1274.e3.

MAMA. *Implementing the Mobile Alliance for Maternal Action Approach.* Available online at: file:///C:/Users/SHREYASHI/Downloads/MAMALessonsLearnedBrief.pdf accessed on 10th December 2019.

Mobile Kunji. Available online at: https://www.itu.int/net4/wsis/archive/stocktaking/Project/Details?projectId=1513945836 accessed on 10th December, 2019.

Modi, D., Gopalan, R., Shah, S., Venkatraman, S., Desai, G., Desai, S., Shah, P. 2015. "Development and formative evaluation of an innovative mHealth intervention for improving coverage of community-based maternal, newborn and child health services in rural areas of India." *Glob Health Action.* **8**: 26769.

Modi, D., Desai, S., Dave, K., Shah, S., Desai, G., Dholakia, N., Gopalan, R., Shah, P. 2017. "Cluster randomized trial of a mHealth intervention "ImTeCHO" to improve delivery of proven maternal, neonatal, and child care interventions through community-based Accredited Social Health Activists (ASHAs) by enhancing their motivation and strengthening supervision in tribal areas of Gujarat, India: study protocol for a randomized controlled trial." *Trials.* 18(1): 270.

Modi, D., Dholakia, N., Gopalan, R., Venkatraman, S., Dave, K., Shah, S., *et al.* 2019. "mHealth intervention 'ImTeCHO' to improve delivery of maternal, neonatal, and child care services—A cluster-randomized trial in tribal areas of Gujarat, India." *PLoS Med.* **16**(10): e1002939.

MOTHER app. Available online at: https://apps.mgov.gov.in/descp.do?appid=531andparam=app accessed on 10th December, 2019.

mSakhi: Award-winning Mobile Phone App for Frontline Health Care. Available online at: https://www.intrahealth.org/msakhi-award-winning-mobile-phone-app-frontline-health-care accessed on 10th December, 2019.

Nayak, B.S., Lewis, L.E., Margaret, B., Bhat, Y.R., D'Almeida, J., Phagdol, T. 2019. "Randomized controlled trial on effectiveness of mHealth (mobile/smartphone) based Preterm Home Care Program on developmental outcomes of preterms: Study protocol." *J Adv Nurs*. **75**(2): 452-460.

Nimmagadda, S., Gopalakrishnan, L., Avula, R., Dhar, D., Diamond-Smith, N., Fernald, L., Jain, A., Mani, S., Menon, P., Nguyen, P.H., Park, H., Patil, S.R., Singh, P., Walker, D. 2019. "Effects of an mHealth intervention for community health workers on maternal and child nutrition and health service delivery in India: protocol for a quasi-experimental mixed-methods evaluation." *BMJ Open*. **9**(3): e025774.

Operationalisation of ICDS–CAS to address problem of undernutrition. Press Information Bureau, Government of India: Ministry of Mother and Child Development. Available online at: https://pib.gov.in/Pressreleaseshare.aspx?PRID=1557644 accessed on 11th December 2019.

Pai, N., Supe, P., Kore, S., Nandanwar, Y., Hegde, A., Cutrell, E., Thies, W. 2013. Using automated voice calls to improve adherence to Iron supplements during pregnancy: A pilot study Proceedings of the Sixth International Conference on Information and Communication Technologies and Development: Full Papers, 1: 153-163.

Patel, A.B., Kurhe, K., Prakash, A., Bhargav, S., Parepalli, S., Fogleman, E.V., Moore, J.L., Wallace, D.D., Kulkarni, H., Hibberd, P.L. 2019. "Early Identification of Preterm Neonates at Birth With a Tablet App for the Simplified Gestational Age Score (T-SGAS) When Ultrasound Gestational Age Dating Is Unavailable: Protocol for a Validation Study." *JMIR Res Protoc*. **8**(3): e11913.

Preterm Care: Do Not Harm. Available online at: https://www.healthynewbornnetwork.org/blog/smartphone-app-for-learning-best-practices-for-preterm-care-potential-point-of-care-tool-for-blended-learning/ accessed on 10th December, 2019.

ReMiND project. Available online at: https://www.crs.org/sites/default/files/tools-research/a4_case_study_remind_final_online.pdf accessed on 10th December, 2019.

Sankaranarayanan, J., Sallach, R.E. 2014. "Rural patients' access to mobile phones and willingness to receive mobile phone-based pharmacy and other health technology services: a pilot study." *Telemed J E Health*. **20**(2): 182-185.

Schweers, J., Khalid, M., Underwood, H., Bishnoi, S., Chhugani, M. 2016. "mLabour: Design and Evaluation of a Mobile Partograph and Labor Ward Management Application." *Procedia Eng*. **159**: 35-43.

Sharma, R., Hebbal, M., Ankola, A.V., Murugabupathy, V. 2011. "Mobile-phone text messaging (SMS) for providing oral health education to mothers of preschool children in Belgaum City." *J Telemed Telecare.* **17**(8): 432-436.

The Safe Delivery app. Available online at: https://www.maternity.dk/safe-delivery-app/ accessed on 11th December, 2019.

Trai Telecom Subscription Data as of 31st May 2019. Available online at: https://main.trai.gov.in/sites/default/files/PR_No.49of2019.pdf accessed on 10th December, 2019.

Vinekar, A., Gilbert, C., Dogra, M., Kurian, M., Shainesh, G., Shetty, B., Bauer, N. 2014. "The KIDROP model of combining strategies for providing retinopathy of prematurity screening in underserved areas in India using wide-field imaging, tele-medicine, non-physician graders and smart phone reporting." *Indian J Ophthalmol.* **62**(1): 41-49.

22

Ovarian Endometriosis with or without Allied Adenomyosis Exert Differential Pain Responses

Pramathes Das Mahapatra, Kasturi Chatterjee, Sayantan Jana, Snehasikta Swarnakar and *Amlan K. Ray*

1. Introduction

Pelvic pain and its association with endometriosis has baffled clinicians and gynaecologists. It is believed to be a complex syndrome for endometriosis and concomitant adenomyosis (Berkley *et al.*, 2005; Taylor *et al.*, 2012), but the underlying mechanism is still unclear. Occurrence of endometriosis associated pelvic pain among women was found to be about 10 per cent (Nasir and Bope, 2004). Endometriosis is defined by the endometrial lesions outside the uterus, commonly on the peritoneum. The clinical expressions of endometriosis are pain in the pelvis like dysmenorrhea, dyspareunia, dyskezia and chronic pelvic pain (CPP)(Berkley *et al.*, 2005). However, epidemiological studies hardly show any consistency between types of pain and stages of endometriosis specific location (Fedele *et al.*, 1990; Vercellini *et al.*, 1996). On the other hand, adenomyosis is a benign condition in the uterine musculature (Leyendecker *et al.*, 2009), sharing similar pathogenesis with endometriosis (Di Donato and Seracchioli, 2014). Similar to any other chronic pain conditions, neuronal innervations in endometriotic lesions are believed to be the cause of pain responses (Berkley *et al.*, 2005). Zhang *et al.* claimed endometriosis as a 'neurovascular condition'; because endometriosis is inextricably associated with unpleasant and emotional sensation of pain, which is linked with tissue inflammation, vasculogenesis, and as well as innervations (Zhang *et al.*, 2009). Thus, pelvic pain manifested with endometriosis may arise from combinatorial effects of systemic and local hormonal environment; local pool of growth factors, such as nerve growth factor and vascular endothelial growth factor; vascularity and sensory and sympathetic innervations.

Quantification of pain requires detailed descriptions about the intensity, location and affectivity of pain which is to be expressed by the patient (Dworkin *et al.*, 2005). Most of the studies classify pelvic pain in terms of absent, mild, moderate and severe stages, including the degree of debility experienced using different pain scales (Breivik *et al.*, 2008). There are several scales for pain that had a positive outcome of responsiveness and pain score sensitivities, especially for endometriosis treatments; however, the Visual Analogue Scale (VAS) has been used extensively worldwide by virtue of the 'most precise pain evaluation' measurement (Hjermstad *et al.*, 2011; Bourdel *et al.*, 2015). In the present study, we have utilized VAS for assessment of Endometriosis-Related Pain Symptoms (ERPS) which belong to five physiological/ phenotypical pains, pulsatile, shifting, muscle contractile, steady and sudden pain. We have further incorporated three psychometric properties to ERPS to support our argument over psychological domain. These are weakness, illness and scaring. The psychiatric conditions of pain is a part of somatization disorder (Eisendrath, 1995; Birket-Smith 2001) like weakness (Reiter and Gambone, 1991), illness behaviours (Wesselmann and Czakanski, 2001) and scaring, pertaining to ERPS. The newer approach of ERPS has been attempted to get further insight and focus upon the objective and subjective nature of pain. The physical pain is the biological/ objective event and the psychological pain is the subjective response of the woman. In the present study, besides dysmenorrhoea and dyspareunia, we have actually looked into the pain status of early and late stages of endometriosis patients with or without adenomyosis by utilizing these specific and unique pelvic pain responses. The purpose of the study is to elucidate pain symptoms delineated in eight pain sub-types, which may work out as an upgrade in VAS tool for differentiating endometriosis from its allied complications (here, adenomyosis). Our study also tried to understand whether psychological stress like illness, weakness and scaring, has any exacerbated effects over endometriosis-associated adenomyosis.

2. Methods

2.1. Clinical Study

The study was conducted at Spectrum Clinic and Endoscopy Research Institute (SC-ERI), Kolkata in collaboration with Cancer Biology and Inflammatory Disorder Division, CSIR-Indian Institute of Chemical Biology, Kolkata. The study was conducted at SC-ERI from April 2013 to January 2015, in a total population of 145 women with the patient consent and approval from SC-ERI Human Ethical Committee. All women met the following inclusion criteria: Age 18-45 years, laparoscopic diagnosis of ovarian endometriosis with and without adenomyosis, pain symptoms were more than 6 months and had a history of infertility. Exclusion criteria include extensive use of pain killers, pelvic anomalies, hysterectomy and malignant gynaecological diseases. The pain questionnaire was given to fill-up before diagnostic surgery during the hospital stay (SC-ERI) in presence of physician and laparoscopic details were documented to correlate with the self-reported pain description.

Pain descriptive demographic data and assessment of pain using visual analogue scale (VAS) for four different groups: (i) Early endometriosis (stage I-II, n=27); (ii) Early endometriosis (stage I-II)+adenomyosis (n=21); (iii) Late Endometriosis (stage III-IV, n=56); (iv) Late endometriosis (stage III-IV)+adenomyosis (n=41) were analyzed. Ovarian endometriosis was staged according to the revised American Society of Reproductive Medicine (rASRM) guidelines. In addition to dysmenorrhoea, chronic pelvic pain, and dyspareunia; eight specific types of pain were studied in detail. Questionnaire was used to accumulate data pertaining to five physiological pains (pulsatile pain, shifting pain, sudden pain, muscle contractile pain, steady pain) and three psychological pains (weakness, illness, scaring). The quantitative pain measurement using visual analogue scale was to identify pains that were self-reported by women by simply putting tick mark in 10-point scale of all eight pain types. In our study, 0-3 was categorized as low pain; 4-7, moderate pain; and 8-10 severe pain, while 0 was considered as no pain, and 10 point considered as 'worst pain imaginable'.

2.2. *Characterization*

Different physiological pains have been characterized and classified according to the following properties. *Pulsatile pain* defines an alteration of weak and strong beats of pain pertaining to the length of menstrual cycle based on the severity of disease stage. It might originate below the umbilicus, or at the right or left side of the pelvis. *Shifting pain* defines such discomfort which seems to move from the site of origin (preferably below the umbilicus) to the other part of the pelvis followed by both the lower limbs and centred in the suprapubic area but may radiate to the back of the legs or the lower back (Nasir and Bope, 2004). This is also to pertaining to the length of the menstrual cycle. *Sudden pain* appears irrespective of menstrual period with high intensity followed by appears-to-get collapsed. *Muscle contractile pain* attributes a stiffness of muscle in lower abdomen felt during the passing of urine, during the period. *Steady pain* denotes a persistent pain from moderate to severe irrespective of menstrual period.

Weakness, in the present study, is a state of mind marked by mild to severe loss of physical strength when suffering from endometriosis and allied complications. *Illness* is a state of mind where woman may mentally accept the present level of endometriosis and allied complications which helps in mitigating the negative impact of psychosocial stage related to the disease (Chmaj-Wierzchowska *et al.*, 2015). *Scaring* is a state of mind where woman feels apprehensive of sensing danger for not knowing or gets scared for being operated.

2.3. *Statistical Analysis*

The degree of pain intensity was assessed by pain-specific type using visual analogue scale. Statistical analyses of the data were performed using GraphPad Instat3 software. Graphs were prepared using Sigma plot and Origin pro8 software. ***$p<0.001$ corresponds highly significant; **$p<0.01$ corresponds significant; *$p<0.05$ corresponds less significant; NS corresponds not significant. Data obtained from $p < 0.05$ was accepted as level of significance. Comparison between groups was made using one-way analysis of variance (ANOVA) followed by Student-Newman-Keuls test.

3. Results

3.1. Characterization of Patient Population for Endometriosis and Allied Adenomyosis

Out of total population (n=145), 27(18.62%) women had endometriosis only at early stages and 56 (38.62%) women had late stages endometriosis. About 21 (14.48%) women had early endometriosis with adenomyosis and corresponding to 41 (28.27%) women were at late stage endometriosis with adenomyosis. The presence of dysmenorrhea is predominant in all four groups. Endometriosis with early and late stages had reported positive for dysmenorrhea pain ~70.3% and 94.6% of cases respectively, whereas early and late stage endometriosis with adenomyosis showed ~95.2 and 87.8% positive cases for dysmenorrhea pain respectively. As endometriosis is associated with infertility, we investigated infertility status among the population. Women with early and late stages of endometriosis had 66.6 per cent and 43.3 per cent cases of infertility, whereas early and late stages of endometriosis with allied adenomyosis had 47.6 and 67.5 per cent infertility rate (Table 22.1).

Table 22.1: Association of ovarian endometriosis with dysmenorrhea and infertility

Characteristics	*Early endometriosis*	*Early endometriosis with adenomyosis*	*Late endometriosis with adenomyosis*	*Late endometriosis*
Case numbers (N_{total} =145)	N=27	N=21	N=56	N=41
Age (Mean±SD)	29.92±5.56	31.25±6.50	31.1±7.51	32.25±5.83
Dysmenorrhoea (present)	19/27(70.3%)	20/21(95.2%)	53/56(94.6%)	36/41(87.8%)
Associated with Infertility	18/27(66.6%)	10/21(47.6%)	23/53(43.3%)	27/40(67.5%)

3.2. Assessment of five Phenotypical Endometriosis-related Pain Symptoms in Patients with Endometriosis only and Endometriosis-Allied Adenomyosis

The full spectrum of pain has been classified into three levels of pain scores: low pain score (0-3), moderate pain score (4-7) and high pain score (8-10) in five phenotypes of pain, e.g. pulsatile, shifting, sudden, muscle contractile and steady pain and three psychological categories of pain, e.g. weakness, illness and scaring. Population under individual categories do not express any pain so far in all eight categories of pain are kept under 0 score, means no pain.

3.2.1. Pulsatile Pain

In **pulsatile pain,** severe pain (8-10 score) has been observed 18.51 per cent and 37.5 per cent in early and late stages of endometriosis respectively, and 42.85 per cent and 65.85 per cent in early and late endometriosis with adenomyosis population. Correspondingly, moderate pain (4-7 score) was observed in 25.92 per cent and 41 per cent in early and late stages of endometriosis respectively, 38 per cent and 19.51 per cent in early and late endometriosis with adenomyosis of population. Almost 55.55 per cent for early endometriosis, 21.42 per cent for late endometriosis, 19 per cent for early endometriosis with adenomyosis and 14.63 per cent for late endometriosis with adenomyosis of population showed no-to-low pain scores (0-3 score). However, substantial number of population that had no pulsatile pain (0 score) were 48.14 per cent for early endometriosis, 16 per cent for late endometriosis, 14.29 per cent for early endometriosis with allied adenomyosis, and 12.19 per cent for late endometriosis with allied adenomyosis out of the population. Although, the pulsatile pain was present in four groups showed an incremental depiction of high pain score from early stages to late stages of endometriosis with or without adenomyosis, no significant ($p>0.05$) up regulation for total pain score was observed between early endometriosis stages with and without adenomyosis. However, late stage endometriosis with adenomyosis showed significant ($p<0.05$) up regulation of total pain score than only late stage endometriosis (Fig. 22.1A).

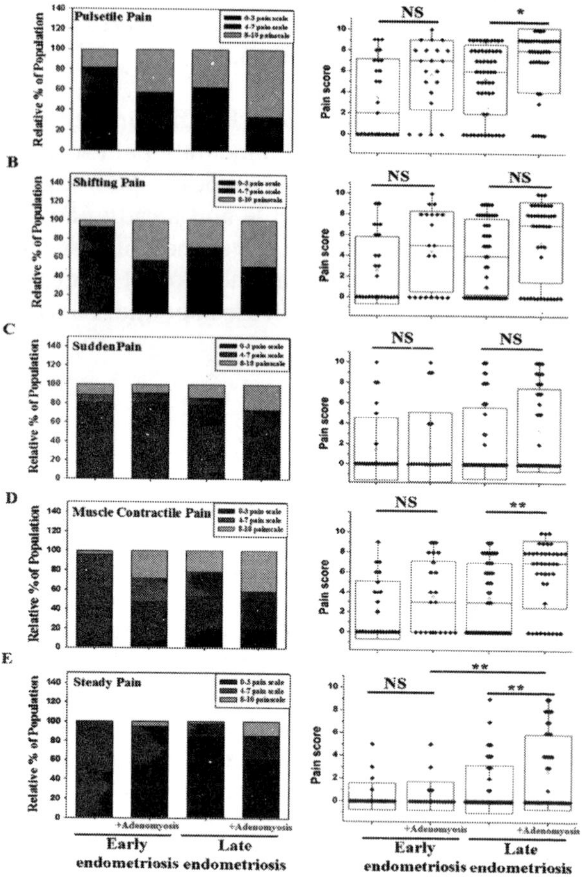

Fig. 22.1: Different physiological pain responses in ovarian endometriosis with and without adenomyosis. [A total of 145 ovarian endometriosis patients were studied with or without adenomyosis: (i) Early endometriosis (I-II) n=27; (ii) Early endometriosis (I-II) with adenomyosis n=21; (iii) Late Endometriosis (III-IV) n=56 (iv) Late endometriosis (III-IV) with adenomyosis (n=41). The population was studied for five different pain symptoms: (A) Pulsatile pain, (B) Shifting pain, (C) Sudden pain, (D) Muscle contractile pain, (E) Steady pain. The first figure in each pain responses showed the relative population percentage distribution for no-to-mild (0-3), moderate (4-7) and severe pain (8-10) in four groups. The second figure in each pain responses showed the distribution of pain scores for all patients from different groups. **p<0.01 corresponds significant; *p< 0.05 corresponds less significant; NS corresponds not significant p>0.05.]

3.2.2. Shifting Pain

In **Shifting pain**, severe pain (8-10 score) was observed in 42.85 per cent and 48.78 per cent population respectively for early and late stages of endometriosis with adenomyosis, whereas only 7.4 per cent and 28.57 per cent population showed severe pain in early and late stages of only endometriosis respectively. Moderate pain levels (4-7 score), was observed in 25.92 per cent for early stages of endometriosis, 23.21 per cent for late stages of endometriosis, 23.8 per cent for early stages of endometriosis with adenomyosis, and 19.51 per cent for late stages of endometriosis with adenomyosis. The major population of shifting pain resides within no-to-low pain scores (0-3). The low pain score populations were 66.66 per cent for early endometriosis for early endometriosis; 48.21 per cent for late endometriosis; 33.33 per cent for early endometriosis with adenomyosis; 31.7 per cent late endometriosis with adenomyosis respectively. The total pain score values for early and late stage in association with respective adenomyosis stages are not statistically significant (p>0.05) (Fig. 22.1B).

3.2.3. Sudden Pain

Severe sudden pain (8-10 score) was not much found in early endometriosis (11.11%), early endometriosis with adenomyosis (9.52%) and late endometriosis (14.28%) populations, however, 26.82 per cent of the late endometriosis with adenomyosis, the population were suffering with severe sudden pain. Population for moderate sudden pain (4-7 scores) were observed in 7.4 per cent of early endometriosis, 7.14 per cent of late endometriosis, 9.52 per cent of early endometriosis with adenomyosis and 17.07 per cent of late endometriosis with adenomyosis. Rest of the population, which also consists of the most of population, resides within the no-to-low pain score regions (0-3 scores). The total pain score values for early and late stage in association with respective adenomyosis stages are not statistically significant(p>0.05) (Fig. 22.1C).

3.2.4. Muscle Contractile Pain

Higher per cent of population were found suffering with severe muscle-related contractile pain in the endometriosis with adenomyosis groups (Fig. 2D). Whereas severe pain was observed 28.57 per cent and 41.46 per cent populations respectively for early and late stages of endometriosis with adenomyosis, only 3.7 per cent and 21.42 per cent population were suffering with severe muscle contractile pain for early and late stage endometriosis respectively. Population per cent in moderate pain scales (4-7 score) were 33.33 per cent for early endometriosis, 25 per cent for late endometriosis, 23.8 per cent for early endometriosis with adenomyosis and 39.02 per cent late endometriosis with adenomyosis. Most of population had no-to-low pain scores (0-3): 62.96 per cent for early endometriosis, 53.57 per cent for late endometriosis, 47.61 per cent for early endometriosis with adenomyosis, except for late endometriosis with adenomyosis population (19.51%). However, no statistically significant change ($p>0.05$) in pain levels were observed among early endometriosis with or without adenomyosis groups; late stage endometriosis with adenomyosis showed significantly increased ($p<0.01$) muscle contractile pain levels than only late-stage endometriosis patients (Fig. 22.1D).

3.2.5. Steady Pain

Most of the studied population showed no-to-low steady pain responses, which is 96.29 per cent for early endometriosis, 83.92 per cent for late endometriosis, 90.47 per cent for early endometriosis with adenomyosis, 60.97 per cent for late endometriosis with adenomyosis (Fig. 22.2E). Population with moderate and severe pain respectively were 3.7 and 0 per cent for early endometriosis, 14.29 per cent and 1.78 per cent for late endometriosis, 4.76 and 4.76 per cent for early endometriosis with adenomyosis, 24.39 per cent and 14.63 per cent for late endometriosis with adenomyosis respectively. The total pain score for late endometriosis with adenomyosis significantly ($p<0.01$) increased in comparison to the early endometriosis with adenomyosis patients. Furthermore, significant difference ($p<0.01$) was observed between late stages of endometriosis without and with adenomyosis, however, no significant change ($p>0.05$) was observed between early stages of endometriosis *vs.* endometriosis with adenomyosis (Fig. 22.1E).

3.3. Assessment of Three Psychological Endometriosis-related Pain symptoms in Patients with Endometriosis only and Endometriosis-allied Adenomyosis

The presence and severity of three **psychological pains** such as weakness (Fig. 22.2A), illness (Fig.2B) and scaring (Fig.2C) were analyzed within the populations.

3.3.1. Weakness

Weakness with high (8-10) score has been observed in 11.11 per cent for early endometriosis, 3.57 per cent for late endometriosis, 9.52 per cent for early endometriosis with adenomyosis, and 26.82 per cent for late endometriosis with adenomyosis of population. Weakness with moderate (4-7) score has been observed in 18.51 per cent for early endometriosis, 60.71 per cent for late endometriosis, 47.61 per cent for early endometriosis with adenomyosis, and 56.09 per cent for late endometriosis with adenomyosis showing a trend of increased population density at late stage of the disease. Low scores for weakness has been observed in 70.37 for early endometriosis, 42.85 for early endometriosis with adenomyosis, 35.71 per cent for late endometriosis and 17.07 per cent for late endometriosis with adenomyosis of population. For total population of pain scores, endometriosis in late stage exhibited significantly elevated ($p<0.01$) weakness responses in comparison to early endometriosis only (Fig. 22.2A).

3.3.2. Illness

Illness is a state of mind where woman may mentally accept the diseased state which helps in mitigating the negative impact or stress of psychosocial stage related to the disease. Illness with high (8-10) score has been observed in 11.11 per cent for early endometriosis, 1.78 per cent for late endometriosis, 9.52 per cent for early endometriosis with adenomyosis, and 19.51 per cent for late endometriosis with adenomyosis of population. Illness with moderate (4-7) score has been observed in 14.81 per cent for early endometriosis, 50 per cent for late endometriosis, 33.33 per cent for early endometriosis with adenomyosis, and 58.53 per cent for

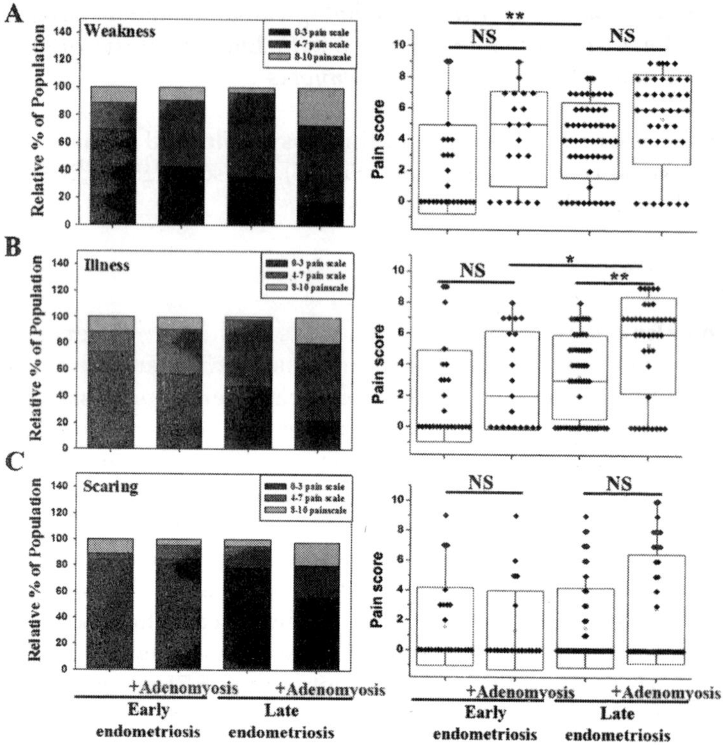

Fig. 22.2: Different psychological pain responses in ovarian endometriosis with and without adenomyosis. [A total of 145 ovarian endometriosis patients were studied with or without adenomyosis: (i) Early endometriosis (I-II) n=27; (ii) Early endometriosis (I-II) with adenomyosis n=21; (iii) Late Endometriosis (III-IV) n=56; (iv) Late endometriosis (III-IV) with adenomyosis (n=41). The population was studied for three different psychological pain symptoms: (A) Weakness, (B) Illness, (C) Scaring. The first figure in each pain responses showed the relative population percentage distribution for no-to-mild (0-3), moderate (4-7) and severe pain (8-10) in four groups. The second figure in each pain responses showed the distribution of pain scores for all patients from different groups. **$p<0.01$ corresponds significant; *$p< 0.05$ corresponds less significant; NS corresponds not significant $p>0.05$.]

late endometriosis with adenomyosis showing an incremental population density. Low scores for weakness has been observed in 74.07 per cent for early endometriosis, 48.21 per cent for late endometriosis, 57.14 per cent for early endometriosis with adenomyosis, and 21.95 per cent for late endometriosis with adenomyosis of population (Fig. 22.2B). For total pain scores in groups, late stage endometriosis-associated adenomyosis exhibited significantly elevated ($p<0.05$) illness responses than early endometriosis-associated adenomyosis. For late stages, endometriosis-adenomyosis group showed highly significant ($p<0.01$) elevated illness-responses than only endometriosis.

3.3.3. Scaring

In **scaring**, majority of the population with high (8-10) score has been observed in 11.11 per cent for early endometriosis, 9.52 per cent for early endometriosis with adenomyosis, 1.78 per cent for late endometriosis and 19.51 per cent for late endometriosis with adenomyosis of population. Illness with moderate (4-7) score has been observed in 14.81 per cent for early endometriosis, 33.33 per cent for early endometriosis with adenomyosis, 50 per cent for late endometriosis and 58.53 per cent for late endometriosis with adenomyosis showing an incremental population density. Low scores for weakness has been observed in 74.07 per cent for early endometriosis, 57.14 per cent for early endometriosis with adenomyosis, 48.21 per cent for late endometriosis and 21.95 per cent for late endometriosis with adenomyosis of population. For total pain scores in different groups, scaring does not have any significant changes irrespective of endometriosis severity with or without adenomyosis (Fig. 22.2C).

4. Discussion

Pain is involved with nociceptive, inflammatory, or neuropathic mechanisms, and these mechanisms are relevant to endometriosis-associated pelvic pain. The expressivity of discomfort in *in vivo* endometriotic models represented associated innervations and inflammatory mechanisms (Zhang *et al.*, 2009). This phenomenon is involved in generating neuronal responses (Tokushige *et al.*, 2006) which might transmit throbbing and pain in the pelvis (Choi *et al.*, 2015). In accordance with the other findings, our results revealed that the shifting pain from the pelvis to both the lower limbs reflects nociceptive innervations in respective location (Stratton and Berkley, 2011).

The present study was focused on different forms of pain sensation in the presence of ovarian endometriosis and associated adenomyosis. The eight categories of pains showed that population for both physiological and psychological pain levels had an incremental signature of pain with advancement of the disease, irrespective of absence or presence of adenomyosis. Even though, majority of the population for sudden and steady pains lied within low pain zone. However, occurrences of pain were more pronounced in the advanced stage of endometriosis and endometriosis-adenomyosis combine. In pulsatile, muscle contractile and steady pain, the late stage endometriosis with adenomyosis for late endometriosis with adenomyosis showed significant increased pain responses ($p<0.05$, $p<0.01$, and $p<0.01$ respectively) than without adenomyosis. The results of three physical/phenotypical pains could be a part of the strong regimen in diagnosing and clinical decision making. Prevalence of pulsatile and shifting pain ranges to correlating with menstrual symptoms, whereas muscle contractile pain is an associated complication irrespective of menstruation.

Accumulated evidences on women affected with endometriosis from this quantitative study suggested that level of psychological pains include weakness, illness and scaring were almost progressively higher with the stages of diseases in the present population. Weakness, illness and scaring incorporated in three psychological pain forms could be interpreted as a psychological phenomenon in tandem with other phenotypical pain forms. With the elucidation of physical pains and associated three psychological phenomenon considered in this study, it might be plausible to assess the 'diagnosable psychopathology' that result due to exacerbated effects of endometriosis and concomitant adenomyosis (Dersh *et al.*, 2002). In psychological response-based scales, weakness increased significantly ($p<0.05$) with an advancement of only endometriosis for early endometriosis, whereas illness increased significantly with an advancement of endometriosis with adenomyosis for early endometriosis with adenomyosis ($p<0.05$) to the extent of late stages of endometriosis with adenomyosis for late endometriosis with adenomyosis. Furthermore, illness was highly significant in endometriosis-allied adenomyosis than only endometriosis in late stages of the disease ($p<0.01$). The results suggested the detrimental effects of disease as psychological stress that plays a major role in patient conditions which warrants further management. Weakness almost appeared with every episodic pain since the age of symptom. With the consistent follow-up treatment along with acquiring the knowledge about endometriosis, women used to be the almost inclined to the therapeutic procedures for strengthening the quality of life. Most interestingly, our findings showed that the scaring level is not as pronounced as women are quite ignored about the disease. Nevertheless, some populations are featured in the figure irrespective of the stages.

Moreover, previous studies support psychiatric conditions of pain as a part of the somatization disorder (Eisendrath, 1995; Birket-Smith, 2001) like weakness to the illness behaviours—providing an excuse, towards "legitimate and accepted disease" to discourage gossip and scaring, pertaining to ERPS (Wesselmann and Czakanski, 2001). Such conditions are the revelation of consciousness or lack of awareness of the basis of algogenic mechanism (Chapron, Fauconnier *et al.*, 2003; Vercellini, Fedele *et al.*, 2007) and the chances of this development are more pronounced with the prolonged clinical management. This process, on the contrary, might strengthen the self-knowledge among women to accept the great extent of responsibility for their own betterment (Albert, 1999).

Dysmenorrhoea with its severity and dyspareunia act as a sort of alarm, from where clinicians diagnose the disease beforehand, however, our study further explored as a supportive diagnostic tool for identification of endometriosis and allied complications. Thus, detailed study with pain could be a 'wakeup call' against endometriosis-allied complications. Our data pertaining to eight types of pain could not only updating our understanding on pain in patient conditions, i.e. associated with only endometriosis and allied complications but has opened a new vista to corroborate our findings with the inflammatory mechanisms. If a simple measurement (VAS) of pain intensity could be the logical outcome variable, then the focus could plausibly be shifted from lesions (due to endometriosis) to pain sensation (Stratton and Berkley, 2011), as it might equate subjective feedback from the patient's side with objective data (Flaherty, 1996).

In conclusion, our study has considered VAS for measuring endometriosis-related pain in five physical and three psychological scales to understand its potentiality for identification of endometriosis-allied adenomyosis. We identified significant changes between endometriosis and associated adenomyosis for pulsatile pain, muscle contractile pain, steady pain and illness; thus, these pain scales can be utilized as potential tools for better prognosis of endometriosis from endometriosis-allied adenomyosis. Out of three psychological pains studied, an understanding of illness perceptions is essential for effective evaluation of pain management, and we hope that this psychological component has enormous potential for research and practice in psychosomatic disorders. However, more comprehensive investigations, enriched with large population data, are warranted to clarify further links between etiology of pelvic pain and ectopic pathogenesis.

Acknowledgement: The authors are thankful to Prof. Joydeb Roy Choudhury and Dr. Ansuman Sarkar for their sincere comments and discussions.

REFERENCES

Albert, H. (1999). "Psychosomatic group treatment helps women with chronic pelvic pain." *J Psychosom Obstet Gynaecol* **20**(4): 216-225.

Berkley, K.J., A.J. Rapkin and R.E. Papka (2005). "The Pains of Endometriosis." *Science.* **308**(5728): 1587-1589.

Birket-Smith, M. (2001). "Somatization and chronic pain." *Acta Anaesthesiologica Scandinavica.* **45**(9): 1114-1120.

Bourdel, N., J. Alves, G. Pickering, I. Ramilo, H. Roman and M. Canis (2015). "Systematic review of endometriosis pain assessment: how to choose a scale?" *Hum Reprod Update.* **21**(1): 136-152.

Breivik, H., P. C. Borchgrevink, S. M. Allen, L.A. Rosseland, L. Romundstad, E. K. Hals, G. Kvarstein and A. Stubhaug (2008). "Assessment of pain." *Br J Anaesth.* **101**(1): 17-24.

Chapron, C., A. Fauconnier, M. Vieira, H. Barakat, B. Dousset, V. Pansini, M. C. Vacher-Lavenu and J.B. Dubuisson (2003). "Anatomical distribution of deeply infiltrating endometriosis: surgical implications and proposition for a classification." *Hum Reprod.* **18**(1): 157-161.

Chmaj-Wierzchowska, K., M. Kampioni, M. Wilczak, S. Sajdak and T. Opala (2015). "Assessment of pain and stress intensity among women with ovarian endometriomas versus teratomas." *Pain Research and Management : The Journal of the Canadian Pain Society* **20**(3): 133-136.

Choi, Y.J., J.A. Chang, Y.A. Kim, S.H. Chang, K.C. Chun and J.W. Koh (2015). "Innervation in women with uterine myoma and adenomyosis." *Obstet Gynecol Sci.* **58**(2): 150-156.

Dersh, J., P.B. Polatin and R.J. Gatchel (2002). "Chronic pain and psychopathology: research findings and theoretical considerations." *Psychosom Med.* **64**(5): 773-786.

Di Donato, N. and R. Seracchioli (2014). "How to evaluate adenomyosis in patients affected by endometriosis?" *Minim Invasive Surg.* **2014**: 507230.

Dworkin, R.H., D.C. Turk, J.T. Farrar, J.A. Haythornthwaite, M.P. Jensen, N.P. Katz, R.D. Kerns, G. Stucki, R.R. Allen, N. Bellamy, D.B. Carr, J. Chandler, P. Cowan, R. Dionne, B.S. Galer, S. Hertz, A.R. Jadad, L.D. Kramer, D.C. Manning, S. Martin, C.G. McCormick, M.P. McDermott, P. McGrath, S. Quessy, B.A. Rappaport, W. Robbins, J.P. Robinson, M. Rothman, M.A. Royal, L. Simon, J.W. Stauffer, W. Stein, J. Tollett, J. Wernicke and J. Witter (2005). "Core outcome measures for chronic pain clinical trials: IMMPACT recommendations." *Pain.* **113**(1-2): 9-19.

Eisendrath, S.J. (1995). "Psychiatric aspects of chronic pain." *Neurology.* **45**(12 Suppl 9): S26-34; discussion S35-26.

Fedele, L., F. Parazzini, S. Bianchi, L. Arcaini and G.B. Candiani (1990). "Stage and localization of pelvic endometriosis and pain." *Fertil Steril.* **53**(1): 155-158.

Flaherty, S.A. (1996). "Pain measurement tools for clinical practice and research." *AANA J.* **64**(2): 133-140.

Hjermstad, M.J., P.M. Fayers, D.F. Haugen, A. Caraceni, G.W. Hanks, J.H. Loge, R. Fainsinger, N. Aass and S. Kaasa (2011). "Studies comparing Numerical Rating Scales, Verbal Rating Scales, and Visual Analogue Scales for assessment of pain intensity in adults: a systematic literature review." *J Pain Symptom Manage.* **41**(6): 1073-1093.

Leyendecker, G., L. Wildt and G. Mall (2009). "The pathophysiology of endometriosis and adenomyosis: tissue injury and repair." *Arch Gynecol Obstet.* **280**(4): 529-538.

Nasir, L. and E.T. Bope (2004). "Management of pelvic pain from dysmenorrhea or endometriosis." *J Am Board Fam Pract.* **17 Suppl**: S43-47.

Reiter, R.C. and J.C. Gambone (1991). "Nongynecologic somatic pathology in women with chronic pelvic pain and negative laparoscopy." *J Reprod Med.* **36**(4): 253-259.

Stratton, P. and K.J. Berkley (2011). "Chronic pelvic pain and endometriosis: translational evidence of the relationship and implications." *Hum Reprod Update.* **17**(3): 327-346.

Taylor, R.N., L. Hummelshoj, P. Stratton and P. Vercellini (2012). "Pain and endometriosis: Etiology, impact, and therapeutics." *Middle East Fertility Society Journal.* **17**(4): 221-225.

Tokushige, N., R. Markham, P. Russell and I.S. Fraser (2006). "High density of small nerve fibres in the functional layer of the endometrium in women with endometriosis." *Hum Reprod.* **21**(3): 782-787.

Vercellini, P., L. Fedele, G. Aimi, G. Pietropaolo, D. Consonni and P.G. Crosignani (2007). "Association between endometriosis stage, lesion type, patient characteristics and severity of pelvic pain symptoms: a multivariate analysis of over 1000 patients." *Hum Reprod.* **22**(1): 266-271.

Vercellini, P., L. Trespidi, O. De Giorgi, I. Cortesi, F. Parazzini and P.G. Crosignani (1996). "Endometriosis and pelvic pain: relation to disease stage and localization." *Fertil Steril.* **65**(2): 299-304.

Wesselmann, U. and P. Czakanski (2001). "Pelvic pain: A chronic visceral pain syndrome." *Current Pain and Headache Reports.* **5**(1): 13-19.

Zhang, X., B. Lu, X. Huang, H. Xu, C. Zhou and J. Lin (2009). "Endometrial nerve fibers in women with endometriosis, adenomyosis, and uterine fibroids." *Fertil Steril.* **92**(5): 1799-1801.

23

Maternal Inheritance Deficiency of Glucose-6-Phosphate Dehydrogenase Enzyme in Human

Ramie H. Begum

Introduction

Maternal inheritance means the inheritance of a genetic trait with or without its associated phenotypes exclusively from the mother. The inheritance may be through the DNA of the X chromosome or by the mitochondrial DNA present in the mother's egg cytoplasm. Many genetic defects of human are maternally inherited. Glucose-6-Phosphate dehydrogenase (G6PD) is a housekeeping enzyme vital for the life of every cell of the body. This enzyme catalyzes the first step of the oxidative phase of the pentose phosphate pathway (PPP) (Fig. 23.1), a cascade of biochemical reactions that convert glucose to another form of sugar, the ribose-5-phosphate. Ribose-5-phosphate is the building block of nucleic acid molecules, precisely DNA and RNA that function as the genetic material in all living organisms. The G6PD is a primeval evolved enzyme ubiquitous in nature and found in all organisms from prokaryotes to yeast to protozoa, plant and animals.

The first step of the pentose phosphate pathway produces the molecule NADPH which plays a fundamental role of protecting the cells from oxidative stress created by reactive oxygen species (ROS) produced during normal cellular metabolic processes or during usage of certain drugs. Reactions involving NADPH produce compounds that stop the ROS to build up to toxic levels as to harm the cell.

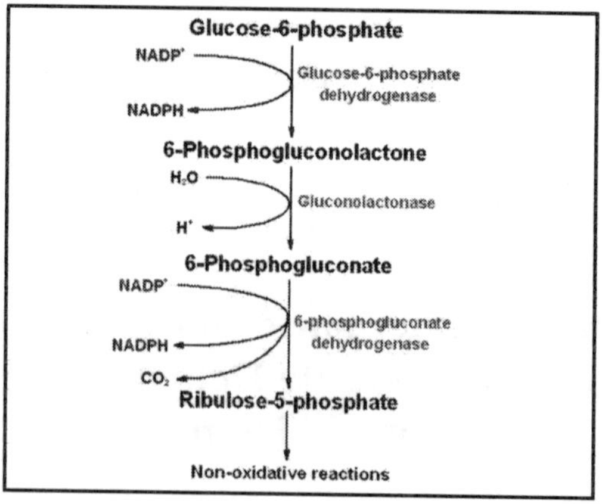

Fig. 23.1: Oxidative Stage of Pentose Phosphate Pathway.

The G6PD enzyme is coded by the corresponding G6PD gene located in the telomeric region of the distal arm of the X chromosome (xq28) in human and is thus maternally inherited (Fig. 23.2). The G6PD gene was cloned and sequenced in 1986 by Persico *et al.* (1986). It spans 18.5 kb in the X chromosome and consists of 13 exons and 12 introns coding for a product of 1545bp. Interestingly the first 600bp of the 5′ of the G6PD gene corresponding to the exon 1 and part of exon 2 are not translated, therefore, the gene is translated from the 127bp of exon 2. The product is a 59 Kilo Dalton (KD) protein with 514 amino acids (aa) molecules. The G6PD promoter was found to be embedded in a CpG island that is conserved from mice to humans. The promoter of the G6PD gene contains a TATA-like sequence, TTAAAT, and numerous stimulatory protein 1 (Sp1) elements, but no CAAT element. The number of exons and introns and the size and sequence of the exons are conserved in higher eukaryotes.

Any change in the base pairs of the coding region of the G6PD gene results in mutation which can further be transcribed into a non-functional or faulty G6PD enzyme with reduced activity resulting in a state commonly known as G6PD deficiency (G6PDd). Almost all G6PDd are caused by a point mutation of the genomic DNA resulting in an amino acid substitution (Beutler and Vulliamy, 2002).

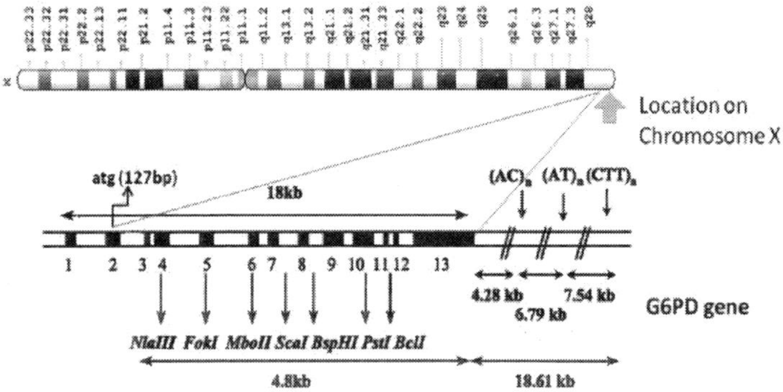

Fig. 23.2: Location and coding structure of the G6PD gene on the X chromosome.

Inheritance and Implications of G6PDd

Deficiency of G6PD is an X-linked recessive disorder, with an inheritance pattern similar to that of hemophilia and colour blindness: males usually manifest the abnormality having a single copy of the X chromosome and females are mostly carriers (Fig. 23.3). Females may be symptomatic if they are homozygous or if inactivation of their normal X chromosome occurs.

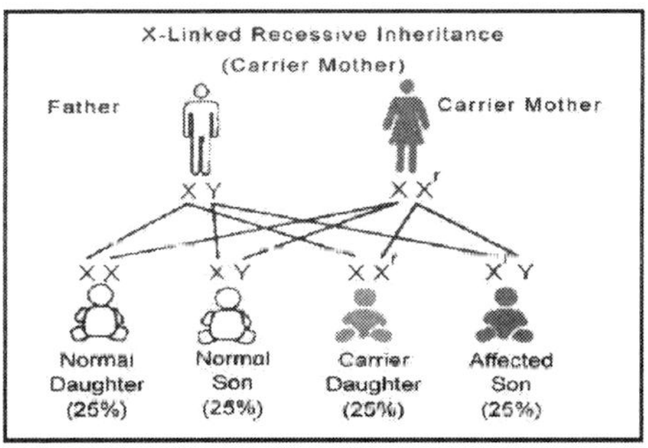

Fig. 23.3: Inheritance of G6PD deficiency.

Mature Red Blood Cells (RBCs) which carry oxygen from lungs to tissues throughout the body are the only non-nucleated cells of the human body. In the RBCs, the production of NADPH by G6PD is crucial for protecting them from oxidative damages since they lack other NADPH producing enzymes. The β-chain of hemoglobin is particularly susceptible to oxidation. Protection of oxidation is mediated by glutathione which is actively synthesized and present in RBCs.

The deficiency of G6PD mainly affects the erythrocytes or red blood corpuscles (RBCs) to break down prematurely, clinically known as hemolysis. The most common problem associated with this disorder is hemolytic anaemia, which occurs when RBCs are broken down faster than the body can replace them. The symptomatic manifestations are paleness, yellowing of the skin and eyes, dark urine, fatigue, shortness of breath and a rapid heart rate to supply the required oxygen. Deficiency of G6PD is often also implicated as a cause of severe neonatal jaundice (Isa *et al.*, 2017).

Hemolytic anaemia in G6PD deficient individuals is often activated by three principal triggers; infections, or as response to certain food or drugs.

Historically, G6PDd was also referred to as 'favisim' coined after the observed hemolytic affect in patients with G6PDd after consumption of fava beans (*Vicia fava*), a type of legume consumed widely containing high contents of divicine, convicine and isouramil-molecules suspected to be highly oxidative (McMillan *et al.*, 1993).

Infections are often implicated as cause of hemolytic anaemia in G6PD deficient patients since during infections the immune system generates an inflammatory reaction releasing considerable amount of ROS. Erythrocytes of the G6PD deficient patients often cannot cope with the high levels of ROS leading to cell lysis.

Several drugs have been reported to be associated with the hemolytic anaemia of G6PD deficient individuals. Few drugs to be avoided by G6PD deficient patients are listed along with considerably safer options to be taken with supervision in Table 23.1, though higher doses may not be advisable. Case by case evaluation is always advisable to assess the potential risk and the benefits of the drugs while since in many cases it is difficult to relate the adverse outcome of the diseases to the drug affect or disease severity.

Table 23.1: Drugs to be avoided or taken with supervision by G6PD-Deficient Patients

Drugs to be Avoided by G6PD-Deficient Patients	*Drugs to be Used with Caution in Therapeutic Doses for Patients with G6PDD*
Diaminodiphenyl sulfone (Dapsone)	Acetaminophen (Tylenol)
Flutamide (Eulexin)	Acetylsalicylic acid (Aspirin)
Furazolidone (Furoxone)	Antazoline (Antistine)
Isobutyl nitrite	Antipyrine
Methylene blue	Ascorbic acid (Vitamin C): intravenous doses only
Niridazole (Ambilhar)	Benzhexol (Artane)
Nitrofurantoin (Furadantin)	Chloramphenicol
Phenazopyridine (Pyridium)	Chlorguanidine (Proguanil, Paludrine) Chloroquine
Primaquine	Colchicine
Rasburicase (Elitek)	Diphenyldramine (Benadryl)
Sulfacetamide	Glyburide (glibenclamide, Diabeta, Glynase)
Sulfanilamide	Isoniazid
Sulfapyridine	L-Dopa
	Quinine
	Streptomycin
	Sulfacytine
	Sulfadiazine
	Sulfaguanidine
	Sulfamethoxazole (Gantanol)
	Sulfisoxazole (Gantrisin)
	Trimethoprim
	Tripelennamine (Pyribenzamine)
	Vitamin K

Source: Luzzatto *et al.*, (2014).

The time frame and the clinical presentation of drug induced hemolysis in G6PD deficient patients has been described fairly well (Youngster *et al.*, 2010). Fatigue is the most common symptom arising due to decrease in RBCs which in advanced state may present as back or abdominal pain. In acute phase jaundice may occur.

Drug induced hemolysis present a typical time frame with hemolysis beginning within 24 hours and continuing up to 10 days after drug discontinuation in some cases. Jaundiced state results after about 50 per cent of the RBCs are haemolysed while onset of haemoglobinuria sets in within the first week. The severity of the haemolysis is dependent on the drug dose and the allelic variant of the G6PD. In severe cases, haematocrit levels can drop to less than 50 per cent of normal. Severe hemolysis may result in acute kidney injury (Youngster *et al.*, 2010).

Generally, the prognosis for G6PD-deficient patients is quite good. Most patients live relatively normal lives as long as they avoid triggers. Many people never experience any symptoms or signs of the presence of this condition. Molecular genotyping methods for epidemiological assessments have predominated in recent years but most estimates of G6PDd prevalence are based on enzyme activity studies in males. Genotyping assessments inform risks for males, but they are less informative for females as the majority of those carrying the G6PDd allele will be heterozygotes and most of these females will test as G6PD normal with the usual screens (detecting <30% of normal activity) but may still be at risk of significant hemolysis (Santana *et al.*, 2013).

Detection of G6PD Deficiency

Several tests can be carried out to detect the prevalence of G6PDd, but only a few tests can detect the G6PDd in heterogygous females reliably. Measuring the production capacity of G6PD by measuring the concentration of NADPH is commonly used for detection of all the variants. The most frequently used test to detect the amount of NADPH production is the fluorescent spot test, spectrophotometric assay and the cytochemical assay. All these tests are based on the production of fluorescence (the fluorescent spot test and the spectrophotometric assay) or colour (cytochemical assay). NADPH fluorescence when it is excited with light of a wavelength of 340 nm, whereas $NADP^+$ does not, and NADPH converts colourless tetrazolium salt into coloured formazan, whereas $NADP^+$ does not. The Brilliant Cresyl Blue (BCB) dye test, based on the reduction of BCB to a colourless state by NADPH, was previously a commonly used test but has largely been replaced by the fluorescent spot test (Beutler, 1994). Metosulfate-3-(4,5-dimethylthiazal-2-yl)-2,5-diphenyltetrazolim bromide test (PMS/MTT test) is commonly used in Asia (Nkhoma *et al.*, 2009).

The Fluorescent Spot Test (FST).

When erythrocytes contain enough functional G6PD, $NADP^+$ is converted into NADPH. A blood spot on filter paper fluoresces when excited at 340 nm after addition of G6P and $NADP^+$ (Beutler, 1984). The fluorescent spot test is reliable for the detection of hemizygous males and homozygous females, but is unreliable for the detection of heterozygous females. The population of healthy erythrocytes converts enough NADP+ into NADPH in heterozygous females (on average 50% of the erythrocytes) to produce fluorescent spots, and then the heterozygous deficiency is missed. A sensitivity of 32 per cent and specificity of 99 per cent has been found for the detection of heterozygously-deficient women. The fluorescent spot test requires a black light (a lamp that emits light of 340 nm only).

The Spectrophotometric Assay

This test requires the use of a spectrophotometer to assess the intensity of the developed colour. It is a reliable test for the detection of hemizygous males and homozygous females. The detection of heterozygous females raises problems, because the population of healthy erythrocytes in these women produces NADPH in a way similar to that seen in the fluorescent spot test. The sensitivity of this test for the detection of heterozygous women is 11, whereas the specificity is 99 per cent.

DNA-based Tests

It became apparent early in the study of G6PDd that there were differences in the characteristics of the residual enzyme in different deficient individuals. Fortunately, the development of a number of PCR-based methods for the detection of known mutations of G6PD has made it possible to detect G6PDd and to identify the specific mutation responsible with relative ease (Lin *et al.*, 2005) and can be used to diagnose homozygous, hemizygous, and heterozygous-deficient patients. The advantage of the method is that DNA samples are much more stable than the enzyme in blood samples, and that very small volumes suffice for diagnosis. Methods of detection include uses specific primer to amplify the exon sequences and the use of restriction endonucleases to cleave naturally occurring restriction sites (Tiskoff *et al.*, 2001) and then analyzing the numbers of DNA segments produced by the specific restriction enzymes. The numbers of DNA segments produced by normal sequence is different than that of mutated sequences. Sequencing of the amplified sequences can also be done to detect individual DNA base mutation detection. The big limitation for this kind of detection is one set of primer being able to detect only one specific mutation. For any novel mutation, the existing primers may not be able to detect it if the mutation is beyond the length of amplified sequence. At the moment, DNA tests can only be used for screening of prevalent mutations. Moreover, DNA-based detection also require expensive sophisticated equipments with skilled personnel to operate them, which makes them unsuitable for use in Third World countries where the problem persist more.

Cytochemical Assay

This test utilizes the staining capacity of individual erythrocytes with G6PD activity by conversion of exogenous G6P and $NADP^+$. The assay is based on the reduction of water-soluble colourless tetranitro blue tetrazolium to its water-insoluble dark-coloured formazan by NADPH via the electron carrier 1-methoxyphenazine methosulfate (Van Noorden *et al.*, 1982). Erythrocytes that contain G6PD activity will have dark-purple granules, whereas G6PD-deficient erythrocytes will remain unstained. The percentage of stained and unstained cells can be determined by light microscopy. However, the drawback is the unreliability caused due to the leakage of coloured end-products from healthy erythrocytes and unstained cells into the medium. Optimization of the staining procedure improves the reliability of the test.

The cytochemical assay can be used for detection of hemizygously, homozygously, and heterozygously-deficient patients reliably because it shows G6PD activity in individual erythrocytes. This assay is time consuming and manual intensive, however, with the development of flow cytometric methods evaluation of stained and unstained cells can be determined objectively. Even though the assay is expensive and technically difficult and not convenient for routine use.

The Deficiency of G6PD and Its Relationship with Malaria

Malaria is a major killer disease worldwide with high mortality rates among children. Of the five malarial species of *Plasmodium; P. falciparum, P. vivax, P. malariae, P. ovale* and *P. knowlesi*, identified for infections in human, *P falciparum* is the deadliest. *P falciparum* kills >1 million children in Africa alone every year. It approximately kills one person every 30 second. At least 500 million people are currently infected with *P. falciparum*. It is estimated to cause about half a billion episodes of disease each year and at least two billion people are at risk. The emergence of agriculture is associated with the epidemic spread of malaria (especially *P. falciparum*). Thus malaria is the strongest known selective force in the recent history of mankind. A number of polymorphisms associated with erythrocyte cell surface oligoproteins (blood groups), globin genes (HbS, HbC, HbE, thalassemias, oxidative stress (G6PDd), cytoadherence and immune system have been associated with protection against malaria (Kwiatkowski, 2005).

The geographical prevalence pattern of G6PDd correspondence with that of malarial endmicity or previously malaria endemic regions. G6PDd is seen geographically dominant in Africa, Middle East, Asia and Mediterranean. A prevalence of more than 10 per cent has been summarized in Africa and Southeast Asian countries where *Plasmodium falciparum* is endemic. The prevalence of G6PDd in malaria-endemic countries range from very low (e.g., the Democratic Republic of Korea) to over 30 per cent (Recht *et al.*, 2018). In many cases, it is also observed to be site specific, e.g. in Indonesia. A positive correlation occurred between the prevalence of malaria and G6PDd: coastal (5.9%) *versus* inland (0.2%) for malaria ($p<0.001$), and 6.7 per cent and 3.1 per cent for G6PDd ($p<0.001$) at coastal and inland sites, respectively (Satyagraha *et al.*, 2015). In contrast, places like Japan, Northern China and Northern Europe where malaria was historically not endemic; the recorded prevalence is less than 0.1 per cent (Matsuoka *et al.*, 2005). Although a prevalence of 10 per cent is recorded in the USA, but the affected men are of African or Mediterranean origin (Nkhoma *et al.*, 2009).

The geographical overlap of G6PD with malarial endemicity has led to hypothesis that the prevalence of G6PDd provides partial protection to malarial infection, although it predisposes deficient individuals to hemolysis (Ruwende *et al.*, 1995). Homogygous deficient females and hemigygous deficient males were observed to be less sick while infected with the malaria parasite than the G6PD normal individuals which possibly is due to the fact that *Plasmodium* can proliferate less competently in the erythrocytes (Roth *et al.*, 1988). A negative association between G6PDd and hypreparasitemia has been observed while such observations were not made in cases with cerebral malaria. African populations exhibit a negative association of malaria and G6PDd as compared to Asian and other continents (Mbanefo *et al.*, 2017) which may be due to the reason that in Africa, G6PD deficient patients having higher enzyme activity and milder consequences than the patients from the Mediterranean or Asia (Scriver *et al.*, 2001). Malaria infection involving the *P. vivax* in general have no association with G6PDd, however, exceptional isolated cases exist (Louicharoen *et al.*, 2009, Khim *et al.*, 2013).

Deficiency of G6PD can prevent malaria infection but as the infection continues the parasite can adapt itself to produce its own G6PD which then renders the patient susceptible to malarial infection. *Plasmodium* protozoans preferentially attack immature RBC but *P. falciparum* can invade RBC of all ages. *Plasmodium* oxidizes RBC NADPH from the Pentose Phosphate pathway for its metabolism. This results in a deficiency of RBC GSH, most severe in G6PD deficient individuals, leading to peroxide-induced hemolysis which curtails the development of *Plasmodium* (Ruwende *et al.*, 1995). However, after several cell cycles the *Plasmodium* can adapt to produce its own G6PD, reducing the adaptive benefit of G6PDd. Chronic acute malaria causes anaemia and in case of individuals with G6PDd, the malarial infection can be complicated due to usage of antimalaria drugs like primaquine or dapsone leading to life threatening acute intravascular hemolysis followed by acute renal failure and anaemia (Wickramasinghe and Adballa, 2000). These drugs produce severe reactions in severely deficient individuals and can also cause the oxidation of haemoglobin, making it lose the ability to be a reversible oxygen carrier (Tripathy and Reddy, 2007).

Several countries of Central and South America like Mexico, Belize, Costa Rica, Dominican Republic, Ecuador, El Salvador are already in the process of malaria elimination. While Argentina is in the path of elimination of reintroduction phase, Paraguay is pushing for malaria free certification and malaria has re-emerged in Venezuela as public health services weakened. With the exception of French Guiana, all countries currently prescribe primaquine as the *P. falciparum* gamaetocytocide. Primaquine though not frequently used for malaria management may be used as combination therapy with artemisin derivatives leading to undetected G6PD deficient individual to go through hemolytic anaemia in malaria endemic areas. WHO recommends that G6PD deficient patients with *P. ovale* or *P. vivax* malaria should not be given daily dose of primaquine, these patients may receive primaquine once weekly @ 0.75 mg/kg for 8 weeks instead to prevent relapse, provided close medical supervision is available for managing any signs of acute hemolytic anaemia (WHO, 2015). The majority of G6PDd cases are reported from the Amazon region and a heterogenous number of variants with majority being the G6PD A-variant. There are limited data on the distribution of G6PDd variants in areas where malaria is endemic. In Brazil as revised guidelines comes up, this will be lowered to 0.25 mg/kg while Colombia has just updated the national malaria treatment guidelines to include primaquine single dose.

In regions of East Asia and Oceania, where malaria relapse rate is high (>50%) radical cure effectively halves the incidence of vivax malaria which is a considerable advantage. WHO (2015) recommends a higher dose of primaquine (0.5 mg/kg/day) dose in most countries except for Malaysia, Myanmar and the Phillipines where a lower dose of 0.25 mg/kg/day is still practiced. Sri Lanka was certified malaria free in 2016 and is currently engaged in prevention of the re-introduction phase. China, Malaysia, Bhutan, the Republic of Korea and the Democratic People's Republic of Korea, Iran and Saudi Arabia are in the elimination phase. Except the Indian subcontinent where many countries use primaquine as the major anti-malarial drug, primaquine is rarely used by the private practitioners (Phok *et al.*, 2017). The adherence of 14 day radical treatment regime is dependent on circumstance and education practices and have been observed in Thailand, Indonesia, Pakistan, India, Brazil (Recht *et al.*, 2018).

Although typical Asian variants would be expected to have a high haemolytic anaemia risk during radical cure treatment with primaquine, apart from the A-, Mahidol, Viangchan, and

Mediterranean variants, there is very limited quantitative information on hemolysis in the different G6PDd variants. Although use of primaquine in radical treatment regime involves a great risk of hemolysis for individuals with G6PDd, but at the same time the treated patients do have substantial benefits (Luzzato and Seneca, 2014). The risks are analytically overestimated due to results derived from studies mostly on healthy subjects. The testing of G6PDd is officially although recommended in many countries before administration of malaria treatment, in reality, due to lack of infrastructure and inadequate logistics the practice is not regular, leaving clinicians to make their own decisions. Places where testing for G6PDd is not available, the patient management approach should then be considered taking the patients ethinicity and origin into account, the degree of anaemia and the availability of provision of blood transfusion in case of severe hemolysis (WHO, 2015).

Epidemiology of G6PDd and Its Variants

The deficiency of G6PD is recognized as the most common enzymopathy and affects around 400 million people worldwide (Vulliamy *et al.*, 1998). It is, however, very difficult to identify the deficient individuals since most deficient individuals are asymptomatics till they are exposed to triggers. Females are homogygously deficient or heterogygously deficient but males are hemigygously deficient and thus it is expressed commonly in males. The severity of G6PDd is categorized in four classes (WHO, 1989; Beutler, 1994); Class I or severe (chronic non-spherocytic anemia), Class II or intermediate (less than 10% of normal enzyme activity), Class II or mild (10%-60% of normal enzyme activity) and Class IV or asymptomatic (60%-100% of normal enzyme activity). A fifth class with higher enzyme activity may also be considered (Beutler, 1996).

The frequency of this disorder varies greatly among different populations. G6PD A which is a Class III mutation with a gene frequency of 11 per cent is recorded more frequently in African and Afro-Americans, Asians and Colombians (Valencia *et al.*, 2016). The large region of Middle East with its large diverse populations harbours a wide selection of G6PDd variants. Although the prevalence of G6PDd is lower in the region than the malaria endemic countries of Africa, it ranges from 10 per cent to 17 per cent. A severe form of Class II variant, G6PD B is observed more among the Mediterranean and the Middle Eastern.

The severe G6PD Mediterranean, another Class II variant predominates over much of Europe, the Middle East, and West and Central Asia. Patients with this variant are at risk of aggressive hemolysis if repeated doses of primaquine are administered (Beutler, 1996). Frequency of G6PD Mediterranean, varies between 2-20 per cent in Greece, Turkey and Italy and the highest prevalence of 70 per cent is recorded among the Kurdish Jews (Nkhoma *et al.*, 2009).

The G6PDd A-variant, the most prevalent in Africa and the Americas is generally considered mild though it may sometimes cause severe hemolysis. In Asia and Oceania, numerous variants have been recorded which are more severe than the G6PD A-. Though less prevalent, these variants are more severe in manifestation. Several of the common Asian variants like the Viangchan, Kaiping, Coimbra, Mediterranean, Vallodolid, Union and Gaohe have been categorized as severely deficient groups (Howes *et al.*, 2013).

The Indian Neighbourhood

The Indian neighbourhood generally shows an influence of genetic makeup, ethnicity and geographical area on the distribution of the G6PDd variants. Almost all of the G6PD-deficient cases detected in Laos, Cambodia, Vietnam and Malaysian are G6PD Viangchan, while in many other countries G6PD Mahidol dominates the share (Table 23.2).

In Vietnam, the incidence of G6PDd varies between the northern and southern areas and ethnicities. In southern Vietnam, there is a high prevalence of G6PDd among ethnic Kinh (8.7%) and S'tieng (14%), living in areas which are or were highly endemic for malaria. In Northern Vietnam, where malaria transmission is lower, G6PDd is virtually absent. At least ten variants have been detected (Matsouka et al, 2007, Heu *et al.*, 2009) in which eight different polymorphisms were identified of which six resulted in an amino acid substitutions and three were novel mutations. The major G6PD variants present are G6PD Viangchan and G6PD Mahidol. Two of the novel mutations; Vietnam1 and Vietnam2 exist among the ethnic Kinh Vietnamese. G6PD Viangchan, common throughout South-East Asia, accounted for 77 per cent of the variants and is significantly associated with haemoglobinuria (Heu *et al.*, 2009).

Table 23.2: G6PDd prevalence in India and its neighbouring malaria endemic countries (Modified from Recht *et al.*, 2018)

Countries	*Estimated G6PDd*	*Prevalence for common G6PDd variants*
Thailand	>13%–17%	Mahidol, Viangchan, Canton, Kaiping, Mediterranean, Songklanagarind, Union, Vanua Lava, Chinese-5, Gaohe, Kerala Kalyan, Quing Yan
Malayasia	>7%–10%	Andalus, Canton, Chatham, Coimbra, Kaiping, Mediterranean, Namouru, Nankang, Union, Vanua Lava, Viangchan Jammu, Chinese-5, Gaohe, Mahidol, Orissa, Quing Yan
Myanmar	>3%–7%	Mahidol, Canton, Coimbra, Viangchan Jammu, Kaiping, Mediterranean, Union, Valladolid, Kerala Kalyan
Lao People's Democratic Republic	>13%–17%	Viangchan
Cambodia	>13%–17%	Viangchan, Kaiping, Canton, Valladolid, Mahidol, A-
Vietnam	>7%–10%	Viangchan, Canton, Kaiping, Union, Bao Loc, Coimbra,Chinese-5, Gaohe, Mahidol, Quing Yan
Bangladesh	>3%–7%	
Nepal	>3%–7%	Mediterranean
India	>7%–10%	Mediterranean, Kerala-Kalyan, Odisha, Chatham, Coimbra, Namouru, Nilgiri, Odisha
Pakistan	>13%–17%	Mediterranean, Chatham, Odisha
Afghanistan	7%–10%	Mediterranean
Iran	>10%–13%	Mediterranean, Chatham, Cosenza
China	>3%–7%	Kaiping, Canton, Gaohe, Chinese-5, Quing Yan, Chinese-1,Coimbra, Fushan, Haikou, Hechi, Liuzhou, Miaoli, Nankang, Songklanagarind, Taipei, Taipei Hakka, Union, Valladolid, Viangchan, A, Guangzhou, Keelung, Mahidol, Nanning, Quing Yan, Ube Konan

G6PD mutations are often found to be ethnic-specific in Thailand. A prevalence rate of 14.2 per cent is recorded in the Thai population, G6PD Mahidol being the most common at 38.1 per cent, followed by G6PD Vaingchan (19%), G6PD Chinese 4 (14.3%), G6PD Canton (9.5%), G6PD Union (9.5%), G6PD Kaiping (4.8%) and G6PD Gaohe (4.8%) (Phompradit *et al.*, 2011; Kanchanavithayakul *et al.*, 2017).

In Indonesia, variant prevalence exhibits geographical and ethnic specification. In the Flores and Palue Islands, the prevalence rate of G6PDd is lower in five ethnic groups, namely Manggarai, Bajawa, Nage-Keo, Larantuka, and Palue than the native Sikka or non-native Riung. On the islands of West Timor, Sumba, Sulawesi, Muna and Bangka, G6PD Vanua Lava of Melanesian origin was more commonly detected among the natives Timorese, Sumbanese, Savunese, Kendari, Buton, Muna, Minahasa, and Sangirese (Tantular *et al.*, 2010). In the Sumba Island in eastern Indonesia, G6PDd was observed to be site specific for coastal at 6.7 per cent *versus* inland at 3.1 per cent for the dominant variants of G6PD Vanua Lava, Viangchan, and Chatham, accounting for 98.5 per cent (Satyagraha *et al.*, 2015).

G6PD Viangchan is the predominant variant in Cambodia, among the migrant Cambodian labourers with a prevalence rate of 26.1 per cent while among the native Cambodians, it accounts for the 82.4 per cent of the deficient populations followed by G6PD Union, and G6PD Coimbra (Louicharoen *et al.*, 2009).

Nearer home, in Myanmar, G6PD Mahidol is the predominant variant (68%) among the different populations of Myanmar, followed by Kaiping (18%), Viangchan (6%), Mediterranean (4%), Union (2%) and Canton (2%) (Lee *et al.*, 2018). Among the native Burmese of the country, G6PD Mahidol is encountered almost 96.2 per cent of the time among the deficient population, rest shared by G6PD variants Canton, Coimbra, Viangchan Jammu, Kaiping, Mediterranean, Union, Valladolid, Kerala-Kalyan (Phompradit *et al.*, 2011). In the border regions of China-Myanmar, the ethnic Kachin are 9.6 per cent G6PD deficient and G6PD Mahidol was most frequent variant at 89.7 per cent, followed by Kaiping at 8.0 per cent and Viangchan at 2.2 per cent. G6PD Canton and Chinese 4 are also present among 1.1 per cent of the population (Li *et al.*, 2015). Although, G6PD Mahidol is classed as moderate (Class III; 10%–60% residual activity), it indicates severity similar to the G6PD Viangchan variant (common in Lao PDR and Eastern Thailand (Bancone *et al.*, 2019).

The prevalence of G6PDd among the different ethnicities in Nepal is 3 per cent to 7 per cent. In the malaria endemic districts, G6PDd among the ethnic Rajbanshi and Tharu is 11.7 per cent and 5.6 per cent respectively. On geographical assessment, higher prevalence of G6PDd was also found in Jhapa (9.8%) and Morang districts (8%) (Ghimire *et al.*, 2017)

G6PDd Status in India

G6PDd was reported from India more than 50 years ago from the Parsi population of Mumbai in the year 1963 (Baxi *et al.*, 1963). The prevalence of G6PDd varies from 2.3 per cent to 31.4 per cent among different castes, ethnic and linguistic groups with an overall rate of 7.7 per cent and the highest prevalence of 31.4 per cent recorded among the Gamit tribe of Western India. The government has tried to map G6PDd more accurately in the highly diverse Indian population. The distribution of G6PDd, when assessed according to natural regions and climatic regions, the frequency was recorded high in the Himalayan regions (0.087) as compared to non-Himalayan region (0.043). In general, the frequency of G6PDd is comparatively higher in North and West India, indicating substantial stability of the allele in these areas; while in the Southern India it is uniformly low except in the states of Andhra Pradesh and Tamil Nadu, not much data are available from the East. So far several different G6PD variants are reported from India, including G6PD Mediterranean, G6PD Odisha, G6PD Andhra Pradesh, G6PD Cutch, G6PD Jammu, G6PD Kerala-Kalyan, G6PD Porbandar, G6PD Chatham, G6PD Insuli, G6PD Coimbra, and G6PD West Bengal.

The frequency of G6PD is reported to be higher among the tribal communities (0.055) in India as compared to other ethnic groups and social stratifications (Bhasin and Walter, 2001; Sukumar *et al.*, 2004; Bhasin 2006; Kumar *et al.*Odisha 2016). The ethnic tribal groups in India form a major fraction of the Indian population at 8.01 per cent. A total of 461 tribal communities have been identified (Singh and Rajyalakshmi, 1993) and are believed to be the earliest settlers or inhabitants of the region. Tribals in India are classified based on their ethnic, racial and linguistic origin, socio-economic status and cultural prototype. This group of the population speak about 750 dialects belonging to one of the four larger language groups, Indo-European, Austro-Asiatic, Tibeto-Burman and Dravidian (Kosambi 1991, Singh and Rajyalakshmi, 1993). Comparatively a higher prevalence rate (>10%) of the G6PDd is observed among the tribal groups of Nagaland, Chhattisgarh, West Bengal, Odisha, Dadra and Nagar Haveli and Gujarat followed by Himachal Pradesh, Uttarakhand, Andhra Pradesh and Madhya Pradesh with a uniformly low frequencies (<5%). In the western India in the states of Rajasthan, Gujarat, Dadra and Nagar Haveli and Maharashtra. The prevalance rate of G6PDd ranges from 1.4 to 31.4 among the different tribal groups with considerable heterogeneity of the variants. The ethnic Gamit has the highest recorded prevalence of India (31.4%), followed by the Dhelki Kharia (30.4%), Dhankas (20.4%), Warlis (19.6%), Dhodias (17.8%), Bhils (16.3%), Garasiyas (15.2%) and Madia (14.4%). A complete absence of the gene was observed among the Mahadev Kolis from Ahmadnagar district in Maharashtra (Jain *et al.,* 1981; Rao and Gorakshar, 1990; Mukherjee *et al.,* 1993; Gupte *et al.,* 2005; Choubisa, 2009, ICMR, 2010). A highest prevalence is among the Vataliya Prajapati (27.9%) when stratified along caste and language. The Kutchi Bhanushalis recorded at 13 per cent and the Parsis at 15.7 per cent (Gupte *et al.,* 2005; Kumar at al., 2016)

In the states of Central India comprising Madhya Pradesh and Chattisgarh, the prevalence of G6PDd among the major tribal Gonds varies from 13.0 per cent to 21.3 per cent. Among the Bhils, the prevalence is 3.4 per cent to 6.7 per cent (Mukherjee *et al.,* 2015) Higher prevalence rate is also detected amongst the Kawars (21.5%), Baiga (14.2%) and Oraons (13.4%) (Kaeda *et al.,* 1995.).

Data from Northern India and Southern India is unexpectedly low and does not present a comprehensive picture. Few studies available report the prevalence among the Meghwal-Chamar and the Punjabi Khatris at 15.1 per cent and 14 per cent respectively. In the Southern India, in the state of Andhra Pradesh, G6PDd prevalence range from 6.1 per cent to 13 per cent. Tribals in the Nilgiris show a prevalence of 10.6 per cent and Kurumba tribe of Kerela records a 11.9 per cent (Kumar *et al.,* 2016)

In the state of West Bengal in Eastern India, G6PDd has been recorded among the Santals from Midnapore district. The deficiency of G6PD is very high (6-16%) among the tribal populations in districts of Chhattisgarh and Odisha. In Odisha, the overall prevalence rate varies within 1.3 per cent to 17.4 per cent. Very high frequency is recorded among the Parajas (17.4%), Juangas (17.6%), Kondhas (12.5%), Bhumizs (12.2%) and Kolhas (10.7%) (Mukherjee *et al.*, 2015).

Among the different tribal population of the North East India, the incidence of G6PD deficiency is found to be 17.5 per cent among the Mizos of Mizoram, 8 per cent among the Khasis of Meghalaya, 6 per cent among the Nishis, 5 per cent among the Apatani and 3 per cent among the Adi tribes of Arunachal Pradesh. Prevalence of 15 per cent is found among the mixed group of other Arunachal tribes (Tripathy and Reddy, 2007). In the state of Assam, the Bodo tribe showed a prevalence of 19 per cent followed by the Rabhas (15.8%) and Mikirs (15.6%). In the Angami Nagas, a tribal group of Nagaland, prevalence of G6PDd was found to be high at 27.1 per cent (Seth and Seth, 1971). A recent unpublished data from the author showed a low overall G6PDd prevalence rate of 3.06 per cent among the different tribes of Assam ranging between 7.69 per cent among the Ahoms, 5.21 per cent among the Assamese caste, 2.7 per cent among the tribe Dimasa and 1.59 per cent among the Bodos.The prevalence of G6PDd in India is not related closely to malaria endemicity; in central India, where 50 per cent of *P. falciparum* malaria cases occur, the prevalence of G6PDd is 6.1 per cent (Bhasin and Walter, 2001). G6PD variants exhibit ethnic specificity as well and different variants may dominate in different groups. Overall, G6PD Mediterranean appears to be the most common deficient variant (60.4%), followed by Kerala-Kalyan (24.5%) and Odisha (13.3%) (Sukumar et. al., 2004). G6PD Namoru is the major polymorphic variant in the tribal populations in southern India (Chalvam *et al.*, 2007). The prevalence of G6PDd as well as molecular variants of the G6PD gene is highly heterogeneous among the tribal population of Odisha (Nishank *et al.*, 2008). Lesser known variant, like the G6PD Kalyan among tribal population inhabiting Bombya and G6PD Kerela among the Indians living in Pacific North-west of America have also been reported (Ahulwalia *et al.*, 1992). G6PD Jamnagar was found to be associated with drug-induced haemolytic anaemia whereas G6PD Rohini was also described during a population survey (Sukumar *et al.*, 2005).

Novel Variants from India

Molecular analysis of the variants among the deficient population revealed a number of novel variants from India. The variant G6PD Jammu with substitution at nt 871 (G > A) (Beutler *et al.*, 1991) and variant Chatnam (aa 335 Ala > Thr)(Vulliamy *et al.*, 1998) were reported first from India. A variant reported among males of Indian decent in South Africa was designated as G6PD Porbandar (Cayanis *et al.*, 1977). The variant G6PD Namoru (208 T > C) was characterized from tribal population of Southern India (Chalvam *et al.*, 2008). G6PD Kalyan was described from a Koli male (Ishwad and Naik, 1984) and G6PD Rohini from a Marathi male (Sayyed *et al.*, 1992) , both from the state of Maharashtra. However, later it was found that four variants Kerala, Kalyan, Rohini and Jamnagar are same in terms of nucleotide substitutions (nt 949 G > A, resulting in the same amino acid substitution (aa 317 Glu > Lys) and is now designated as Kerala-Kalyan. A very polymorphic variant co-existing among the tribes of Odisha living in hyper endemic zones of malaria and similar to or with more or less 10-20 per cent of the normal enzyme activity and normal electrophoretic mobility was named, G6PD Odisha (Kaeda *et al.*, 1995). A novel G>A mutation in the nt 593 of the exon 6 with a frequency 10 per cent among the Tribals in the Nilgiri hills was designated G6PD Nilgiri (Chalvam *et al.*, 2008). A new variant G6PD Insuli was also reported from India (Sukumar *et al.*, 2003).

The globally dominant G6PD Meditarrean variant differs in India than the European population. The Indian sub-variant is characterized by mutation at nt 563 C > T, whereas in the European population it is characterized by nt 1311 C > T. Because of this difference in the mutation of the nucleotide position, it is theorized that G6PD Mediterranean is evolved independently in Asia and Europe though both the mutation are found in India (Sukumar *et al.*, 2004). The deficiency of G6PD is maternally inherited and mostly male children are effected and rarely homogygous females. The effected individual is often at great risk of haemolytic anaemia in certain stress condition regarding certain food items and drug usage. Enforcement of a mandatory screening for G6PD along with other routine blood test for neonates may reduce the risk factor tremendously. The record of the medical history would be very handy for future references for prescription of drugs in course of disease treatment and more so in malaria endemic areas though in India G6PDd prevalence is not found related to malaria endemicity. The population of India being so diverse in terms of origin and ethnicities, a detailed study of the G6PD variant prevalence is also felt necessary since not many studies have been done. Variant studies may present a more comprehensive data in relation to the severity of the disorders among the different ethnicities and social background.

REFERENCES

Achoubi, N., Asghar, M., Meitei, S.Y., Sachdeva, M.P. *et al.* 2010. "Haemoglobinopathies and glucose-6-phosphate dehydrogenase deficiency in a malaria endemic region of Manipur, Northeast India." *Anthropol Sci.* **118**(3): 201-204.

Ahluwalia, A., Corcoran, C.M., Vulliamy, T.J., Ishwad, C.S., Naidu, J.M., *et al.* 1992. "G6PD Kalyan and G6PD Kerala; two deficient variants in India caused by the same 317 Glu—>Lys mutation." *Hum Mol Genet.* **1**(3): 209–210.

Bancone, G., Menard, D., Khim, N., Kim, S., Canier, L. et al, 2019. "Molecular characterization and mapping of glucose-6-phosphate dehydrogenase (G6PD) mutations in the Greater Mekong Subregion." *Malar J.* **18**(1), 20. https://doi.org/10.1186/s12936-019-2652-y

Baxi, A.J., Balakrishnan, V., Undevia, J.V., Sanghvi, L.D. 1963. "Glucose-6-phosphate dehydrogenase deficiency in the Parsee community, Bombay." *Indian J Med Sci.* **17**: 493-500.

Beutler, E. and Vulliamy, T.J. 2002. "Hematologically Important Mutations: Glucose-6-phosphate Dehydrogenase." *Blood, Cells, Mol, Dis.* **28**: 93-103, https://doi.org/10.1006/bcmd.2002.0490.

Beutler, E., Westwood, B., Kuhl, W. 1991. "Definition of the Mutations of G6PD Wayne, G6PD Viangchan, G6PD Jammu, and G6PD 'Lejeune'." *Acta Haematol.* **86**: 179-182. doi: 10.1159/000204830.

Beutler, E. 1994. "G6PD deficiency." *Blood.* **84**: 3613–3636.

Beutler, E. 1996. "G6PD: population genetics and clinical manifestations." *Blood Rev.* **10**(1): 45-52.

Beutler, E. 1984. *Red Cell Metabolism: A Manual of Biochemical Methods*, 3rd edn. Grune and Strattan, New York.

Bhasin, M.K. 2006. "Genetics of castes and tribes of India: glucose- 6-phosphate dehydrogenase deficiency and abnormal haemoglobins (HbS and HbE)." *Inter J Hum Gen.* **6**(1): 49–72.

Bhasin, M.K., Walter, H. 2001. *Genetics of castes and tribes in India.* Kamla-Raj Enterprises: Delhi.

Cayanis, E., Lane, A.B., Jenkins, T., Nurse, G.T., Balinsky, D. 1977. "Glucose-6-Phosphate Dehydrogenase pobandar: A new slow variant with slightly reduced activity in a South African family of Indian descent." *Biochem Genet.* **15**: 765-773. https://doi,org/10.1007/BF00484102.

Chalvam, R., Kedar, P.S., Colah, R.B., Ghosh, E.K., Mukherjee, B. 2008. "A novel R198H mutation in the glucose-6-phosphate dehydrogenase gene in the tribal groups of the Nilgiris in Southern India." *Hum Genet.* **53**: 181–184.

Chalvam, R., Mukherjee, M.B., Colah, R.B., Mohanty, D., Ghosh, K. 2007. "G6PD Namoru (208 T'! C) is the major polymorphic variant in the tribal populations in southern India." *British Journal of Haematology.* **136**: 512-513. doi:10.1111/j.1365-2141.2006.06463.x.

Choubisa, S.L. 2009. "Sickle cell haemoglobin, thalassaemia and G-6-PD enzyme deficiency genes in Garasiya tribe inhabited malaria endemic areas of Sirohi district, Rajasthan (India)." *J Commun Dis.* **41**: 13-18.

Ghimire, P., Singh, N., Ortega, L. *et al.* 2017. "Glucose-6-phosphate dehydrogenase deficiency in people living in malaria endemic districts of Nepal." *Malar J.* **16**: 214.

Gupte, S.C., Patel, P.U., Ranat, J.M. 2005. "G6PD deficiency in Vataliya Prajapati community settled in Surat." *Indian J Med Sci.* **59**(2): 51-56.

Howes, R.E., Dewi, M., Piel, F.B., Monteiro, W.M., Battle, K.E., *et al.* 2013. "Spatial distribution of G6PD deficiency variants across malaria-endemic regions." *Malar J.* **12**(1): 418–419.

Hue, N.T., Charlieu, J.P., Chau, T.T. *et al.* 2009. "Glucose-6-phosphate dehydrogenase (G6PD) mutations and haemoglobinuria syndrome in the Vietnamese population." *Malar J.* **8**: 152. https://doi.org/10.1186/1475-2875-8-152.

Indian Council of Medical Research (ICMR). 2010. Report of the ICMR Multicentric Task Force on Intervention programme for nutritional anaemia and haemoglobinopathies amongst some primitive tribal populations of India.

Isa, H.M., Mohamed, M.S., Mohamed, A.M., Abdulla, A., Abdulla, F. 2017. "Neonatal indirect hyperbilirubinemia and glucose-6-phosphate dehydrogenase deficiency." *Korean J Pediatr.* **60**(4): 106–111. doi:10.3345/kjp.2017.60.4.106.

Ishwad, C.S. and Naik, S.N. 1984. "A new glucose-6-phosphate dehydrogenase variant (G-6-PD Kalyan) found in a Koli family." *Hum Gen.* **66**(2-3): 171-175.

Jain, R.C., Mehta, J., Mehta, N.L., Joshi, K.C., Gupta, O.P., Andrew, A.M. 1981. "Sickle cell trait, thalassaemia and glucose-6-phosphate dehydrogenase deficiency in the Bhil tribe of Southern Rajasthan." *Indian J Med Res.* **73**: 548–53.

Kaeda, J.S., Chhotray, G.P., Ranjit, M.R., Bautista, J.M., Reddy, P.H., Stevensm J., *et al.* 1995. "A new glucose-6-phosphate dehydrogenase variant G6PD Orissa (44 Ala→Gly) is the major polymorphic variant in tribal populations in India." *Am J Hum Genet.* **57**: 1335-1341.

Kanchanavithayakul, A., Prasittisa, K., Kiat-Amornrak, P., Chanda, M. Nuchprayoon, I., Cheepsunthorn, C.L. 2017. "Prevalence of glucose 6-phosphate dehydrogenase deficiency and genetic mutations among

Karen and Lao Populations in Thailand." *The Southeast Asian J Trop Med Pub Hlth.* **48**(6): 1308-1317.

Khim, N., Benedet, C., Kim, S., Kheng, S., Siv, S. et al. 2013. "G6PD deficiency in *Plasmodium falciparum* and *Plasmodium vivax* malaria-infected Cambodian patients." *Malar J.* **12:** 171 https://doi.org/10.1186/1475-2875-12-171.

Kosambi, D.D. 1991. *The culture and civilization of ancient India in historical outline.* New Delhi: Vikas Publishing House.

Kumar, P., Yadav, U., Rai, V. 2016. "Prevalence of glucose-6-phosphate dehydrogenase deficiency in India: An updated meta-analysis." *Egyptian Journal of Medical Human Genetics.* **17**(3): 295-302. https://doi.org/10.1016/j.ejmhg.2016.01.004.

Kwiatkowski, D.P. 2005. "How malaria has affected the human genome and what human genetics can teach us about malaria." *Am J Hum Genet.* **77**: 171-90.

Lee, J., Kim, T.I., Kang, J., Jun, H., Giang, H., *et al.* 2018. "Prevalence of glucose-6-phosphate dehydrogenase (G6PD) deficiency among malaria patients in Upper Myanmar." *BMC Infect Dis.* **18**:131 https://doi.org/10.1186/s12879-018-3031-y.

Li, Q., Yang, F., Liu, R., Luo, L., Yang, Y., Zhang, L., *et al.* 2015. "Prevalence and Molecular Characterization of Glucose-6-Phosphate Dehydrogenase Deficiency at the China-Myanmar Border." *PLoS ONE* **10**(7): e0134593. https://doi.org/10.1371/journal.pone.0134593.

Lin, Z., Fontaine, J.M., Freer, D.E., Naylor, E.W. 2005. "Alternative DNA-based newborn screening for glucose-6-phosphate dehydrogenase deficiency." *Molecular Genetics and Metabolism.* **86**: 212-219. https://doi.org/10.1016/j.ymgme.2005.05.008.

Louicharoen, C., Patin, E., Paul, R., Nuchprayoon, I., Witoonpanich, B. *et al.* 2009. "Positively selected G6PD-Mahidol mutation reduces Plasmodium vivax density in Southeast Asians. Science." **326**: 1546–1549.

Luzzatto, L. and Seneca, E. 2014. "G6PD deficiency: a classic example of pharmacogenetics with on-going clinical implications." *Br J Haematol* **164**(4): 469–480.

Luzzatto, L. and Seneca, E. 2014. "G6PD deficiency: a classic example of pharmacogenetics with on-going clinical implications." *Brit J Hematol.* **164**(4): 469–480. https://doi.org/10.1111/bjh.12665

Matsuoka, H., Nguon, C., Kanbe, T. *et al.* 2005. "Glucose-6-phosphate dehydrogenase (G6PD) mutations in Cambodia: G6PD Viangchan (871G>A) is the most common variant in the Cambodian population." *J Hum Genet.* **50**: 468-472. https://doi.org/10.1007/s10038-005-0279-z.

Mbanefo, E.C., Ahmed, A.M., Titouna, A., *et al.* 2017. "Association of glucose-6-phosphate dehydrogenase deficiency and malaria: a systematic review and meta-analysis." *Sci Rep.* **7**:45963. doi:10.1038/srep45963.

McMillan, D.C., Bolchoz, L.J., Jollow, D.J. 2001. "Favism: effect of divicine on rat erythrocyte sulfhydryl status, hexose monophosphate shunt activity, morphology and membrane skeletal proteins." *Toxicol. Sci.* **62**: 353-359.

Mukherjee, M.B., Colah, R.B., Martin, S., Ghosh, K. 2015. "Glucose-6-phosphate dehydrogenase (G6PD) deficiency among tribal populations of India—Country scenario." *Ind J Med Res.* **141**(5), 516–520. https://doi.org/10.4103/0971-5916.159499.

Mukherjee, M.B., Gangakhedkar, R.R., Sathe M.S. 1993. "Abnormal haemoglobin, G6PD deficiency and their pattern of interaction in the tribal population of Valsad district (Gujarat)." *Indian J Hematol Blood Transf.* **11**: 227-31.

Nishank, S.S., Chhotray, G.P., Kar, S.K., Ranjit, M.R. 2008. "Molecular variants of G6PD deficiency among certain tribal communities of Orissa, India." *Ann Hum Biol.* **35**: 355-61.

Nkhoma, E.T., Poole, C., Vannappagari, V., Hall, S.A., Beutler, E. 2009. "The global prevalence of glucose-6-phosphate dehydrogenase deficiency: A systematic review and meta-analysis." *Blood Cells, Mol, Dis.* **42**(3): 267-278. https://doi.org/10.1016/j.bcmd.2008.12.005.

Persico, M.G., Viglietto, G., Martini, G., *et al.* 1986. "Isolation of human glucose-6-phosphate dehydrogenase (G6PD) cDNA clones: primary structure of the protein and unusual 5' non-coding region [published correction appears in Nucleic Acids Res 1986 Oct 10;14(19):7822]." *Nucleic Acids Res.* **14**(6): 2511–2522. doi:10.1093/nar/14.6.2511

Phok, S., Phanalasy, S., Thein, S.T., Likhitsup, A. 2017. "Private sector opportunities and threats to achieving malaria elimination in the Greater Mekong Subregion: Results from malaria outlet surveys in Cambodia, the Lao PDR, Myanmar, and Thailand." *Malar J.* **16**(1): 180.

Phompradit, P., Kuesap, J., Chaijaroenkul, W. *et al.* 2011. "Prevalence and distribution of glucose-6-phosphate dehydrogenase (G6PD) variants in Thai and Burmese populations in malaria endemic areas of Thailand." *Malar J.* **10**:368 https://doi.org/10.1186/1475-2875-10-368.

Rao, V.R., Gorakshakar, A.C. 1990. Sickle cell hemoglobin, β- thalassemia and G6PD deficiency in tribes of Maharashtra, India." *Gene Geogr.* **4**: 131-134.

Recht, J., Ashley, E.A., White, N.J. 2018. "Use of primaquine and glucose-6-phosphate dehydrogenase deficiency testing: Divergent policies and practices in malaria endemic countries." *PLoS Negl Trop Dis.* **12**(4): e0006230. https://doi.org/10.1371/journal.pntd.0006230.

Roth, E.F. Jr, Calvin, M.C., Max-Audit, I., Rosa, J., Rosa, R. 1988. "The enzymes of the glycolytic pathway in erythrocytes infected with Plasmodium falciparum malaria parasites." *Blood.* **72**(6): 1922-1925.

Ruwende, C., Khoo, S., Snow, R. *et al.* 1995. "Natural selection of hemi- and heterozygote for G6PD deficiency in Africa by resistance to severe malaria." *Nature.* **376**: 246–249. https://doi.org/10.1038/376246a0.

Santana, M.S., Monteiro, W.M., Siqueira, A.M., Costa, M.F., Sampaio, V. *et al.* 2013. "Glucose-6-phosphate dehydrogenase deficient variants are associated with reduced susceptibility to malaria in the Brazilian Amazon." *Trans R. Soc Trop Med Hyg.* **107**: 301-306. 10.1093/trstmh/trt015.

Satyagraha, A.W., Sadhewa, A., Baramuli, V., *et al.* 2015. "G6PD deficiency at Sumba in Eastern Indonesia is prevalent, diverse and severe: implications for primaquine therapy against relapsing Vivax malaria." *PLoS Negl Trop Dis.* **9**(3): e0003602. doi:10.1371/journal.pntd.0003602.

Sayyed, Z., Mukherjee, M.B., Mudera, V.C., Colah, R., Gupte, S. 1992. "Characterization of G6PD Rohini—a new class III Indian Variant." *Ind. J Med Res.* **96**: 96-100.

Scriver, C.R., Sly, W.S. and Childs, B. 2001. *The Metabolic and Molecular Bases of Inherited Disease.* 8th edit McGraw-Hill. New York (2001).

Seth, P.K. and Seth, S. 1971. "Biogenetical studies of Nagas: glucose-6-phosphate dehydrogenase deficiency in Angami Nagas." *Hum Biol.* **143**(4): 557-61.

Singh, A.K. and Rajyalakshmi, C. 1993. "Status of Tribal Women in India." *Social Change.* Dec. 1993. **23**(4): 3-18.

Sukumar, S., Mukherjee, M., Colah, R.B. and Mohanty, D. 2003. "Molecular characterization of G6PD Insuli—a novel 989 CGC → CAC (330 Arg → His) mutation in the Indian population. Blood Cells, Molecules, and Diseases." May-June: 246-247.

Sukumar, S., Mukherjee, M.B., Colah, R., Mohanty, D. 2004. "Molecular basis of G6PD deficiency in India." *Blood Cells Mol Dis.* **33**: 141-145.

Sukumar, S., Mukherjee, M.B., Colah, R.B., Mohanty, D. 2005. "Two distinct Indian G6PD variants G6PD Jamnagar and G6PD Rohini caused by the same 949 G→A mutation." *Blood, Cells, Mol, Dis.* **35**(2): 193-195. https://doi.org/10.1016/j.bcmd.2005.03.001.

Tantular, I.S., Matsuoka, H., Kasahara, Y., Pusarawati, S. *et al.* 2010. "Incidence and Mutation Analysis of Glucose-6-Phosphate Dehydrogenase Deficiency in Eastern Indonesian Populations." *Acta Med.* Okayama, **64**(6): 367-373.

Tishkoff, S.A., Varkonyi, R., Cahinhinan, N., Abbes, S., Argyropoulos, G., *et al.* 2001. "Haplotype diversity and linkage disequilibrium at human G6PD: recent origin of alleles that confer malarial resistance." *Science.* **293**: 455-462.

Tripathy, V. and Reddy, B.M. 2007. "Present status of understanding on the G6PD deficiency and natural selection." *J Post Grad Med.* **53**(3): 193-202.

Valencia, S.H., Ocampo, I.D., Arce-Plata, M.I., et al. 2016. "Glucose-6-phosphate dehydrogenase deficiency prevalence and genetic variants in malaria endemic areas of Colombia." *Malar J.* **15**: 291. https://doi.org/10.1186/s12936-016-1343-1.

Van Noorden, C.J., Vogels, I.M., James, J., Tas, J. 1982. "A sensitive cytochemical staining method for glucose-6-phosphate dehydrogenase activity in individual erythrocytes. I. Optimalization of the staining procedure." *Histochemistry.* **75**: 493–506.

Vulliamy, T.J., Kaeda, J.S., Ait Chafa, D., Mangerini, R., Roper, D., Barbot, J., *et al.* 1998. "Clinical and haematological consequences of recurrent G6PD mutations and a single new mutation causing chronic non-spherocytic haemolytic anaemia." *Brit J Haematol.* **101**: 670-675. doi:10.1046/j.1365-2141.1998.00763.x.

Wickramasinghe, S.N. and Abdalla, S.H. 2000. "Blood and bone marrow changes in malaria." *Best Pract and Res Clin Haematology.* **13**(2): 277-299. https://doi.org/10.1053/beha.1999.0072.

World Health Organisation (WHO). 2015. *World Malaria Report 2015.* Geneva, Switzerland: World Health Organization.

World Health Organization (WHO). 1989. "Working group glucose-6-phosphate dehydrogenase deficiency." *Bull World Health Organ.* **67**: 601–611.

Youngster, I., Arcavi, L., Schechmaster, R., Akayzen, Y., Popliski, H., Shimonov, J. *et al.* 2010. "Medications and glucose-6-phosphate dehydrogenase deficiency: an evidence-based review." *Drug Safety.* **33**: 713–726.

24

Maternal Health Disorders and Diseases Among the Brahmin Women

Tiluttoma Baruah

Introduction

Maternal health problem is related to health complications of women seen during pregnancy, childbirth and the post-partum period. It can also term as pregnancy complications which involves the mother's health, baby's health or both. Some women have health problems before they become pregnant that could lead to complications. Other problems arise during the pregnancy. Post-partum complications are also seen among some women. Pregnancy complications can range from mild and annoying discomforts to severe, sometimes life threatening, illness. Problems during pregnancy may include physical and mental conditions that affect the health of the mother or the baby. Maternal mortality is also seen due to such complications related to pregnancy. Maternity problems can be classified as of many types, such as—

1. Maternal Problems

These types of problems originate mainly in the mother:

- *(a)* *Gestational diabetes:* It occurs when some women without diabetes develops high blood sugar levels during pregnancy.
- *(b)* *Hyperemesis gravidarum:* It is characterized by severe vomiting, weight loss and feeling faint.

(c) *Pelvic girdle pain:* It causes pain, instability and limitation of morbidity and functioning in any of the three pelvic joints.

(d) *High blood pressure:* Chronic poorly controlled high blood pressure before and during pregnancy puts a pregnant women and her baby at risk for problems. It is associated with such as pre-eclampsia, placental abruption and gestational diabetes.

(e) *Anemia:* It is characterized by lower levels of haemoglobin during pregnancy. Diagnosis in women is based on haemoglobin of less than 120 to 130 g/l (12 to 13 g/dl). Women with pregnancy related anemia are helped by taking iron and folic acid supplement.

(f) *Infectious disease:* A pregnant women is more susceptible to certain infectious diseases. Pregnant women are more severely affected by influenza, UTI etc.

(g) *Hypothyroidism:* Hypothyroidism is an autoimmune disease that affects the thyroid in women. This condition can move a profound effect during pregnancy and on the field.

(h) *Low blood pressure:* Low blood pressure during pregnancy is a normal occurrence fluctuating hormones and changes in circulation can often lower the blood pressure, especially in the first and second trimester of pregnancy. Most commonly, symptoms of low blood pressure in pregnancy include dizziness and even fainting.

2. *Foetal and Placental Problems*

(a) *Ecotopic pregnancy:* When a fertilized egg implants outside the uterus, usually in the fallopian tube as ectopic pregnancy. It could lead to abdominal pain, shoulder pain or vaginal bleeding.

(b) *Miscarriage:* Loss of a pregnancy prior to 20 weeks. As many as 20 per cent of pregnancies end in miscarriage. In most cases, miscarriage cannot be prevented. Sometimes, a woman undergoes treatment to remove pregnancy tissue in uterus.

(c) *Placental abruption:* Placental separates from uterine wall before delivery known as placental abruption. It leads to vaginal bleeding, cramping, abdominal pain etc. It means the foetus does not get enough oxygen. Severe cases require immediate medical attention and early delivery of the baby.

3. *Complications Following Childbirth*

(a) *Haemorrhage:* Haemorrhage or post-partum bleeding is a serious complication. Primary post-partum haemorrhage is blood loss following childbirth of more than 500 ml or 1000 ml is risk factor. On the other hand, secondly, Haemorrhage may refer to abdominal or excessive bleeding after 24 hrs and before 12 weeks of post-natal. It may lead to miscarriage or maternal mortality.

(b) *Psychological trauma:* Post-partum depression is a moderate to severe repressive episode starting anytime during pregnancy or within the four weeks following delivery. It occurs in 4 per cent-20 per cent pregnancies.

(c) *Obesity and weight gain:* Recent studies suggest that the heavier a woman is before she becomes pregnant, the greater her risk of pregnancy complications including pre-eclampsia, still birth etc.

4. *Overview of Disease during Pregnancy*

(a) *Asthma:* It is a condition in which a person's airways become inflamed, narrow and swell and produce extra mucus, which makes it difficult to breathe. Effect of asthma on pregnancy also varies. But, if asthma is severe and poorly controlled it increases the risk of preterm delivery, pre-eclampsia etc.

(b) *Fever:* During the 1st trimester of pregnancy, a temperature higher than 103°F increases risk of miscarriage, defects of the brain or spinal cord in the baby. Preterm labour etc.

(c) *Liver or Gallbladder:* Liver or Gallbladder problems may result from normal changes during pregnancy. Gallstones appear to be more common during pregnancy. Pregnant women, who develop gallstones, may block the gallbladder or causes infection. Surgery may be necessary; it is usually safe for pregnant women and foetus.

(d) *Appendicitis:* During pregnancy, appendicitis is the most common and non-obstetric emergency that may entail surgery. It is not a rare disorder and is seen in approximately 1 out of 1500 pregnancies.

5. *Stillbirth*

It is typically defined as foetal death at or after 20 to 28 weeks of pregnancy. It results in a baby born without signs of life. Many stillbirths are linked to complications with the placenta. Other causes may include, such as pre-eclampsia, bacterial infection, maternal/gestatonal diabetes etc.

6. *Infertility*

Infertility is the inability of a person, animal or plant to reproduce by natural means. In humans, infertility is the condition of reproductive system that prevents the conception of children. There are many causes of infertility. The most common cause of female infertility is ovulatory problems which generally manifest themselves by absent menstrual periods. Male infertility is most common due to deficiencies in the semen.

About the Place and the People Under Study

Bamungaon is a small village located in Bihpuria of Lakhimpur district of Assam. It is 1 km from the Bihpuria Town inhabited by Brahmin people. It is located at 27.03°N and 93.90°E. It has an average elevation of 102 m (335 ft). The area is known for its panorama of the charming scenes of nature, verdant agricultural field and numerous exotic plants. The climate of the region is characterized by a subtropical humid climate with hot summer and moderate winter. The flora and fauna of the region under study is mainly influenced by the climate and topography of the region.

Most of the households have running water system, private wells and tube wells present in some households. There is no supply of drinking water facility provided by regional administrative authority. The Bamungaon comprises 45 households, of which 39 households are traditional house type and 6 households are modern type. All these households have the provision of electrification except 3 households where electrification is not there. Sanitation is also improved now-a-days. 37 households preferred *pucca* sanitation. Only 8 households have *katcha* latrine type. They do not prefer open space. Educational status of women in the village of Bamungaon is not bad. No illiterate woman is in the village. In the village 8.33 per cent females are under metric, 19.17 per cent members are matriculate, 27.5 per cent women are intermediate, 31.67 per cent females are graduate and post graduate females are also there 11.67 per cent.

In village Bamungaon transport and communication system is also in a good condition. The villagers use different vehicles like bus, truck, taxi, sumo, private bike and car etc. Networks of BSNL, Reliance, Airtel are also available. For minor ailments, the villagers consult the doctor at the community hospital of the village. For major ailment or for maternal delivery they go to private or civil hospitals of Lakhimpur town. In the village, there are two government health centres which provide free government necessary medicines for health related problems. Activities of 'Asha Karmi' for awareness of child health care and maternal health care among pregnant women is seen in that village.

Assamese Brahmins are the Brahmins present in Assamese society, being one of the four traditional Hindu social divisions along with the Kshatriya, Vaishya and Sudras. Brahmins migrated to Assam many centruries ago and belong to the Indo-Aryan race. There they promoted learning, Vedic religion and astrology, besides imparting general Vedic knowledge to the public. There origin was probably the Indo-Gangetic plain; according to the Nidhanpur Copper plate; around 200 Brahmin families of various gotras and *ved sakhas* moved from there to Assam of the imitation of Bhutibarmana in the 6th century c.c . Another statement is that Brahmins of Assam valley belong to the group of Indo Aryans, who are believed to be having their origins as far West Bengal to Kannauj. There is a myth that the Ahoms brought the Brahmins were present in Assam much earlier to the advent of Ahoms and hence also known as Kamrupi Brahmins. During the reign of Koch Kings, the Kamrupi Brahmins were quite prosperous. In fact one of the earliest Kings of the Ahom dynasty is known as Brahmani Konwar, because he was brought up by a Brahmin family and till date time the Ahom Kings were not Hindu and as such there is no question of Ahoms inviting Brahmins to Assam. Brahmins of Assam are 'Saktra' or worshipper of Shakti and are non-vegetarian. Such Assamese Brahmin family within the community belongs to a specific Gotra (Brahmin identity Surname) which is unique to a family thereby indicating their origin or the lineage. Many of the Brahmins in Assam write the conferred titles either given to them as a gift by the Ahom Kings or else which they have adopted being in Assam for a long time.

Findings

An attempt has been made to present prevalence of various types of diseases or disorders related maternity of 15-65 years of married women in Brahmin population of 'Bamungaon', Bihpuria. Tabulation and analysis were done here to find out afflicted married women by different diseases and disorders.

Table: 24.1: Distribution of Maternal Health disorders and problems

Type	*Frequency*	%
Gestational diabetes	2	1.74
Hyperemesis gravidarum	12	10.43
Pelvic girdle pain	19	16.52
High blood pressure	19	16.52
Anaemia	39	33.92
UTI	5	4.35
Yeast infection	1	0.87
Hypothyroidism	2	1.74
Low blood pressure	16	13.91
Total	115	100

Source: Fieldwork, 2018.

From Table 24.1, it can be said that high prevalence of anaemia and low blood pressure are seen being 39 (33.92%) respectively. Equal frequency of High blood pressure and Pelvic girdle pain are seen, which is 19 (16.52%). The infectious diseases like UTI, yeast infection are found which account for 5 (4.35%) and 1(0.87%) respectively. Prevalence of gestational diabetes, hyperemes is gravidarum and hypothyroidism are found to be 2 (1.74%), 12 (10.43%) and 2 (1.74%) respectively.

Table 24.2: Distribution of Foetal and Placental Problems

Type	*Frequency*	*%*
Ectopic pregnancy	1	11.11
Miscarriage	5	55.56
Placental abruption	3	33.33
Total	9	100

Source: Fieldwork, 2018.

From Table 24.2, it is clear that Foetal and Placental problems with Ectopic pregnancy, Miscarriages and Placental abruption have been found to be 1 (11.11%), 5 (55.56%) and 3 (33.33%) respectively.

Table 24.3: Distribution of Complications following Childbirth

Type	*Frequency*	*%*
Haemorrhage	6	23.08
Obesity or weight gain	20	76.92
Total	26	100

Source: Fieldwork, 2018.

From Table 24.3, it can be said that complications following after childbirth are also found. Haemorrhage or heavy bleeding after 24 hours and 12 weeks of post-natal are recorded to be 6 (23.08%). Prevalence of obesity or weight gain is recorded among 20 (76.92%) of total women.

Table 24.4: Distribution of Diseases occurred during Pregnancy

Type	*Frequency*	*%*
Asthma	1	16.67
Fever	3	50
Liver and Gallbladder	1	16.67
Appendicitis	1	16.67
Total	6	100

Source: Fieldwork, 2018.

From the study conducted various types of diseases like asthma, fever, gallbladder, appendicitis have been found to be 1 (16.67%), 3 (50%), 1 (16.67%) and 1 (16.67%) respectively.

Table 24.5: Distribution of Complications following Childbirth

Type	*Frequency*	*%*
Stillbirth	6	37.5
Infertility	10	62.5
Total	16	100

Source: Fieldwork, 2018.

From Table 24.5, it can be said that prevalence of stillbirth (intrauterine foetal death) and infertility are also have found. Frequency distribution of stillbirths and infertility account for 6 (37.5%) and 10 (62.5%) respectively.

Table 24.6: Distribution of the sample according to age

Age group	*Frequency of afflicted women*	*%*	*Frequency of non-afflicted women*	*%*
15-24	10	9.90	5	26.31
25-34	41	40.59	7	36.84
35-44	35	34.65	5	26.31
45-54	11	10.89	1	5.27
55-64	4	3.97	1	5.27
Total	101	100	19	100

Source: Fieldwork, 2018.

From Table 24.6, it can be said that highest frequency of afflicted women is seen in the age group of 25-34 being 40.59 per cent followed by 35-44, 45-54, 15-24 and 55-64 where percentages are 34.65, 10.89, 9.90 and 3.97 respectively. Frequency of non-afflicted women is highest in the age group of 25-34 being 36.84 per cent followed by 15-24, 35-44, 45-54 and 55-64 where percentages are 26.31, 26.31, 5.27 and 5.27 respectively.

Conclusion

From the study conducted, it was found that gestational diabetes is seen in total 1.74 per cent of total afflicted women. 10.43 per cent women were found to suffer from Hyperemesis gravidarum. Prevalence of pelvic girdle pain and high blood pressure has been found to be 16.52 per cent of total afflicted women. High frequency of anaemia has been found, which accounts for 33.92 per cent of afflicted women. Infectious diseases like UTI and yeast infection account for 4.35 per cent and 0.87 per cent respectively. Hypothyroidism and low blood pressure is also found to be 1.74 per cent and 13.91 per cent respectively. Foetal and placental problems have been found at low frequency. Ectopic pregnancy is found among 11.11 per cent. Miscarriage and placental abruption account for 55.56 per cent and 33.33 per cent respectively. Diverse complications following childbirth such as post-partum bleeding or haemorrhage have been found to be 23.08 per cent after child birth. Obesity during pregnancy also found in 76.92 per cent among pregnant women. Moderate presence of certain types of diseases is reported during pregnancy. Afflictions with asthma, fever, gallbladder and appendicitis accounted for 16.67 per cent, 50 per cent, 16.67 per cent and 16.67 per cent respectively. Stillbirth of foetal death and infertility rate is registered. 37.5per cent are affected because of complications with placenta, pre-eclampsia, bacterial infection etc. 62.55 per cent of total women are estimated to have difficulty conceiving or staying pregnant, which is known as infertility. It has been seen that highest frequency of afflicted women is seen in age group of 25-34 being 40.59, followed by 35-44, 45-54, 15-24 and 55-64 where percentage are 34.65, 10.89, 9.90 and 3.97 respectively. Frequency of non-afflicted women is highest in age group 25-34 being 36.84 per cent followed by age group 15-24, 35-44, 45-54 and 55-64 where percentages are 26.31, 26.31, 5.27 and 5.27 respectively. Total afflicted and non-afflicted women have been found to be 84.17 per cent and 15.83 per cent of total population respectively.

Socio-cultural factors are responsible for affecting pregnancy, Brahmin women performmes some religious ceremonies for pregnant women during the seventh month of foetal stage known as *Bhat Pitha* ceremony by its maternal uncle. This ritual is only done by women of the particular village. In fifth month of foetal stage they also perform *Panchamrit Bhujon* ritual and at the ninth month they also perform *Athu Lua* rituals. These types of ceremonies are believed to be mainly related to wellness of mother and the child.

REFERENCES

Berha, Abadi Kidanemariam, Getachew Mullu Kassa, Achenef Asmamaw Muche. 2018. "Prevelence of Hypertensive Disorder of Pregnancy in Ethiopia." *Journal of Pregnancy Childbirth,* **18**(2) 136-139.

Bhinde, Amarnath, Kaitad R.Damania and Shirish N.Daftary. 2004. *Practical guide to High Risk Pregnancy and Delivery.* Elsevier Publication, Europe.

Iyengar, Kirti, Sharad D. Iyengar and Kalpana Dashora. 2004. "Pregnancy related death in Rural Rjasthan India: Exploring causes, context and caste seeking through Verbal Autopsy." *Journal of Health, Population nad Nutrition.* **30**(4) 234-237.

Singh, Dipti, Srinivas Goli and Sulabha Parsuraman, 2014. "Association between Obstetric complications and previous pregnancy outcomes with current pregnancy outcomes in Uttar Pradesh, India." *The Indian Journal of Medical Research.* **25**(2) 215-223.

Vanders, Kathrine F., Andrej M. Grjibovski and Nathalie C. Store. 2015. "Hyperemesis Gravidarum and Maternal Cancer risk, a Scandinavian nested case control study." *International Journal of Cancer.* **137**(5) 246-250.

http://www.ede.gov./reproductivehealth/maternalhealth/pregnancycomplication/DOA: 10/04/2018

http://www.pregnancybirthbaby.org.all/commonpregnancyproblems/ DOA: 15/04/2018

25

Metabolic Syndrome and Menopause
A Study among Adult Females

Ramanpreet Randhawa and *Sharda Sidhu*

Introduction

Metabolic Syndrome (MS) is a clinical and pathological entity which represents the presence of combination of interrelated metabolic abnormalities, including obesity, high blood pressure, elevated levels of Fasting Blood Glucose (FBG) and abnormal level of lipids, that promotes the development of Type 2 Diabetes Mellitus (T2DM) and cardiovascular diseases (Ford, 2005). Menopause in women leads to numerous vicissitudes in hormonal and other physiological factors. It is found to be adversely associated with all the cardiometabolic risk parameters in women manifesting menopause is an independent predictor of metabolic syndrome among females (Eshtiaghi *et al.*, 2010; Pandey *et al.*, 2010; Arthur *et al.*, 2012; Strand *et al.*, 2014; Mandob *et al.*, 2015; Marchi *et al.*, 2016). The biological prospect of this association is illuminated by the fact that menopausal women experience changes confined to metabolic syndrome, including increased abdominal obesity, hyperglycemia, and dyslipidemic changes (Arthur *et al.*, 2012). This is accredited to declined levels of estrogen which promotes reduction in fat free mass and elevation in visceral abdominal fat accumulation independently of age, race and ethnicity at menopause. Numerous investigators (Carr, 2003; Park *et al.*, 2003; Ainyet *et al.*, 2007; Chedrauiet *et al.*, 2007) threw spotlight on the notion that the attainment of menopause is associated with unfavourable changes in body composition accompanied by greater amounts of intra-abdominal fat, lipid imbalances, disturbance in the insulin levels, fluctuations in blood pressure status and most dominantly metabolic aberrations resulting in web of chief components of metabolic syndrome (Grundy *et al.*, 2005; Alberti *et al.*, 2006). The objectives of the present study are to find out the associations of metabolic syndrome among Menopausal women.

Materials and Methods

The present cross-sectional data was collected from adult upper middle class Jat-Sikh females ranging in age 40-65 years and residing in various urban and rural areas of Amritsar district. The study group included 1520 females, out of which, 791 females were pre-menopausal and 729 females were post-menopausal. An effective sample size was estimated through statistical power analysis by conducting a pilot study. Those women who were having irregular menstruation, pregnant, lactating and experienced cessation of menstruation due to hysterectomy or any other surgical cause were excluded from the study. Ethical clearance from the Institutional Ethics Committee of Guru Nanak Dev University, Amritsar was obtained prior to carry out the study. After fully explaining the nature, procedure, aims and objectives of the study to all the females in Punjabi language, verbal as well as written informed consent was obtained. The participation of women was voluntary. First of all, women were taken into confidence and then contacted for the study according to their convenience and prior appointment. The anonymity and confidentiality of participants' information was guaranteed. The data on age at menopause was taken from those subjects who stopped menstruating completely by asking them to recall their age at the time of last menstrual period. The anthropometric measurements were taken on each subject using standard methodology. In addition to this, abdominal obesity was assessed by measuring Waist Circumference (WC). The blood pressure of each subject was recorded by auscultatory method using mercury sphygmomanometer and stethoscope to identify women with hypertension according to JNC-VII (2003) guidelines. Fasting blood glucose (FBG) of each subject was checked in the fasting stage with capillary finger prick method using a standardized digital Contour TS Glucometer (Bayer Healthcare, USA) and compatible strips to diagnose T2DM as per American Diabetes Association (ADA) guidelines in 2017. For studying lipid profile, 3 ml of venous blood was withdrawn from the median cubital vein of each subject in the morning after 8-10 hours overnight fast using a standard protocol (WHO, 2010) with the assistance of a phlebotomist. Various biochemical tests were performed using commercially available Erba kits on semi-automatic Erba Mannhein Biochromatic Analyzer to predict the levels of Triglycerides (TGL), and High Density Lipoproteins-Cholesterol (HDL-C). From this information, assessment of Metabolic Syndrome (MS) was assessed using internationally renowned and valid criteria named as Joint Interim Statement (JIS, 2009) also known as Harmonized Asian-Specific Diagnostic Criterion among adult pre-menopausal and post-menopausal females of Amritsar.

Results

The percentage prevalence of metabolic syndrome among adult females of Amritsar was assessed after stratification of females according to menstrual status (Table 25.1 and Fig. 25.1A). In the present study, internationally recognized diagnostic criterion namely, Joint Interim Statement (JIS, 2009) also known as harmonized Asian-specific criterion was applied to identify the females who satisfy this criterion for diagnosis of metabolic syndrome. In the pooled sample, the prevalence of metabolic syndrome was found as 44.7 per cent and 60.1 per cent among pre-menopausal and post-menopausal women using JIS (2009) criterion. The difference in the percentage prevalence of metabolic syndrome between pre-menopausal and post-menopausal females was statistically significant (χ^2=111.4, df=1; p<0.001).

Table 25.1: Percentage prevalence of Metabolic Syndrome (MS) using international diagnostic criterion among adult pre-menopausal and post-menopausal females of Amritsar

Diagnostic criterion	*Adult females (1520)*		
JIS (2009)	*With MS*	*Without MS*	*χ^2 value*
Pre-menopausal (791)	44.7 (354)	55.3 (437)	111.4***
Post-menopausal (729)	60.1 (438)	39.9 (291)	

Figures in parentheses indicate the number of subjects.
***Significant at p<0.001.
Joint Interim Statement (JIS).

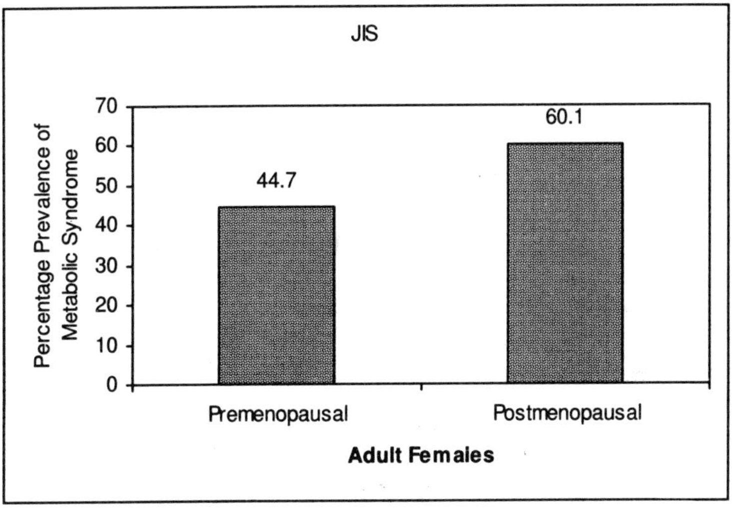

Joint Interim Statement (JIS).

Fig. 25.1: A Histogram showing the percentage prevalence of metabolic syndrome among adult pre-menopausal and post-menopausal females using international diagnostic criterion.

Discussion

Menstrual status is a fundamental key factor while determining the prevalence of metabolic syndrome among females. Present study documented increased prevalence of metabolic syndrome among post-menopausal females than pre-menopausal females. The switch from pre-menopausal phase to post-menopausal status is associated with the emergence of many features of the metabolic syndrome including (i) increased abdominal body fat, (ii) a shift towards a more unbalanced lipid profile accompanied with elevated triglycerides and low-density lipoprotein-cholesterol levels and reduced high density lipoprotein-cholesterol, and (iii) deranged insulin levels (Lloyd-Jones *et al.*, 2009). The emergence of such metabolic anomalies may be accredited to loss of estrogen due to ovarian failure related to attainment of menopause. Similar observations were laid down by Ainy *et al.* (2007), Eshtiaghi *et al.* (2010), Heidari *et al.* (2010) and Jesmin *et al.* (2013). In a study done by Neto *et al.* (2012) on Brazilian women, it was determined that compared to pre-menopausal counterparts (mATP-III 24.0% and IDF 37.0%), the post-menopausal females depicted two times more prevalence of metabolic syndrome (mATP-III 44.0% and IDF 61.5%). An epidemiological study conducted in Ghana (Arthur *et al.*, 2012) postulated that post-menopausal females had almost two times higher estimates of metabolic syndrome as compared to pre-menopausal females according to IDF and mATP-III definitions. Marchi *et al.* (2016) studied 958 Brazilian women, including 277 pre-menopausal women and 681 post-menopausal women and observed 9.4 per cent of premenopausal women yielded metabolic syndrome while 22.2 per cent of post-menopausal women diagnosed with metabolic syndrome as per ATP-III criterion. In agreement to pre-menopausal and post-menopausal disparity, 40.2 per cent and 49.5 per cent prevalence of metabolic syndrome was noticed in pre-menopausal and post-menopausal females of China using mATP-III criterion (Strand *et al.*, 2014). The frequency of metabolic syndrome increases from the beginning of the menopausal transition to post-menopause because the components of metabolic syndrome are more dominant in post-menopausal women compared to pre-menopausal women (Polotsky and Polotsky, 2010). Among females of Tehran, the prevalence of metabolic syndrome was 53 per cent in pre-menopausal women and 69 per cent in post-menopausal women (Ainy *et al.*, 2007).

In the published literature, few national studies were available on the prevalence of metabolic syndrome among pre-menopausal and post-menopausal females. Among 200 Indian females residing in urban and rural areas Chhabra *et al.* (2014) estimated the prevalence of metabolic syndrome as 27.0 per cent and 43.0 per cent in pre-menopausal and post-menopausal females, respectively. Pandey *et al.* (2010) identified that the prevalence of metabolic syndrome was 45.0 per cent and 44.0 per cent among pre-menopausal females whereas it was 55.0 per cent and 56.0 per cent in case of post-menopausal females according to IDF and JIS criteria, respectively. Similarly, a study done on north Indian women in the age group of 45-35 years assessed 59.4 per cent pre-menopausal females and 65.7 per cent of post-menopausal females satisfying mATP-III standard of metabolic syndrome (Sharma *et al.*, 2016). Among females of Odisha, 52.2 per cent prevalence of metabolic syndrome was assessed using JIS definition by Prasad *et al.* (2012). Deedwania *et al.* (2014) carried out a multicentric study (located in all geographic areas) among urban subjects and applied three diagnostic criteria. They observed the prevalence of metabolic syndrome using Harmonized Asian-specific criterion (JIS) as 40.4 per cent and 34.5 per cent using mATP-III criterion and 22.8 per cent as per the ATP-III standard among women. An another study carried out by Mangat *et al.* (2010) showed that 44.8 per cent and 59.6 per cent females had metabolic syndrome on the basis of ATP-III and JIS guidelines, respectively. Based on mATP-III standard, 9.4 per cent and 22.2 per cent prevalence of metabolic syndrome was observed among Brazilian women by Marchi *et al.* (2016). It is apparent from the complied results of present study that postmenopausal females depicted higher figures of metabolic syndrome than pre-menopausal females.

Several investigators (Heidari *et al.*, 2010; Neto *et al.*, 2010; Pandey *et al.*, 2010) demonstrated higher prevalence of metabolic syndrome among post-menopausal females than pre-menopausal women. A study accomplished among women (age group 40-65 years) of Argentina (South America) encountered a relative risk of 1.61 of developing metabolic syndrome during post-menopausal phase (Coniglio *et al.*, 2009). A meta-analysis confirmed this fact by estimating higher estimates of metabolic syndrome among women who stopped menstruating than those who still menstruate, regardless of population (Mendes *et al.*, 2012). The third National Health and Nutrition Examination Survey (NHANES III) emphasized the relationship between metabolic syndrome and increased mortality among women during menopausal approach as compared to pre-menopausal women (Lin *et al.*, 2006). The results of various previous studies have been inconsistent, some studies have observed that there is no dissimilarity in cardiovascular risk factors when comparing pre-menopausal with post-menopausal women (Kannel *et al.*, 1976; Peters *et al.*, 1999). Few studies revealed that there was dominance of metabolic syndrome among post-menopausal women, which varies from 32.6 per cent to 41.5 per cent (Chedraui *et al.*, 2007; Ding *et al.*, 2007). Estrogen promotes the accumulation of gluteo-femoral fat (Krotkiewski *et al.*, 1983), and the loss of estrogen with menopause is associated with an increase in abdominal fat (Poehlman *et al.*, 1995). The higher prevalence of metabolic syndrome in the post-menopausal women can be ascribed to estrogen induced body fat redistribution. Metabolic syndrome and cardiovascular diseases are more common in women above 55 years of age with significant increase in individual risk factors in the post-menopausal phase. Changing hormonal milieu with declining estrogen and alteration of its ratio with testosterone has been implicated as a causal factor for the emergence of metabolic syndrome at menopausal transition (Pandey *et al.*, 2010). In nutshell, metabolic Syndrome is increasing massively in the transition phase in every woman's life from pre-menopausal to menopausal phase.

Acknowledgements

We would like to express our profound gratitude to all the female respondents for their cooperation and contribution towards this study. We are wholeheartedly thankful to Miss Jaspreet Kaur for her assistance in the collection of data. The authors deeply acknowledge the funding received from the Guru Nanak Dev University under the scheme University with Potential for Excellence (UPE) and Centre with Potential for Excellence in Particular Area (CPEPA).

REFERENCES

Ainy, E., Mirmiran, P., Zahedi, S. 2007. "Prevalence of metabolic syndrome during menopausal transition in Tehranian women: Tehran Lipid and Glucose Study (TLGS)." *Maturitas* **58:** 150–155.

Alberti, K.G., Eckel, R.H., Grundy, S.M., Zimmet, P.Z., Cleeman, J.I, Donato, K.A. *et al.* 2009. "Harmonizing the metabolic syndrome: a joint interim statement of the International Diabetes Federation Task Force on Epidemiology and Prevention; National Heart, Lung and Blood Institute; American Heart Association; World Heart Federation; International Atherosclerosis Society; and International Association for the Study of Obesity." *Circulation* **120**(16): 1640-1645.

Alberti, K.G., Zimmet, P., Shaw, J. 2006. "Metabolic syndrome—a new worldwide definition. A consensus statement from the International Diabetes Federation." *Diabet Med* **23**: 469-480.

American Diabetes Association (2017). *Diabetes Care* **40**(1): 1-135.

Arthur, F.K.N., Adu-Frimpong, M., Osei-Yeboah, J., Mensah, F.O. and Owusu, L. 2012. "Prediction of metabolic syndrome among post-menopausal Ghanian women using obesity and atherogenic markers." *Lipids in Health and Disease* **11**: 101 www.lipidworld.com/content/11/1/101.

Carr, M.C. 2003. "The emergence of the metabolic syndrome with menopause." *The Journal of Clinical Endocrinology and Metabolism* **88**(6): 2404-2411.

Chedraui, P., Hidalgo, L., Chavez, D., Morocho, N., Alvadro, M. and Huc, A. 2007. "Quality of life among post-menopausal Ecuadorian women participating in a metabolic syndrome screening program." *Maturitas* **56**: 45-53.

Chhabra, N., Sodhi, K., Kukreja, S. *et al.* 2014. "Central obesity and prevalence of metabolic syndrome in post-menopausal women." *Webmedcentral Obesity* **5**(1): WMC004532.

Coniglio, R.I., Nellem, J., Gentili, R., Sibechi, N., Agusti, E., Torres, M. 2009. "Metabolic syndrome in employee in Argentina." *Medicina* **69**: 246-52.

Deedwania, P.C., Gupta, R., Sharma, K.K., Achari, V., Gupta, B., Maheshwari, A. and Gupta, A. 2014. "High prevalence of metabolic syndrome among urban subjects in India: A multiside study." *Diabetes and Metabolic Syndrome: Clinical Research and Reviews* **8**: 156-161.

Ding, Q.F., Hayashi, T., Zhang, X.J., Funami, J., Ge, L., Li, J. *et al.* 2007. "Risks of CHD identified by different criteria of metabolic syndrome and related changes of adipocytokines in elderly post-menopausal women." *J Diabetes Complications* **21**(5): 315-319.

Eshtiaghi, R., Esteghamati, A. and Nakhjavani, M. 2010. "Menopause is an independent predictor of metabolic syndrome in Iranian women." *Maturitas* **65**: 262-266.

Ford, E.S. 2005. "Prevalence of the metabolic syndrome defined by the International Diabetes Federation among adults in the US." *Diabetes Care* **28**: 2745-2749.

Grundy, S.M. 2004. "Obesity, metabolic syndrome and cardiovascular disease." *J Clin Endocrinol Metab* **89**: 2595-2600.

Heidari, R., Sadeghi, M., Talaei, M., Rabiei, K., Mohammadifard, N., Sarrafzadegan, N. 2010. "Metabolic syndrome in menopausal transition: Isfahan Healthy Heart Program, a population based study." *Diabetology and Metabolic Syndrome* **2**(59): 1-6.

Jesmin, S., Islam, R., Islam, S., Sohag, M., Sultana, S.N., Zaedi, S., Yamaguchi, N., Iwashima, Y., Hiroe, M., Watanabe, T. 2012. "Comprehensive assessment of metabolic syndrome among rural Bangladeshi women." *BMC Public Health* 12: 49.

Joint National Committee on detection, evaluation and treatment of high blood pressure. 2003. The seventh report of Joint National Committee on detection, evaluation and treatment of high blood pressure (JNC VII). *Journal of American Medical Association* **289**: 2560-72.

Kannel, W.B., Hjortland, M.C., McNamara, P.M. and Gordon, T. 1976. "Menopause and risk of cardiovascular disease: the Framingham study." *Ann Intern Med* **85**:447-452.

Krotkiewski, M., Björntorp, P., Sjöström, L. and Smith, U. 1983. "Impact of obesity on metabolism in men and women. Importance of regional adipose tissue distribution." *J Clin Invest* **72**: 1150-1162.

Lin, W.Y., Yang, W.S., Lee, L.T., *et al.* 2006. "Insulin resistance, obesity and metabolic syndrome among non-diabetic pre- and post-menopausal women in North Taiwan." *IJO* **30**(6): 912-917.

Lloyd-Jones, D., Adams, R., Carnethon, M., De Simone, G., Ferguson, T.B. *et al.* 2009. "Heart disease and stroke statistics—2009 update. A report from the American heart association statistics committee and stroke statistics subcommittee." *Circulation* **119**: 480-486.

Mandob, D.E., Rosalie, N.K., Marlyse, L.K. 2015. "Prevalence of metabolic syndrome among post-menopausal women Yaounde-Cameroon." *International Journal of Health Sciences and Research* **5**(11): 278-284.

Mangat, C., Goel, N.K., Walia, D.K. *et al.* 2010. "Metabolic syndrome: a challenging health issue in highly urbanized union territory of North India." *Diabetology and Metabolic Syndrome* **2**(19): 1-8.

Marchi, R.D., Dell'Agnolo, C.M., Lopes, T.C.R., Gravena, A.A.F., Demitto, M.D.O., Brischiliari, S.C.R., Borghesan, D.H.P., Carvalho, M.D.D.B.C., Pelloso, S.M. 2016. P"revalence of metabolic syndrome in pre- and post-menopausal women." *Arch EndocrinolMetab* **61**(2): 160-166 doi: 10.1590/2359-3997000000253.

Mendes, K.G., Theodoro, H., Rodrigues, A.D., Busnello, F., Lorenzi, D.R.S., deOlinto, M.T.A. 2013. "Menopausal status and metabolic syndrome in women in climacteric period treated at a clinic in Southern Brazil." *Open J Endocr Metab Dis.* **3**: 31-41.

Neto, J.A.F., Figueredo, E.D., Barbosa, J.B., Fde, F.B., Costa, G.R., Nina, V.J. *et al.* 2010. "Metabolic Syndrome and Menopause: Cross-Sectional Study in Gynecology Clinic." *Brazilian Archives of Cardiology* **95**(3): 339-345

Pandey, S., Srinivas, M., Agashe, S. *et al.* 2010. "Menopause and metabolic syndrome: a study of 498 urban women from western India." *Journal of Midlife Health* **1**(2): 63-69.

Park, Y.W., Zhu, S., Palaniappan, L., Heshka, S., Carnethon, M.R., *et al.* 2003. "The metabolic syndrome: prevalence and associated risk factor findings in the US population from the Third National Health and Nutrition Examination Survey, 1988-1994." *Arch Intern Med* **163**: 427-436.

Peters, H.W., Westendorp, I.C., Hak, A.E., Grobbee, D.E., Stehouwer, C.D., *et al.* 1999. "Menopausal status and risk factors for cardiovascular disease." *J Intern Med* **246**: 521-528.

Poehlman, E., Toth, M., Gardner, A. 1995. "Changes in energy balance and body composition at menopause. A controlled longitudinal study." *Ann Interm Med* **123**: 673-675.

Polotsky, H.N., Polotsky, A.J. 2010. "Metabolic Implications of Menopause." *Semin Reprod Med* **28**(5): 426–443

Prasad, D.S., Kabir, Z., Dash, A.K., Das, B.C. 2012. "Prevalence and risk factors for metabolic syndrome in Asian Indians: A community study from urban Eastern India." *J Cardiovasc Dis Res* **3**: 204-211.

Sharma, M., Mahna, R. 2012. "Metabolic syndrome among Indian adults." *International Journal of Food and Nutritional Sciences* **1**(1): 62-69.

Strand, M.A., Huseth-Zosel, A., He, M., Perry, J. 2015. "Menopause and the risk of metabolic syndrome among middle-aged Chinese women." *Family Medicine and Community Health* **3**(1): 15-22.

World Health Organization. 2010. *WHO guidelines on drawing blood: best practices in phlebotomy:* Press WHO. 125.

Index

INTACT